THE
FOOD BABE
WAY

THE FOOD BABE WAY

**Break Free from the Hidden Toxins in Your
Food and Lose Weight, Look Years Younger,
and Get Healthy in Just 21 Days!**

VANI HARI

Foreword by Mark Hyman, MD

LITTLE, BROWN AND COMPANY
New York   Boston   London

Little, Brown and Company
Hachette Book Group
1290 Avenue of the Americas
New York, NY 10104
littlebrown.com

First Edition: February 2015

Little, Brown and Company is a division of Hachette Book Group, Inc. The Little, Brown name and logo are trademarks of Hachette Book Group, Inc.

The publisher is not responsible for websites (or their content) that are not owned by the publisher.

The Hachette Speakers Bureau provides a wide range of authors for speaking events. To find out more, go to hachettespeakersbureau.com or call (866) 376-6591.

ISBN 978-0-316-37646-4
LCCN 2014954149

10 9 8 7 6 5 4 3 2 1

RRD-C

Printed in the United States of America

To the Food Babe Army — the courageous ones who stand
with me to fight for a better food system

CONTENTS

Foreword by Mark Hyman, MD   ix

Note to the Reader   xiii

Introduction   3

PART I
THOSE TRICKY SONS OF . . .

Chapter 1: We've Been Duped   19

Chapter 2: We Are the Chemicals We Eat—The Sickening 15   38

Chapter 3: Cut Out the Chemical Calories   58

PART II
21 DAYS OF GOOD FOOD AND GOOD HABITS

Chapter 4: Week 1—Fluid Assets for Food Babes   79

    Day 1—Cleanse Daily with My Morning Lemon Water Ritual   80

    Day 2—Be a Lean, Green Drinking Machine   85

    Day 3—Stop Drinking with Your Meals   96

    Day 4—Be Aware of What's in Your Water   103

    Day 5—Ease Back on Dairy Foods   110

    Day 6—No More Big Gulps!   118

    Day 7—Love Your Liver   128

Chapter 5: Week 2 — Food Habits for Food Babes   143

     Day 8 — Pass on Fast Food   145

     Day 9 — Detox from Added Sugar   155

     Day 10 — Eat Meat Responsibly   165

     Day 11 — Eat Raw More Than Half the Time   177

     Day 12 — Break Some Bread — and Other Carbs   181

     Day 13 — Balance Your Healthy Fats   191

     Day 14 — Supplement with These 10 Superhero Foods   201

Chapter 6: Week 3 — Feats of a Real Food Babe   215

     Day 15 — Know Thy GMOs!   216

     Day 16 — Dine Out the Food Babe Way   227

     Day 17 — Do a Kitchen Cleanout   241

     Day 18 — Change Your Little Grocery Shop of Horrors   246

     Day 19 — Cook Outside the Box   259

     Day 20 — Fast Every Day   266

     Day 21 — Travel Organically   270

PART III
THE 21-DAY FOOD BABE WAY EATING PLAN AND RECIPES

Chapter 7: The 21-Day Food Babe Way Eating Plan   281

Chapter 8: The Food Babe Way Eating Plan Recipes   288

Appendix A: Join the Food Babe Army: How to Start a Petition   337

Appendix B: Recommended Reading and Resources   339

*Appendix C: Corporate Bucks Try to Defeat Mandatory
    GMO Labeling*   346

Appendix D: Bibliography   349

Acknowledgments   359

Index   362

FOREWORD

Once or twice in a generation a brave scientist or an ordinary citizen stands up to the status quo and tells the truth about what most of us would rather ignore. It changes everything about how we see the world, about the choices we make and how we live our lives. And sometimes it changes the world. Margaret Mead once said, "Never doubt that a small group of thoughtful, committed citizens can change the world; indeed, it's the only thing that ever has." Vani Hari, the Food Babe, has done what politicians, mothers, doctors, nutritionists, authors, and advocacy groups could not do—single-handedly, with her computer, blog, and very clear voice.

Rachel Carson first alerted Americans to the dangers of pesticides and chemicals in our environment and helped launch the environmental movement. Linus Pauling, at great risk to his career, spoke about the dangers of war and nuclear radiation, and this led to the nuclear test ban treaty and garnered for him the Nobel Peace Prize. Martin Luther King, Jr., endured beatings, jail, and even death to open our eyes to the inhumanity of racism and the abuse of civil rights. And there are thousands of other souls in far corners of the world who are inspired to tell the truth at risk to themselves and their families. Most of them are unsung heroes who quietly stand up for what is right, and we are all better for it.

Vani Hari is a modern-day David, facing the Goliath of the trillion-dollar food industry, which in the guise of fun, colorful, hypertasty, easy-to-eat, convenient foods is creating suffering and sickness around the globe.

Most of us are completely oblivious to what we are eating and its impact on our health and our world. We know little about how our food is grown; how our seeds are engineered; how our farming methods harm the soil, air, and water, and contribute to climate change and dead zones in our oceans. We are mostly unaware of the chemicals that are added to our foods and of how the hormones, antibiotics, plastics, and toxins we eat in our everyday foods harm our bodies. How could we know that we are eating Silly Putty in our French fries and yoga mat softeners in our bread; or cancer-causing preservatives such as BHA and BHT, which have been banned in every country but ours; or that dyes and coloring agents in our macaroni and cheese may cause hyperactivity and behavioral problems in our children; or that natural flavorings are made from ground-up animal parts; or that common foods contain secretions from beavers' anal glands? How could we know that apart from the calories we eat, many of the chemicals in our food are obesogens, contributing to an obesity epidemic that is weighing down our nation and increasingly the world as we create the worst diet on the planet and export it to every other nation except Cuba and North Korea? How could we know that most of the 10,000 additives in our food supply have never been proven safe and are given a free pass by the Food and Drug Administration (FDA)?

There are thousands of health revolutionaries working to change our food system. I consider myself one of them. But very few of us have figured out how to speak truth to power *and* slay Goliath, the food industry, or even make his knees buckle. The beauty and genius of the Food Babe is not simply that she rails against our toxic food system, or educates us about the dangers of industrial food in general. She goes after the Achilles' heel, the one missing scale on the dragon, and shoots an arrow so true and straight, so deadly, that it takes down food giants who otherwise merely laugh at critics, who ignore most of us calling for a change to the food system. Instead, the CEOs and executives of major companies invite her into their inner sanctums and take her advice on how to change for the better. They fear her Food Babe Army, the millions of citizen activists who are sick and tired of being sick and tired.

But Vani Hari doesn't just leave us angry, or save us from azodicarbonamide (the yoga mat ingredient) in Subway sandwiches. No, she goes deep into every aspect of our food system and through tireless, fearless, and stunning detective work uncovers nearly every toxin in our food system. She invites us to take a real look at our food, to read labels like an expert. She has uncovered all the dangerous ingredients in our food and teaches us how to avoid the growth hormones in meat, antibiotics, pesticides, refined and enriched flour, bisphenol A (BPA), high-fructose corn syrup, trans fats, artificial sweeteners, preservatives, artificial and natural flavors, food dyes, dough conditioners, carrageenan, monosodium glutamate (MSG), heavy metals and neurotoxins, and more.

And Vani doesn't just teach us what to avoid. She doesn't leave us hopeless. She has vigorously investigated what we *can* eat, what products and foods give health and life rather than take it away. Her detective skills have uncovered an extraordinary, chemical-free, real-food way of eating that makes sense for everyone. It is the seed of a profound revolution, the type that Congressman Tim Ryan speaks of in *The Real Food Revolution*, a revolution that gets to the root of how our food system destroys our human and natural capital, our health, and our environment.

I am an advocate for a new form of medicine, functional medicine, which addresses the root cause of disease; sees the body as an ecosystem, not a collection of parts; and treats the organism, not just organs—the system, not just the symptoms. One of the fundamental tools of healing is food. If food were just calories, it wouldn't matter where it came from; as long as it had enough energy to sustain us and tasted good, it would be fine.

But the science of nutrition has uncovered a radical new way of looking at food. Food is not just energy. *Food is information.* It contains instructions that communicate messages to your genes, hormones, immune system, gut flora—in fact, to every system of your body. This changes everything we know about food. Health results from the quality of information we put in our bodies. And Vani's "Sickening 15" and the other hidden ingredients and modified food products that make up most of our diet are disease-causing information.

If everyone followed the 21-Day Food Babe Way Eating Plan, the food system as we know it would crumble, and a new era of innovation and creativity would take root. Antiquated industries and food systems would fall apart and new, transformative food systems would arise. Not only would we all be healthier, but we would also reverse the epidemic of chronic disease and obesity globally crippling our citizens, economies, and environment.

And all that begins with one simple question that the Food Babe inspires us to ask, that she has fearlessly asked over and over.

What is in our food?

Is it food? Is it good for us or bad for us? If it is not food, we probably shouldn't eat it. If it is food, we should eat it. That is the guiding principle of the Food Babe Way, a way to live that will lead us into a new era of health and will change the world one fork at a time, one bite at a time, one kitchen at a time, one person at a time. Read this book and you will never think about food, your health, or the world in the same way again. And we will all be better off for it.

—Mark Hyman, MD

NOTE TO THE READER

Neither this eating plan nor any other program should be followed without first consulting a health care professional. If you have any special or medical conditions requiring attention, you should consult with your health care professional regularly regarding possible modifications of the program contained in this book. The author's references to various products are for information purposes only and are not intended as an endorsement for those products from the author, her book, or the publisher. Statements made about products and descriptions of those products are accurate as of the writing of this book, November 2014.

THE
FOOD BABE
WAY

INTRODUCTION

I WANTED TO LUNGE across the table, grab them by their shoulders, and cram their own toxin-laced product down their throats. But I hung on to my cool. I had to be strong. I was there to convince one of the biggest food companies in the world to change their ingredients.

I was sitting in a tiny, claustrophobic conference room at Kraft Foods headquarters in Northfield, Illinois, meeting with some impersonal corporate PR types. I had recently launched an assault on the company for failing to protect consumers, including children, from the toxic colorings in Kraft products—chemicals that pose serious threats to our health.

After being invited to meet with Kraft, I had expected to see the CEO and the top macaroni and cheese product executive. Instead, I was greeted by two soulless employees who had no authority to make any real decisions. I should have known better, especially considering how I was escorted in: by security, and watched like a thief walking into a jewelry store. They even hovered outside the door to the bathroom while I went in. They treated me like a pest and checked my iPhone to make sure I wasn't recording anything.

I explained my position on several issues. At the time of our meeting, more than thirty Kraft macaroni and cheese products laced with artificial dyes were being sold in America. However, in Europe, Kraft removed the dyes and replaced them with natural ingredients like paprika and beta-carotene.

Scientists have confirmed what was already suspected: that these artificial food dyes, which are made from petroleum, can cause allergic reactions, may be tainted with carcinogens (substances that cause cancer), and have been linked in at least one study to hyperactivity in children.

Would Kraft consider a label change to warn consumers? The answer was swift and blunt: No.

How dare they!

I did not let up. I pointed out that Kraft macaroni and cheese is on kids' menus at various chain restaurants like Applebee's, IHOP, and Bob Evans. All the children who order this item are consuming artificial dyes and don't know it because the ingredients are not listed on menus. I asked Kraft if they would consider offering a version without dyes to kids, but they declined to answer.

This was shameless, especially considering they knew how to develop a safer product and were already doing this in other countries.

I grilled them about the Kraft products available in the United Kingdom.

"Why did you reformulate mac and cheese without artificial food dyes overseas but not here in the United States? Artificial food dyes are still allowed in Europe — but you reformulated them there. Why?"

The meeting took on a pathetic tone. They acted as though they hadn't heard me. It was possible they were ruminating on the content of my confrontation. But more likely, they had retreated to some place where denial insulated them from the chill of my words.

Visibly uncomfortable, they stared at me with cold, stuporous eyes. No one took any notes except me.

Kraft is feeding poison to so many families. How can they sleep at night?

Like automatons in lockstep, they stated that they were complying with the FDA laws and look to "scientists and regulators" when formulating their products.

This well-rehearsed company line prompted me to ask: "Why did Kraft spend more than ten million dollars during the last five years lobbying the FDA? And why does Europe require a warning label for these dyes?"

They answered my questions with "We don't know" and "Kraft is making the right choice" and "We have to agree to disagree."

These mega-corporations have chosen to be the primary vendors of the foods that are supposed to fortify families across the country, if not the globe, yet they stuff them full of chemicals not for any nutritional benefit but rather to broaden their reach and fatten their bottom lines. Why aren't these companies doing anything to make our food more nutritious? When we pluck food from the supermarket shelves, we trust that manufacturers have our best interests at heart and that the food is all safe to eat. But we're being conned. Maybe someday food manufacturers will get the message... and we'll all live happily ever after.

I'm Vani Hari, aka the Food Babe. This is what I do—hold food companies accountable for their practices.

Though it pisses off most of the corporate food establishment, I regularly expose the unhealthy ingredients and practices that food companies don't want you to know about. It makes me mad to see how these big corporations have adulterated our foods with trans fats, refined flour, extra sugar, dough strengtheners, fake flavorings, chemical additives, pesticides, hormones, genetically modified organisms, and lots more.

With the help of an army of concerned citizens, I've put the heat on several big food companies—not just Kraft, but also Chipotle, Starbucks, Chick-fil-A, and Subway, to name just a few—to get them to disclose the ingredients in their foods and, where those ingredients are toxins, to remove them. We have rocked the food industry at many different levels.

When I'm not fighting the food establishment, you can find me hanging out at farmers' markets and whole-foods-type supermarkets. I love to eat fresh, additive-free, organically produced food. I like to discover new food products and figure out what sorts of ingredients might be lurking within them. I study food labels intensely. I love to research food and health, in medical journals, university studies, and literature that you can find published only in other countries. I've become friends with the scientists, nutritionists, and experts who aren't afraid to tell the truth about what's happening to our food supply and health. I'm obsessed with knowing what people are putting in their bodies. I've spent entire days, sometimes weeks, doggedly tracing foods and food products back to their roots. I've gone into restaurant chains and grocery stores and quizzed employees, customer service reps, and executives. I've traveled to food factories to learn the processes and meet the makers behind the food we eat. I've made it my mission to educate as many people as I can about how to live an organic lifestyle in an over-processed, contaminated-food world.

I'm just a regular person who got tired of being a victim to big food companies and developed the courage to seek the truth. I'm not a part of the nutrition, dietetics, or medical establishment. And that's a good thing, because many of them have swallowed and passed along industry-funded advice that has made us all sicker, fatter, and more unhealthy than we've ever been in history. We're blighted with increasing rates of obesity, heart disease, diabetes, autoimmune disorders, neurological problems, and many types of cancer. The way these groups—and the government—deny the causes of these epidemics troubles me. They stick their heads in the sand, encourage more of the same behavior that got us in this mess, and just say "We don't know."

I disagree. We do know. They just aren't willing to see—or respond. It's easier for doctors to continue treating symptoms instead of causes and for drug companies to develop new, moneymaking drugs than it is to change the nation's food supply.

I know this because I was just a normal American girl who grew up eating what everyone around me was eating. I loved pizza, fast foods, grocery store birthday cake, candy, anything that came from a box or an industrial deep fryer. I mowed it all down ravenously.

Then I got sick, really sick.

JUNK FOOD AND ME

Before I elaborate, I want to share my life with you—how I was raised, and what led me into food investigations and activism.

My dad was born in India and was the first person in my family to come to America. He came here to study and live the American dream. When his parents (my grandparents) summoned him back to India to get married—in a traditional arranged marriage—he was introduced to my mom and a slew of other women, all in a lineup. He knew my mom was the one right away, and none of the others compared to her. One of my aunts tells me this story all the time.

Thinking she was on a weekend trip to meet a gentleman, my mom had no idea that she would end up married a few days later and be whisked away for the honeymoon to America, where she would live for the rest of her life. She didn't even get to pack up her old room. My dad loves the United States so much that he ended up bringing not only his bride, but every single member of my family here, helping them get their citizenship, jobs, and everything they needed for a comfortable life. My aunt, for example, worked at McDonald's, where we dined frequently.

My parents settled in Charlotte, North Carolina. Like many Southern cities, the town has many famous and popular restaurant chains, serving large plates of foods that are fried, covered in batter, and smothered in gravy. Everyone ate at these chains while I was growing up. They also shopped at the local Harris Teeter and Food Lion. My neighbors were notorious for having the least-healthy snacks on the planet: snack cakes, ice cream sandwiches, every kind of potato and tortilla chip, candy bars, and so forth. But I would gorge nonetheless, never noticing that the boy I was playing with was severely overweight. Kids made fun of him at school. You'd think I'd have known better. But I was ignorant about food back then.

Dad and Mom had my brother first and then, seven years later, me. They named me Vani, a name I hated as a child because my schoolmates made fun of it and no one could pronounce it. But in Indian, it means "voice"—how prophetic, because I've definitely developed one.

When I was a little girl, I loved to go to the grocery store with my mom and stare, mesmerized, at the cereal boxes with their cartoon characters looking back at me. I just knew that the cereal would taste better if there was a cartoon on the box, and I yanked at my mother's skirt, begging her to buy it. I'd steal candy (because she wouldn't buy it for me) and hide it in my pockets until I got home. Then I'd store it in a secret cabinet in a side table next to our living room couch. I'd sneak it as I pleased.

Growing up in the South and being the only Indian kid in the classroom was sometimes challenging. I wanted to fit in with the other girls in my class. I wanted to be just like them, so I ate just like them. I shunned my mother's cooking from the start. She is the most brilliant Indian cook I know—and to think I didn't really taste her food until my early twenties devastates me.

My mom would plan two meals every day: gorgeous fresh vegetarian Indian food for my dad, and for me and my brother, anything we wanted. There were no rules. If we wanted McDonald's, we got it. If we wanted Wendy's, we got it. If we wanted mozzarella sticks from the FryDaddy, she made them. My favorite was the Salisbury steak with mashed potatoes that came out of the freezer and could be heated in minutes in the microwave. Our birthday cakes came from the grocery store freezer section, or from fast-food restaurants, or were made from a box. Having my sixth birthday at Burger King was a highlight for me. My mom wasn't as skilled at making American food from scratch, so she called in the "experts": frozen dinners full of preservatives, cake mixes from Betty Crocker with trans fats and artificial food dyes, premade soups from Campbell's with additives like MSG, among others.

I was a picky child. I ate everything plain, with no sauce. I remember once on a trip with my parents to Chicago, my dad bought me a Burger King croissant sandwich. It was not prepared exactly the way I'd ordered it, and I threw a huge ridiculous fit. The only thing I wasn't picky about was candy. I would eat huge amounts of it with my dad on the couch every evening (a habit which later led to his type 2 diabetes). I was a candy addict. To my family and friends, I was the queen of candy! I knew every brand, every flavor, and always had candy with me. When I look at pictures of me as a child, I find that I was usually gripping candy so no one would take it away from me.

Along with these food habits came problems for me and my brother. We both had severe allergies, asthma, stomach issues, and skin problems. My parents took us in and out of doctor's offices looking for a cure or treatment. We were both on several prescription medications as a result, taking a course of antibiotics and steroids almost every year. I had bad eczema as a child, but in my high school years it was all over my face. When I was eighteen, my brother took me to Europe. We visited the most amazing cities, but in all the pictures we took, there is a large red rash all over my face.

By nature, I'm quite strong-willed and outspoken. However, I dreaded any situation where there might be a camera — weddings, birthdays, or other parties. I look at those pictures now and can see myself hiding in the back. And in every one, my skin looks horrendous. I can't remember a time when my day wasn't determined by how good or bad my complexion was. I never felt beautiful.

I was also beginning to put on weight. Along with my asthma and various types of allergies, the weight gain brought years of absolute misery. At the time, I didn't connect any of these problems to what I was eating. I had no source to consult, no knowledge base to tell me that what I was putting into my body was poisoning me and making me fat.

In high school, I made a decision that would shape my life forever: I quit the cheerleading squad to join the debate team. I spent every waking moment thinking about the year's debate topic. I had to learn to debate both sides of a topic — both affirmative and negative. From this experience, I learned how to argue issues every which way.

As a debater, I spent more time in the library researching the year's debate topic and learning how to beat my opponent than doing my schoolwork. I was obsessed. We didn't have Google back then, so we had to spend countless hours in libraries photocopying journals and newspapers for evidence to use at debate tournaments. Competing on the debate team was one of the most exciting times of my life. I became a nationally ranked debater, placing at Harvard's prestigious debate tournament, attending the Tournament of Champions, and getting recruited to the top debate colleges around the country. Little did I know I was honing skills that would serve me well as a food investigator and activist.

But after my brother and my parents convinced me I was not going to make a living debating, I quit the team in college to concentrate fully on my major: computer science. It was the wave of the future.

After I graduated from college, I received a job offer from Accenture, a major management consulting firm. I was the only woman in my class to get an offer from this prestigious firm, and I thought I had hit the jackpot.

But I was intimidated. Everyone worked long hours—sometimes up to eighty hours a week. Trying to keep up, I followed suit. I continued my childhood pattern of eating to fit in, so I ate what my coworkers ate. Every day, the company catered our meals and snacks from local restaurants—so we could eat quickly and get back to work. I remember spreads with chicken Parmesan, pasta, BBQ, and late-night Krispy Kreme. I ate it all. After working a twelve-hour schedule, alternating between four days of day shift and four days of night shift, plus lots of business travel, I'd gained around thirty pounds in only three months.

Not only was I fat, my eczema was still bad. I thought the condition was incurable. My allergies would not let up. And I was taking several prescription meds, to treat everything from those nasty allergies to my asthma. I was a mess.

After a major project ended, I got an assignment in my hometown, Charlotte, where I didn't have to travel. It was wonderful getting a break from traveling and the late nights, but my poor eating continued. Like so many other people, I'd become addicted to chemically derived food.

Then my life changed.

MY WAKE-UP CALL

It was December 2002. After leaving the gym, I stopped at Chick-fil-A to pick up an under-300-calorie sandwich. Back then I thought this was healthy, and I would eat a Chick-fil-A sandwich three or four times a week, sometimes more.

I got home and collapsed on the floor with knifelike stomach pains of a kind I had never experienced. I first called my brother, who then called my parents. They rushed me to the emergency room. I was so doubled over in pain that I was writhing around on the waiting room floor.

The doctor who treated me pronounced that nothing was wrong and sent me home with instructions to take Advil every four to six hours. This did not work; the pain persisted, relentlessly. The next morning, my parents urged me to see my family doctor. He diagnosed me with acute appendicitis and instructed me to go straight into surgery. I had to have my appendix removed immediately.

During the normally festive, fun-filled month of December, I was home, recovering. It takes the average person one or two weeks to recover from an appendectomy. It took me almost four. Little did I know that this was because my body was so sick and weak from all the processed food I had been ingesting.

Medical experts say that appendicitis happens more or less at random. I believe that in my case, my lifestyle of poor nutrition caused this horrible thing to happen. My whole body was inflamed, so it's easy to understand why an organ in my digestive system was also inflamed.

Those weeks were interminable. Lying in bed recovering, while everyone else was shopping and celebrating the holidays, I made a commitment to myself: to make my health my number one priority.

As soon as I regained my energy, I dug deep into the skills I'd learned as a debater and started researching to identify the most nutritious and healing foods on the planet. I also decided to figure out what was in the food I had been eating—what had made me sick in the first place. I became intoxicated with the process of discovery, and I investigated food issues ferociously: additives we can't pronounce, food coloring made from petrochemicals and the bodies of dried, ground-up insects, cancer-causing preservatives, and much more.

The more I learned, the more outraged I became. I couldn't believe there was beaver's ass in my vanilla ice cream, coal tar in my mac and cheese, yoga mat and shoe rubber in my bread, and the same ingredient used in Silly Putty in my French fries. I never knew that "natural flavorings" were actually created from gross animal parts, or that there was powdered glass (sand) in fast-food chili. I discovered that genetically modified organisms (GMOs) have been added to our food supply. That means some of our food has had foreign genes bred into it—a Frankenfood scenario—to make it last longer, resist pests, and generally be hardier. And for the past fifteen years, many of our meats and dairy products have come from cows injected with hormones and fed antibiotics to increase their meat and milk production.

On another level, I didn't want to believe the facts I read. I wanted to close my eyes, cover my ears, and sing "lalalalalala." I never gave permission for my body to be used as a toxic waste dump or a science experiment. Everything I had been putting in my body was either made from something out of a chemical factory, sprayed with chemicals, or genetically modified to make companies richer and me sicker.

FREEDOM FROM FOOD ADDITIVES: MY TRANSFORMATION

My own chronic health problems led me to make the connection to food, a link that made sense once I started researching the effects of certain chemicals on the body. I learned how to detoxify my very poisoned body, and when I did, all my health problems started to vanish.

I lost those thirty pounds. My so-called incurable eczema totally healed, and my skin glowed. My asthma and allergies became ancient history. My stomach issues vanished. My anxiety was gone; I no longer had to take any drugs, prescription or over-the-counter.

Today, people ask me what I did to transform myself. I didn't go on a diet. I didn't join a gym. I had no special beauty regimen. In fact, my transformation really had nothing directly to do with weight loss, clear skin, or allergy-free health. Those were merely by-products of a single resolution I made: *to break free from my chemical relationship with food.*

My friends and family saw the 180-degree turnaround in my health and my looks. They wanted to know what I had done to change so radically. To this day, my aunt swears I've had work done. There was definitely some work done, but not through cosmetic surgery. It was done through careful research and deliberate thought about what I would put in my body after learning about our polluted food supply.

Everyone I knew begged me to start a blog and join social media so I could share my way of life with them. So I did. I started blogging in 2011 to educate people about the ingredients in their food and teach them how to live an organic, additive-free, healthy lifestyle.

My blog, foodbabe.com, rocketed to popularity because I wasn't afraid to tell the truth. People wanted access to information that was intentionally being kept from them. With a quirky name like the Food Babe, I've been able to battle the biggest food industry giants with attacks they never saw coming. But this wasn't a name I chose for myself. It was given to me by my husband. I had wanted to call the blog something totally different—like "Eat Healthy Live Forever.com." He said no one would remember that, so he came up with "Food Babe."

At first I was skeptical. It's short and sweet but sounded self-centered. Did I have enough guts to call myself the Food Babe?

Despite my doubts, I went with my husband's instinct, and continued with the notion that I would teach everyone to be a Food Babe.

Because I was still working in the corporate world, I kept my identity secret and never put my real name on the blog. Instead, I signed each blog post "Food Babe," until I quit my job and really began to understand my calling in life was to do this work.

My growing distrust of the mainstream food supply has driven me to investigate major food companies. I don't hold back. I write fearlessly on my blog about the injustices I uncover. My blog has attracted millions of people who are willing to hold companies accountable and share important health information with loved ones.

Today, I call my readers the Food Babe Army, because they care not only about what they eat and what their families eat, but also about what everyone eats—and they fight for a healthier food supply. Powerful and amazing, their collective activism is now a very loud voice in our country. Together, we launch petitions against the companies that are poisoning us and raise awareness about food pollution. Today, not only do I have my own health back, but several thousand members of the Food Babe Army have reclaimed their health, too.

With nonstop energy and a strong sense of mission, we will continue to speak up and get corporations to make changes. We cannot be deterred. I discovered that if you believe in something and share the truth, people will take action.

Ironically, I can thank my poor eating habits for opening my eyes to a new way of living that has brought me more fitness, beauty, radiance, and energy than I ever could have imagined.

STOP IMPERILING YOUR HEALTH

When you stop toxic chemicals from invading your body, you'll be thinner, sexier, healthier, and more vital than ever. In fact, let me ask you now:

- Do you have extra pounds to lose that you can't get rid of, no matter what diet you follow?
- Do you struggle with figuring out what to buy and eat?
- Do you find yourself unable to focus during the day?
- Do you eat too many processed foods and not enough real food?
- Do you want a clear, brighter, and more vibrant complexion?
- Do you want to easily create and follow an organic and additive-free diet?

If you answered yes to any of these questions, *The Food Babe Way* is for you.

As we go through this book together, I won't just talk with you about the nasty stuff in our foods. I'll introduce you to an amazing array of foods you can eat. And I'll give you a practical, easy-to-follow twenty-one-day program with delicious, additive-free meal plans that will put you on the path to thin, gorgeous, handsome, energetic, sexy, and healthy.

Amassing more products, diets, regimens, and treatments won't cut it. You've got to rid yourself of polluting foods and reclaim your common sense about what natural, healthy food really is. *The Food Babe Way* is about empowering you—letting you know that the food you eat is, in a sense, creating your future health and well-being. I'm putting all my information, investigative work, and guidance into a real-life plan you can follow daily.

TRANSFORM YOUR WEIGHT, YOUR HEALTH, AND YOUR LIFE IN 21 DAYS

In *The Food Babe Way*, I will show you how to:

- Develop twenty-one positive, everlasting habits, a day at a time, that will get you off chemical-laced food.
- Follow a satisfying, pure diet of real food that will transform your shape, your body, and your health.
- Replace the foods that make you fat, make you look older, and sap your energy with healthful, delicious substitutes.
- Decipher ingredient labels and avoid buying products that could be harming your health.
- Decode the information the food industry is intentionally hiding from you.
- Add certain powerhouse foods to your diet that will help clear the toxins from your body.
- Shop for natural, organic ingredients that won't drain your wallet.
- Prepare additive-free meals with easy and delicious recipes.
- Be prepared for any situation, from shopping at the grocery store to eating at a fancy restaurant.

Trust me, in just twenty-one days, you'll have the knowledge you need to make informed decisions. You'll drop extra pounds along the way. And most important, you'll set up habits for a healthy and organic lifestyle, allowing you to look and feel your best—for life.

I once thought I was a different species from all the beautiful people I went to school with and worked with. But that alien species wasn't me; it was the nasty stuff I was ingesting, care of the food industry. For years I lived a life that disregarded health and common sense. But in the end, I won the long battle against my body, my beauty, and myself.

You, too, can win—if you take food companies to task and gradually rid your body of unnecessary food chemicals. It won't take you ten or twenty years, either—just twenty-one days.

I want this book to be your personal bible. Underline words. Highlight sentences. Dog-ear the pages. You'll learn to be your own food investigator, activist, and nutritionist, so that you can change your relationship with food, become empowered to take charge of your life, and follow a program that delivers dramatic and permanent results.

I invite you on this journey with me. *The Food Babe Way* will be a profound physical and emotional transformation for you.

PART I

THOSE TRICKY
SONS OF . . .

CHAPTER 1

WE'VE BEEN DUPED

EVERY BITE OF FOOD that passes through our lips and every glass of water we drink are potential sources of toxic chemicals, including pesticide residue, preservatives, artificial flavors and colorings, addicting sugars and fats, genetically modified organisms, and more. These toxins can travel to, and settle into, all the organs of your body, particularly the liver, kidneys, gastrointestinal tract, and lungs—and do great damage. Scientists are now blaming chemical-ridden food for the dramatic rise in obesity, heart disease, chronic fatigue syndrome, infertility, dementia, mental illness, and more. Our food system is in dire shape—and so are we.

AN ACCIDENTAL ACTIVIST

Several years ago, after learning that I could live a life beyond the clutch of chemically laced foods, I embarked on a challenging and unforgettable journey. At the time, I was a blogger by night, while my career in business consulting was rocketing up by day. Had it not been for frozen yogurt, I might still be living a double life.

I'm curious by nature. I like to find out all I can about a situation, and I love the process of discovery. I can't imagine anything worse than not experiencing something new, whether it's an organic food, a book, or a foreign country to visit.

So when I discovered Yoforia frozen yogurt, which I found more delicious than other brands, I started eating it like it was going out of style. Yoforia had just opened a new store at my favorite mall; it was the perfect stopping place for a snack.

Yoforia advertised its products as organic. Huge ads stating "organic tastes better" plastered the walls of the store. With that kind of messaging, the frozen yogurt just had to have some yummy, good-for-you stuff in it, right? Plus, you could get your frozen yogurt topped with fresh fruit.

I remember sitting in my cubicle one day talking to my coworker Rachel. She told me she had indulged in a big bowl of Yoforia frozen yogurt the night before while shopping—and that it was to die for. My mouth was watering, and I couldn't wait to start spooning it in.

But I got to thinking: With so many flavors available, what ingredients did Yoforia use for the flavor? I went right into some of the stores and asked. No one would tell me what was in the yogurt; nor were any ingredients posted online.

I tried e-mailing the company. Radio silence. I got suspicious.

I finally convinced one store employee to show me a bag of powdered stuff they were dumping into the yogurt. I investigated more. I found out that there was a dark side to my favorite frozen treat. The primary organic ingredient was the milk. The rest was trans fats, food coloring, and all sorts of other nasty preservatives and additives!

I had been duped. Rachel had been duped. Many innocent people had been duped by Yoforia's marketing. I wanted everyone to know the story, so I blogged about it on foodbabe.com. I emphasized that this was a travesty—to market the product as organic while not disclosing its complete list of ingredients. Unbeknownst to me at the time, my article went viral among a huge community of Yoforia's customers.

There was backlash. The Yoforia CEO got so much grief on the company's customer service hotline that he wrote me a personal letter to apologize and tell me that Yoforia was working to change the ingredients. The letter was rather excuse-ridden, honestly. But a few months later, he met with me personally at a trade show, and we discussed the issues. Using every single debate skill I could muster, I protested that

Yoforia's frozen yogurt wasn't exactly what you'd call healthful or even natural, and that it was misleading, in my opinion, to prominently use the word "organic." As far as I was concerned, Yoforia's marketing was deceptive, and I told him so.

After that meeting, he did pull back on the marketing BS and posted the ingredients online. But as of this writing, Yoforia's ingredients have not changed, and they are still using some misleading marketing messages.

Still, I was floored by the influence my blog had. I thought: "If I can get one company to change for the better, I have the power to hold other food companies accountable, too."

I had stumbled, almost unintentionally, into the world of consumer investigations and citizen journalism. I was convinced that unless food companies changed, we'd continue to be plagued by dangerous additives in our foods. I knew that I, just an everyday girl writing a blog, had a shot at changing the food policies of major corporations. That's when I became a food activist. My passion for exposing the truth about the food industry soared.

IS CHIPOTLE "FOOD WITH INTEGRITY"?

The Yoforia experience shocked me into action. Were other chains with "healthy marketing" pitches telling the truth, or lying through their food wrappers?

I decided to investigate Chipotle because of its slogan: "Food with Integrity." Curious, I looked up the restaurant's website, only to discover that Chipotle had never released its ingredients online. That made me extremely skeptical. I called the company's headquarters to find out why.

"Do you have an allergy to something?" the Chipotle representative asked.

"Why do I have to have an allergy to know what's in your food—don't I have the right to know what I'm eating?"

"Sorry, we can't give you the ingredients."

Undeterred, I went into individual restaurants to find out. No one was willing to talk, except one employee who eventually let me know the truth.

So I said loud and clear on my blog that no one should trust a company that is not willing to disclose their ingredients. I wrote, "How can we trust Chipotle's definition of 'Food with Integrity' when they refuse to post their ingredients or send the information to customers who ask?"

People got so angry and frustrated that they stormed Chipotle's social media pages. Someone even started an online petition on my behalf to pressure the company into being honest about how their food was prepared. We gathered 2,000 signatures almost immediately.

I think what angered people most was the information Chipotle didn't want to share—information that I had uncovered. For example: Hiding out in their famous burrito shell was trans fat. Several of their menu items were full of genetically engineered corn and soy. Almost nothing was organic.

Chipotle got so much negative publicity that they reached out and set up a meeting, where they pledged to start publishing ingredient information. At first I didn't believe them. Nonetheless, I offered to help.

"Listen," I said. "Because you know what's in your food, publishing your ingredients is really very easy. What's taking you so long? I'll help you put them online for free. I know how websites work and can help you do it really quickly—we can get a downloadable PDF up by tomorrow."

"Well, first we want to clean up some of our ingredients before we disclose them on our website," they told me.

That was a good start, I thought.

On March 22, 2013, Chipotle sent me an e-mail that said "Ta dah!" with a link to their much-improved ingredient list online. Not only did they post the full ingredient list, they labeled the genetically engineered (GMO) ingredients on their menu and have vowed to eventually go GMO-free. I heard they are even working to fix that burrito shell. I got the e-mail on my birthday—one of the best gifts I've ever received.

CHICK-FIL-A OR CHEMICAL-FIL-A?

One day, my husband, whom I now affectionately call Mr. Food Babe, came home from work with a nutritional guide from Chick-fil-A. All I could think was "God, please, I hope he did not eat there!"

Instead, he told me about a woman at his office who ate at Chick-fil-A, and that he was trying to convince her not to. (I was very proud of him.) The woman came back to the office after eating there and handed a pamphlet to my husband, saying, "See, not so bad—the sandwich I eat is only three hundred and ninety calories!"

He quickly directed her to the more important information on the sheet: the ingredients, not the calories. There were nearly 100 ingredients in the most popular famous sandwich!

I took a snapshot of that list with my phone and immediately posted it on my personal Facebook page. The reactions I got from close friends and family were everything from horrified to "no one is going to stop me from eating those 100 ingredients of deliciousness."

These wide-ranging reactions inspired me to write one of my most popular posts to date: "Chick-fil-A or Chemical-fil-A?" In fact, I wrote several blog posts during the summer of 2012 about the unholy ingredients in the company's sandwiches, from antibiotics, to MSG, to artificial food dyes, to GMOs and TBHQ.

Let me take a little detour here to say that you can't get much more toxic than TBHQ. It stands for tertiary butylhydroquinone—an ingredient that is listed twice in Chick-fil-A sandwiches, once for the chicken and once for the bun. TBHQ is one scary chemical. It's created from butane (a very toxic gas) and can only be used at a rate of 0.02 percent of the total oil in a product. Why is such a limit imposed? Maybe because eating only 1 gram of this toxic preservative has been shown to cause all sorts of issues, from attention deficit hyperactivity disorder (ADHD) in children to asthma, allergies, dermatitis, and dizziness. It can even cause stomach cancer in laboratory animals.

I interviewed parents and asked them why they took their kids to Chick-fil-A. The top three answers were: "My kids requested it" (who's in charge—you or your kids?); "It's better quality and tastes fresh" (not with nearly fifty additives in one sandwich); and "If I turn in the toy from the kids' meal, I can get an ice cream cone that my kid loves" (that little treat has all sorts of processed sugar, trans fat, and artificial food coloring).

Word got to the company about my posts, and out of the blue came an invitation from Chick-fil-A. I was traveling, living in a tent near the Golden Triangle, where Thailand, Burma, and Laos meet. Suddenly I had a cell phone signal, and an e-mail came through. I woke up my husband, who was half asleep, and screamed, "This is crazy! They're inviting me...me! They must hate what I'm doing and are trying to stop it."

I was scared, nervous, and unsure how to respond at first. I didn't answer the e-mail right away. I waited several days and then decided that to change the world, you have to be willing to meet with your enemies.

In October 2012, I flew to the company's headquarters in Atlanta. I had convinced Chick-fil-A to let me bring a videographer to capture the meeting so I could fully report on what happened. I was chauffeured in a "Cow Mobile," a car outfitted with cow-patterned wrapping. Upon arriving, the first thing I saw was the real Batmobile, the same vehicle used in the blockbuster movies. All I could think was "Damn; they sold a lot of factory-farmed chicken laced with harmful additives to buy that iconic relic."

I spent a whole day there, and they treated me well, presumably to try to win me over. That wasn't going to happen; I was on a mission. I discussed my laundry list of concerns. During the meeting, execs asked me to prioritize the list of requests on a whiteboard. I told them eliminating artificial food dyes would be a quick change to implement. I quizzed them specifically on their vanilla ice cream. "Why do you have Yellow #5 dye in your vanilla ice cream, when that product should be white, anyway, and not yellow?" Their excuse was that they had originally used egg yolk, but it had to come out for processing reasons. I wasn't buying it and insisted that they return to using natural ingredients and making that recipe work.

My number one request, however, was to provide safer and more sustainable chicken raised without antibiotics or GMO feed.

The elimination of antibiotics would be a significant commitment. The more we use antibiotics in our environment, the less effective they are in treating certain superbug infections. The widespread use of antibiotics in animal feed has given rise to new strains of antibiotic-resistant bacteria that could, frankly, wipe out the human race if we don't start doing something about it now.

To date, Chick-fil-A has indicated they will be working with their current suppliers to make the transition, rather than outsourcing antibiotic-free meat that might already be available. But this might take five years — a strategy that gives me some heartache. I'd like to see them influence their suppliers, like Tyson, Perdue, and others, to move faster, or at least consider using other suppliers who are not using antibiotics in the meantime. Regardless, their decision to make this switch will have an enormous impact on the fast-food industry and put pressure on other major chains to finally do the right thing.

My other demands called for the wholesale removal of all artificial ingredients from Chick-fil-A sandwiches. I stressed to the company that they'd be surprised how many people would choose clean, organic food if offered. And if Chick-fil-A did make their menu items additive-free and organic, I promised the company that I'd rent a chicken or cow costume or whatever they wanted and run up and down the street on live TV.

Not long after this meeting, I received an e-mail from Chick-fil-A executives confirming that the company would:

- Remove Yellow #5 and reduce sodium in their chicken soup recipe. The new soup rolled out chain-wide in 2014.
- Remove high-fructose corn syrup and artificial colors from several sauces and dressings. The new, improved condiments were tested and rolled out in 2014.
- Test peanut oil without TBHQ in multiple markets, with plans to roll out the new formulation in 2014.
- Create and test "cleaner" additive-free white buns — without the chemical azodicarbonamide in them. I call azodicarbonamide the yoga mat toxin, because it's found in yoga mats. Commercial bakers love it because it helps keep bread nice and spongy — just as it keeps your yoga mat cushiony. However, this chemical has

been linked to respiratory problems, including asthma in factory workers, and when heated, it produces semicarbazide, a known carcinogen.

Constant pressure on Chick-fil-A for two years had worked.

GMOs, POLITICS, AND ME

While all of this was going on, I ran against 250 people in my district and was elected a delegate to the Democratic National Convention. A delegate is someone who represents the constituents of a voting district at a political convention in order to elect a party's nominees for president and vice-president. Attending these conventions, which are held every four years, are politicians, media, and decision makers from all over the country. I wanted to get their attention.

I ran to be a delegate so I could discuss with key leaders of our government the failure of the Obama administration to pass a law requiring food companies to label foods containing genetically modified organisms (GMOs). President Obama had abandoned this stance. Why? Upsetting Big Agriculture and the chemical industry was not going to help him get reelected in 2012. Protecting the rights of American consumers and keeping his campaign pledge were obviously of secondary importance.

Genetic modification occurs when genes, viruses, or bacteria from one organism are artificially injected into a fruit or vegetable in a process that occurs in a laboratory and not in nature. The result is a GMO, or a genetically modified organism. Genetic modification is done to make a fruit or vegetable more hardy or impervious to the application of specific pesticides. These pesticides are linked to myriad diseases.

GMOs are found in more than 70 percent of processed foods. More than sixty-four countries around the world require GMOs to be labeled or regulated. The United States does not.

At parties and meetings the week of the convention, I had as many conversations as I could about GMO labeling with national Democratic leaders, media, and celebrities. Jesse Jackson, former presidential candidate, and Rahm Emanuel, mayor of Chicago and former chief of staff for President Obama, both said they didn't know anything about the issue and had me repeat the question twice. President Bill Clinton deftly avoided answering the question and instead told me about being vegan. Chris Matthews, talk show host on MSNBC, rolled his eyes at me and asked, "When has that [GMO labeling] ever been an issue brought up on one of my shows?"

I now know why a GMO labeling law has never passed.

To bring attention to this issue, during Michelle Obama's speech, I whipped out my lipstick, a shade called True Blood, and marked the back of my program in big, bold letters: LABEL GMOS!

The next day, I came prepared with real markers. When Secretary of Agriculture Tom Vilsack spoke at the convention, I made sure to get into the front row so that I could protest right in front of his face. It was hard to listen to what he had to say because I was besieged by video cameras and photographers trying to capture what I was doing. For the rest of the convention, a dedicated security guard watched over me, and they banished me to the back row, a punishment that was well worth it in my eyes. If a convention isn't the time to speak up and stand up for your rights, I don't know what is!

Later, when I reread Vilsack's speech, I was reminded that he is a bureaucrat, not a man willing to go against his financial ties to protect the rights and health of American citizens. Despite polls consistently showing that more than 90 percent of the population want GMOs to be labeled, our leaders in Washington refuse to acknowledge this truth and will not implement mandatory GMO labeling at the federal level.

During this time, I was still working at my demanding job as a management consultant. I was successful and earning a good living. The problem was that my passion for food activism was overtaking my life as a corporate wonk. But the die was cast; I realized I had a voice, I had power, and I could change the food world. In the grand scheme of things, I felt a calling to do something greater with my life and have a larger impact on the world. I began to contemplate quitting my job.

Yet I was terrified. I was worried about how I'd make my mortgage, have health insurance, and feed my family. I felt like I was jumping without a net. Nonetheless, I decided to end my thirteen-year management consulting career in December 2012.

As the new year rolled around, I was making no money, and I had no "real job." I was operating in the red, really, because I was putting out money to support the cost of running my blog. But once I made the leap, I was unstoppable.

As soon as I was able to dedicate my full attention to the blog, things started to change dramatically. I plugged away, working from morning until night. My articles went viral. There'd be more than 100,000 Facebook likes on an article, and millions of views, for example.

I realized that my last career had been a bridge to this new path, and frankly, money didn't matter. Everything I had learned up to this point had groomed me to make this transition. I had been able to apply my business acumen and combine it with my passion for food quality. I realized that every good thing that had ever happened to me happened because I had decided to make a change.

CRAFTY KRAFT

Now that I could devote my full attention to activism, I knew I needed to address the prolific use of artificial food dyes in the food system. I had received thousands of letters from parents telling me how their children had gotten healthier after getting off all artificial dyes. Kraft macaroni and cheese, of course, is laced with all sorts of petroleum-based dyes that at least one study has linked to hyperactivity in children. I was shocked that they'd put their consumers, especially kids, at potential risk and that the FDA would allow something like that to be put in products. I wanted Kraft to remove these dyes. They did it with their UK product, why not in the United States?

I started a petition with my friend Lisa Leake on March 5, 2013, targeting Kraft, requesting they remove artificial food dyes from their macaroni and cheese. The petition received more than 24,000 signatures in twenty-four hours, and this response created a media firestorm. Every news agency under the sun called me that week. They wanted to know what had motivated me and why I was petitioning Kraft. I told the news reporters I was sick of Americans getting exploited for profit and that the food industry couldn't hide any longer. When I was invited to appear on *The Dr. Oz Show*, I jumped up on my bed and screamed. I knew *The Dr. Oz Show* would give me the leverage I needed to get Kraft to change. I had stirred up a lot of hornets' nests, for sure.

But my appearance on *The Dr. Oz Show* didn't do anything right away. Kraft sent a statement to the show, saying that the FDA deemed these artificial food dyes safe. In this statement, however, Kraft neglected to say anything about the fact that they had removed these dyes from their European versions. Labeling of food containing dyes is mandatory in Europe. Unless they removed dyes, Kraft would have to label their products like this: "May cause adverse effects on activity and attention in children." It was easier for Kraft to remove dyes from their European products than to have to smack their products with warning labels.

In just a few weeks, I had petitions with more than 270,000 signatures. It wasn't enough just to ship the petitions, I wanted to hand-deliver them—these voices of parents all across the country—to the Kraft headquarters myself. And I did that on April first, April Fools' Day. This was no joking matter, though.

It was a bone-chilling morning in the Windy City. I donned a heavy coat, gloves, and earmuffs to protect me from the freezing weather. Fox News Chicago interviewed me live and invited their medical correspondent, a doctor, to confirm that at least one study has shown a correlation between hyperactivity and the consumption of food dyes.

To prove that the UK version of Kraft macaroni and cheese made with natural dyes was just as yellow and tasty as the US version, I held a taste test on a Chicago street. The media swarmed like fireflies, flashing questions like mad.

A crowd gathered and grew. Holding a tray of macaroni and cheese, I tried to talk to as many people as I could. My fingers went completely numb even with gloves on. Almost everyone, especially the kids, said the UK version tasted great; they loved the color and couldn't tell the difference. It was gratifying to know that so many people, once they understood the issue, would choose the macaroni and cheese product without dyes.

I posted a message on Facebook asking fans to call the headquarters on my behalf to ask Kraft to meet with me. I wasn't the only one who did this; several other food advocates (and personal friends) shared this message with their fans, too: the Center for Science in the Public Interest (CSPI); the Cornucopia Institute; the CEO of Nutiva, John Roulac; Zuri Allen from GMO Inside; Leah Segedie from Mamavation; Cheri Johnson from Label GMOs Hollywood; Max Goldberg from Livingmaxwell; Lisa Leake from 100 Days of Real Food; and countless others.

After our taste-testing stunt, I headed to Northfield, Illinois, where Kraft headquarters was located, to deliver the petitions. I walked the boxes of 270,000 signatures across the street to the corner of the security entrance (technically on Kraft's property) and set up on the sidewalk to give speeches on our mission. Members of Change.org and several supporters of the petition joined me that day in the freezing cold.

After the speeches, we picked up the boxes and headed to the front gate. Immediately, the security guard emerged from the booth and handed me a clipboard on which to sign my name. She said, pointing at me, "You are the only one allowed in," and asked us to put the boxes down so they could be collected.

I looked around, screamed "YES!" and hugged Pulin Modi from Change.org and the other activists and supporters who had come out that day. I was overcome. Our persistence had led Kraft to finally agree to sit down with me. I felt the magnitude of the more than 270,000 voices I was representing. Tears of joy ran down my face, mascara smeared everywhere. This was a monumental opportunity; people had been trying to boot artificial dyes out of food for decades.

Once inside the building, I met with representatives from Corporate Affairs—the soulless meeting I told you about at the beginning of this book.

During the next few months, I kept the pressure on Kraft. I continued media interviews to get the word out. I created charts on ways to boycott Kraft and choose safer brands. Activists around the country helped me spread the message.

People started to reject Kraft and chose Annie's—a product without artificial food dyes. Annie's saw their profits soar by over 14 percent the next quarter. Kraft was feeling the pain financially.

Then, just two months after Kraft reported their quarterly results, bull's-eye. In October 2013, they announced that they would eliminate artificial dyes from three macaroni and cheese products, an action I considered a huge victory. The company now uses spices such as paprika to color the product marketed to children with cartoon characters and all of their deluxe varieties. I'm hoping that Kraft will extend its dye changes to all products. Pressure does yield progress, and I know Kraft will eventually make the switch.

TRICKY MARKETING TACTICS

It was June 2012. A police officer was about to kick me out of a building where Subway had a restaurant, for videotaping the sub-making operation. Thankfully, my best friend, Nicole, had already videoed what we needed on my iPhone. I wanted to show people the "real food" they were eating at Subway.

As a corporate consultant, I ate at Subway all the time while traveling. I considered it healthy road food, even though I had given up other fast food years before.

At the time, I had no idea Subway was using the very same processed foods used by other fast-food joints. I'd typically order a foot-long veggie sub (just like Jared) and eat half at lunch and the other half in my hotel room for dinner.

Eventually, I just got tired of Subway food. But I'd continue to see coworkers sling those clear plastic bags filled with foot-long subs on their desks at lunch. One coworker and a dear friend was Wes. He ate at Subway almost every day with his boss. This is what inspired me initially to investigate Subway. I wanted friends like Wes to have the facts. I researched the ingredient lists, with all the additives and preservatives, and wanted everyone to see the truth about what they were ingesting.

Food companies use a lot of marketing sleight of hand to make you think they're serving up something fresh and nutritious. Subway is one of the best examples. As taken from Subway's website, *"We've become the leading choice for people seeking quick, nutritious meals that the whole family can enjoy."*

Subway wants you to believe they serve healthy food. They use many marketing tactics to drive this point home. The tactics that bother me the most are their partnerships with medical associations and our government leaders, because many people take their endorsements as credible and rely on them.

Here's the reality:

Let's start with the American Heart Association's endorsement of Subway as "heart-healthy." This is a farce.

Subway was the first restaurant to obtain the American Heart Association's Heart-Check certification on certain menu items, namely, just a few sandwiches without any cheese or sauce. Subway, however, prominently displays this little logo all over their marketing materials and in their commercials, along with a disclaimer that could lead one to believe that everything on the menu is heart-healthy.

As for salads, the certification applies only to those served with fat-free sweet onion dressing. But that dressing is loaded with sugar and dimethylpolysiloxane, an additive found in Silly Putty and breast implants. I guess the American Heart Association thinks it's heart-healthy to eat this additive, which is sometimes preserved with formaldehyde.

You may also notice that "Doctor's Associates Inc." appears on Subway's menu, napkins, and packaging. What is this group, anyway?

Well, it's simply the corporation that owns Subway restaurants and is in no way associated with any medical organization. Instead of naming their corporation like other restaurants do (e.g., McDonald's Corporation, Arby's Restaurant Group, Inc.), they chose a name that implies they are a medical organization. How do they explain the reasoning behind this? According to their employee guide:

"The name was chosen by Dr. Peter Buck and Fred DeLuca in 1966.

Dr. Buck was a nuclear physicist by profession, and Fred had aspirations of attending medical school to become a doctor. So, the name Doctor's Associates Inc. seemed to fit their situation."

Can you believe it?

There's more. First Lady Michelle Obama's endorsement of Subway as a "healthy choice" for kids saddens me. Our First Lady is now on the record stating that "Subway's kids' menu makes life easier for parents, because they know that no matter what their kids order, it's going to be a healthy choice" and "Every single item meets the highest nutrition standards." This came after a huge announcement that Subway was launching a $41-million "Pile on the Veggies" advertising campaign using the Muppets, aimed at kids, in cooperation with Michelle Obama's Let's Move initiative.

I got so fed up with Subway's "Eat Fresh" advertising campaign that I targeted the company in my petition to remove azodicarbonamide from their bread (the yoga mat chemical I mentioned above). Subway was serving Americans this ingredient, but not citizens in Europe, Australia, and Asia. Why were we eating yoga mat chemicals, while they were not?

Subway had completely ignored my investigation into their ingredients in 2012, further pressure in 2013 when I filmed a video of myself eating a yoga mat to drive the point home, and repeated phone calls and requests to their corporate headquarters. More than 97,000 people signed the petition.

Finally, on February 6, 2014, Subway announced that they would remove azodicarbonamide from their bread. Subway food still has a lot of other unhealthy ingredients. Clearly, they have a lot more work to do, but I remain hopeful.

Getting a company to remove a single ingredient is certainly a victory. But the real victory is that bringing awareness of one ingredient brings awareness of all the toxic ingredients in a food product. People start to see that our entire food supply is tainted—and they mobilize. Mobilizing concerned consumers to take action in order to change our food is truly at the heart of the Food Babe Way.

DON'T JUST BLAME THE FOOD COMPANIES...

Many people ask me why I choose to target specific companies in my campaigns. They've asked why I don't go after the government agencies that approve the ingredients in our food. Unfortunately, because of the screwed-up system we live with, much of the food is controlled not by the government, but rather by the food corporations that are selling it to us. Food companies spend millions of dollars lobbying government officials to influence votes on laws, rules, and regulations, and sometimes they are able to avoid the system altogether.

You'd think our Food and Drug Administration (FDA) would protect us from all of this, wouldn't you? Hell, no. They're part of the problem. Most decisions about what goes in our food are made without the FDA's knowledge—or ours.

A little history lesson: Back in 1958—the same year the Hula-Hoop was invented, Elvis joined the army, and Pizza Hut was founded—Congress enacted a law that was meant to guarantee that chemicals intentionally added to foods were safe. It was called the Food Additives Amendment, and it was a positive move for the health of all Americans. But Congress and the FDA had no way of knowing how food science and technology would transform our food supply in the future. Around the time the law was passed, there were approximately 800 food additives. A decade later, that jumped to 3,000. Today, an estimated 10,000 chemicals can make their way into our foods, many without any FDA review for safety.

Here's why: The Food Additives Amendment exempts certain common food ingredients from FDA review as long as they are "generally recognized as safe," or GRAS. In 1958, Congress believed that certain additives—like vinegar and oil—were so obviously safe that they weren't worth reviewing or testing. However, this amendment—and its enforcement—created a loophole so big I could park a semitruck inside it. The loophole allows companies to claim that their new chemicals and additives are GRAS without even notifying the FDA.

Today, the FDA allows food manufacturers to do their own testing to determine whether an additive is safe. If the company deems it safe, they go ahead and use it without any input from the agency or the public. This testing is generally performed on animals, where doses are questionable and given in a relatively short time. The whole process screams blatant conflict of interest!

In fact, the FDA has never reviewed the safety of more than 3,000 food chemicals. Most companies don't even notify the agency. An estimated 1,000 chemicals are known only to the companies that use them.

What's even more outrageous is that we can't rely on the ingredient lists on labels to help us fully understand what we're eating. More than 5,000 substances aren't required to be listed.

If the FDA doesn't know what's in food, how can we?

We can't, as long as the FDA is lax on the health dangers posed by additives.

> "We simply do not have the information to vouch for the safety of many of these chemicals. . . . We do not know the volume of particular chemicals that are going into the food supply."
> —Michael Taylor, the FDA's deputy commissioner for food

In 1959, for example, the food additive carrageenan was officially granted GRAS status by the FDA. Despite its being rubber-stamped as healthy by the FDA, there's still argument over the safety of carrageenan. Much of the doubt comes from a University of Iowa review published in *Environmental Health Perspectives* in 2001. Based on animal and laboratory research, this study revealed that carrageenan could cause ulcers in the colon and perhaps even cancer. The review indicated that FDA-approved food-grade carrageenan can be contaminated with non-food-grade carrageenan (degraded carrageenan), which is a known carcinogen. To me, the continued status of carrageenan as GRAS is troubling.

In 1993, the FDA granted approval to Monsanto for its genetically engineered recombinant bovine growth hormone (rBGH), brand-named Posilac, for use by the nation's dairy farmers. It increases milk production by about 10 percent over a cow's life cycle. It's the largest-selling cattle pharmaceutical in the United States.

But Posilac has always been controversial. More and more cancer specialists are apprehensive, because it may increase the risk for breast, colon, and prostate cancers in humans. Unless the milk you're drinking is clearly marked "organic" or "rBGH free," it probably contains this hormone. Incidentally, Posilac is banned in Europe, Canada, Australia, and Japan. This should tell us something.

Even cows get sick from this drug. Just check the label on this hormone, and you'll see a long list of toxic side effects inflicted on these poor cows. One is mastitis, an inflammation of the udders. The inflammation is then treated with antibiotics. Unfortunately, trace levels of these antibiotics may remain in the cow's milk and other dairy products that end up on grocery store shelves.

Other scary GRAS chemicals include the preservatives butylated hydroxyanisole (BHA) and butylated hydroxytoluene (BHT), used to keep the fats and oils in foods from going rancid. They're found in boxed cereals, canned frostings, dessert mixes, instant potatoes, microwave popcorn, baked goods, meat products, and chewing gum. BHA has been found to cause cancer in various animal studies, leading the National Institutes of Health's National Toxicology Program to describe it as "reasonably anticipated to be a human carcinogen." At least the FDA puts limits on BHA and BHT in foods; the preservatives can't exceed 0.02 percent of a product's fat content. But because these chemicals are found in so many foods, how do you know how much you're ingesting? You don't, not really.

Nitrites and nitrates (which turn into nitrites in the body) also are controversial GRAS additives. These chemicals are widely used in cured meats to prevent botulism. But cooking these products at high heat and, to a lesser degree, digesting them, produce nitrosamines— which cause cancer in laboratory animals.

Smoke and mirrors. It just makes me sick.

And now we're finding out that filthy politics have entered the picture.

In 2013, an alarming report was published in the *Journal of the American Medical Association Internal Medicine* by a group of top food additive researchers led by Tom Neltner. They looked at 451 GRAS notifications submitted voluntarily by companies to the FDA between 1997 and 2012, and they found "ubiquitous" conflicts of interest in GRAS approvals. Almost two-thirds of those safety assessments were made by "experts" selected by the food company or a consulting firm. About a fifth of those assessments were made by an employee of an additive manufacturer!

The FDA isn't looking after you. They're looking after food companies. Make no doubt about it, the food industry is in bed with the FDA.

SAVE YOURSELF NOW!

I know you might be upset about what's happening in the food industry, and I don't blame you. After reading about my investigations and finding out you're being duped, you're probably wondering how to avoid being a victim of these circumstances. I can totally relate, and I have a solution.

If you want to be healthy and in shape, you've got to take control. No government agency, big food company, or anyone else is going to do it for you. You can't trust anyone but yourself.

Be fussy about your food choices. Get savvy about what you're eating. The less a food has been processed, the more it benefits your health. Read labels — not so much the calories or carbs in a product, but the list of ingredients. Eat organic, real food; it's the best way to protect yourself. Remember that there are more than 10,000 ingredients added to our food, thousands of which are untested. You don't have to know them all. But there are 15 ingredients I want you to recognize. Let's talk about them now.

CHAPTER 2

WE ARE THE CHEMICALS WE EAT — THE SICKENING 15

You've heard the expression "You are what you eat." Let me rephrase it: You are the chemicals you eat. They make you tired. They put you through skin dramas like rashed, blemished, or dry skin. They make you feel fat and miserable, even though you've been dieting and exercising like crazy. They put you at risk for scary, life-shortening diseases like cancer.

These problems aren't your fault. An entire industry exists whose interest is to obscure or conceal the potential effects of food chemicals you're ingesting on a daily basis. It's not just that there are good foods and bad foods. It's not just that you should eat this and not that. It's also that there are foods that can help you, and foods that can harm you. I'll show you where some of these problems lie — and what to do about them. Let's talk first about what's making you sick.

THE SICKENING 15

Exactly where are these scary chemicals? You're in for a surprise. They're probably in every meal or snack or beverage you had today. Take a look at my Sickening 15.

1. GROWTH HORMONES IN MEAT

When you eat conventional meat, you're probably eating hormones, antibiotics, steroids, and chemicals created by the fear and stress suffered by the animal during slaughter and in its inhumane living conditions.

In 2009, two Japanese researchers published a startling study in *Annals of Oncology*. They pointed out that there has been a surge in hormone-dependent cancers that roughly parallels the surge of beef consumption in Japan. Over the last twenty-five years, hormone-dependent cancers such as breast, ovarian, endometrial, and prostate cancer rose fivefold in that country. More than 25 percent of the beef imported to Japan comes from the United States, where livestock growers regularly use the growth hormonal steroid estradiol. The researchers found that US beef had much higher levels of estrogen than Japanese beef because of the added hormones. This finding led them to conclude that eating a lot of estrogen-rich beef could be the reason for the rising incidence of these life-threatening cancers.

Injected hormones like estrogen mimic the activity of our natural hormones and prevent those hormones from doing their jobs. This situation creates chaos. Growth hormones may alter the way in which natural hormones are produced, eliminated, or metabolized. And guess what? Hormone impersonators can trigger unnatural cell growth that may develop into cancer.

The United States is one of the only industrialized countries that still allows their animals to be injected with growth hormone. Australia, New Zealand, Canada, Japan, and the entire European Union have banned rBGH and rBST because of their dangerous impact on human and bovine health.

US farmers fatten up their livestock by injecting them with estrogen-based hormones, which can migrate from the meat we eat to our bodies—and possibly stimulate the growth of human breast cancer, according to the Breast Cancer Fund, an organization committed to preventing breast cancer by eliminating our exposure to toxins linked to the disease.

Farms in America also dose their livestock with certain growth-stimulating drugs, namely, the feed additive ractopamine, marketed as Paylean for pigs, as Optaflexx for cattle, and as Topmax for turkeys—all banned in other countries, by the way. Ractopamine is a beta-agonist. When animals consume feed, they channel the extra energy into fat cells. But when given beta-agonists, they partition the extra energy into muscle instead of fat.

Supposedly, beta-agonists are safe in food animals because the compounds do not last long in animal tissue. They break down quickly and are excreted before the animal is slaughtered. Of course, these drugs then get into our soil through animal poop.

The Russian consumer protection agency, Rospotrebnadzor, backed a study on ractopamine. In 2014, the agency issued findings showing that eating products with traces of ractopamine leads to an unacceptable level of risk of diseases of the cardiovascular system. This tells me—again— that there is just no acceptable level of any chemical to ingest, ever.

Drink a glass of conventional pasteurized milk, and you might as well be drinking a hormone cocktail. Some dairy farmers inject their animals with hormones so that they pump out more milk. A *Nutrition and Cancer* study reported in 2011 that cow's milk stimulated the growth of prostate cancer cells in lab dishes, while almond milk suppressed the growth of these cells. Interesting, isn't it?

It's important to choose organic dairy. It's healthier than conventional milk. A recent study from Washington State University analyzed the nutrient content of both types of milk and found that organic milk is higher in heart-healthy omega-3 fatty acids and protein than conventional milk.

The Food Babe Way: I'm not against eating meat or dairy. I'm against eating it if you don't know how it was grown or produced. Fortunately, there are lots of farms specializing in drug-free and humanely, organically, and sustainably raised livestock. Look for organic, grass-fed and/or pasture-raised meat, as well as poultry, and dairy.

2. ANTIBIOTICS

Antibiotics are routinely given to livestock to make them fat. Well, they just might do the same thing to you. How is this possible? Antibiotics kill off healthy bacteria in the gut—beneficial bugs called probiotics that influence how we absorb nutrients, burn off calories, and stay lean. Scientists have found that lean people have more of the good, antiobesity bacteria in their guts, compared to people who are overweight.

According to Dr. Martin J. Blaser, in his groundbreaking book *Missing Microbes*, antibiotic use is changing our metabolism and body composition. In experiments conducted with rats, Blaser determined that high-calorie diets alone do not explain the rapid increase in the rate of obesity. This increase could also be attributed to the high use of antibiotics—especially at an early age.

On average, children get as many as twenty antibiotic treatments while they're growing up. In a study of children in Britain, researchers showed that kids who were prescribed a lot of antibiotics were fatter at age seven and age fifteen than children who did not receive many of these drugs.

Antibiotics have been given a free ride for decades, with millions and millions being prescribed. This overexposure is a growing concern. National surveys reported by the US Department of Health and Human Services have shown antibiotic residues in meat, in milk, and, in some cities, in drinking water. That means even if you avoid unnecessary antibiotics from your doctor, you could be getting them from the grocery store and faucet. An estimated 80 percent of antibiotics used in this country are for livestock. This overuse is creating superbugs that could threaten the entire human population.

Antibiotics in food are hard to escape. Unless a package is labeled accordingly, you can pretty much guarantee that antibiotics have been used to produce meat and dairy products such as cheese, milk, sour cream, and ice cream.

The Food Babe Way: Always buy antibiotic-free meat and dairy. Meat that is certified organic is also antibiotic-free. Don't eat the meat or dairy at a restaurant unless you know it's antibiotic-free.

On a personal health note, I take antibiotic medicine only when absolutely necessary—and not for the common cold. The cold is a virus; antibiotics treat bacterial infections. Make sure you absolutely need antibiotics before asking your doctor to prescribe them.

And stop using so much of that alcohol-based hand sanitizer. This product is killing off all the good bacteria you need to stay healthy. Soap works just as well. Finally, consider taking a probiotic supplement to help fill your gut with good bacteria. I take one every day.

3. PESTICIDES

Pesticides, fungicides, and herbicides are sprayed on fruits, vegetables, grains, nuts, and seeds—virtually everything grown in nature—and they're among the most toxic substances on earth, doing untold damage to our bodies.

For one thing, they imitate estrogen (a fat-forming hormone) and disrupt thyroid function—two side effects that encourage weight gain.

According to the Environmental Working Group, apples are the most heavily sprayed fruit. Could these pesticides on an apple be making you fat? Quite possibly, especially if you consider the exposure and accumulation of pesticides over time in our body.

Studies have also linked pesticides to cancer. When you're exposed to pesticides, your body can't properly defend itself against carcinogens from other sources. So your cancer risk goes up. If you're overweight, watch out: Pesticides love to camp out in fat tissue and stay there. There they begin to mimic estrogen; this can lead to estrogen-related health problems such as breast cancer.

One of the worst pesticides is glyphosate, commonly known by the trade name Roundup, produced by the chemical biotech company Monsanto. This company patented seeds and created crops that are resistant to glyphosate through genetic engineering. Because of this, many US farmers started using more of it. We now know from research that glyphosate found in genetically modified foods is a toxin that can accumulate in your body the more you are exposed to it. It has been linked to kidney disease, breast cancer, and some birth defects. It compromises your immunity. And it slows down your metabolism. This is bad, bad stuff.

One thing that totally baffles me is that the word "conventional" is used to describe produce that is grown with pesticides. There's nothing conventional about using toxic chemicals to grow food.

The Food Babe Way: Aren't you supposed to eat more produce to stay healthy? Yes, but not if your fruits and veggies are covered in pesticide residue. So purchase certified organic. Organic foods haven't been sprayed or treated with synthetic pesticides, fungicides, or other harmful chemicals. If you don't have access to organic foods, purchase local and seasonal fruits and vegetables at farmers' markets. The reason I say that is that produce that's transported over long distances or preserved because it's out of season is often sprayed with even more chemicals. Avoid common genetically engineered foods like corn, soy, canola, sugar beets, cottonseed, papaya, zucchini, and squash. Only buy these if they are organic. Wash your produce well, too.

> **Organic 101**
>
> I'll be using the word "organic" throughout this book. But what does the term really mean? Here are some definitions:
>
> *Certified organic:* This means that 95 percent of all ingredients in a product, except salt and water, are organic. According to the USDA: "Organic food is produced by farmers who emphasize the use of renewable resources and the conservation of soil and water to enhance environmental quality for future generations. Organic meat, poultry, eggs, and dairy products come from animals that are given no antibiotics or growth hormones. Organic food is produced without using artificial ingredients, most conventional pesticides, fertilizers made with synthetic ingredients or sewage sludge, bioengineering, or ionizing radiation. Before a product can be labeled 'organic,' a Government-approved certifier inspects the farm where the food is grown to make sure the farmer is following all the rules necessary to meet USDA organic standards. Companies that handle or process organic food before it gets to your local supermarket or restaurant must be certified, too." These products may display the USDA Organic seal.
>
> *100% certified organic:* This means that 100 percent of all ingredients in a product, except salt and water, are organic. These products may use the USDA Organic seal.
>
> *Made with organic ingredients:* This means that 70 percent of all ingredients in a product, except salt and water, are organic. These products might contain genetically modified ingredients or other chemical additives. These products may not use the USDA Organic seal.

4. REFINED AND ENRICHED FLOUR

I'm talking about flour that has been stripped of nutrients and fiber with none put back. Manufacturers "enrich" their dead flour by putting synthetic nutrients back into the product. Thanks a lot. Many flours are even bleached with chlorine or peroxide to make them look white, because some people associate whiteness with quality. Mmmmmmm. A Clorox sandwich for lunch?

What's more, a number of breads are loaded with added sugar to make them taste better. Do we really need this? Sugar is so bad for your waistline, skin, and complexion and increases the chances of diabetes, heart disease, and other illnesses. White flour—well, you might as well eat a box of sugar.

The Food Babe Way: If you buy bread, check the labeling. Make sure it's made with sprouted "whole wheat" flour or "whole grain" flour. Either one should be the first ingredient on the list. Also, avoid enriched, bleached, and white wheat flour. Choose whole wheat and whole grain, whole oats, rye, buckwheat, almond, or quinoa flour instead. By the way, this standard also applies to other flour-based products, like crackers, rolls, bagels, and any commercially baked food.

5. BISPHENOL (BPA)

This isn't a food per se. It's a toxic chemical found in food packaging and in the linings of cans that contain canned foods and soft drinks. BPA disrupts hormones that govern metabolism, growth, reproduction, and other crucial bodily processes.

BPA is banned in Canada and the European Union. It is not banned in the United States, with the exception of baby bottles and infant formula packaging. The FDA has banned the use of this chemical in these types of containers.

Chronic BPA exposure is linked not only to obesity, but also to prostate and breast cancer, and thyroid problems. It is also associated with infertility, diabetes, early puberty, and behavioral changes in kids.

A 2011 Harvard study found that people who ate a single serving of canned soup a day for five days had ten times the amount of BPA in their bodies as they did when they ate fresh soup daily. Soup's on? Not for me if it's BPA-canned.

The Food Babe Way: Thousands of chemicals are allowed in food packaging, the effects of which we still don't know. For this reason, I stay away from plastic as much as possible and go clean with glass and stainless steel.

An easy fix is to buy food in BPA-free cans. Certain companies like

Eden Foods, Native Forest, and Vital Choice Wild Seafood & Organics don't use BPA in their cans. Like soup? Make it from scratch. Check out my soup recipes in Chapter 8. Also, choose BPA-free plastic for food and drink storage.

Another tip: Instead of buying tomato products in cans, try buying

---

Don't Pop This!

If you or someone you know is still eating microwave popcorn, listen up! I can't tell you how many times I used to eat microwave popcorn when I worked in an office. My coworkers would buy one of those packs from the vending machine in the break room and pop that sucker right into the microwave, and the whole floor would smell delicious. I just couldn't help myself. It was the one thing in the vending machine that had to be refilled week after week — way before the stale peanuts. I'm so glad I broke that habit, because let me tell you, this stuff is horrible for your health, and here's why...

The bags holding most microwave popcorn varieties are lined with perfluorooctanoic acid (PFOA). This chemical is the same toxic stuff found in Teflon pots and pans. It can stay in the environment and in the human body for long periods. When heated, it has been linked to infertility, cancer, and other diseases in lab animals. No long-term studies have been conducted on humans, but the Environmental Protection Agency (EPA) lists this substance as a carcinogen.

The contents of the popcorn include processed oils, artificial flavorings (like diacetyl, which causes popcorn lung), natural flavorings, sodium, preservatives (including the highly toxic TBHQ), and trans fats.

Even though no genetically modified popcorn kernels are being produced, several other GMO ingredients in oils or emulsifiers are found in this popcorn. Few microwave popcorns use organic corn, either, so you can be sure they contain harmful pesticides.

If you still love popcorn, don't worry. I won't leave you in the lurch. Check out my Superfood Popcorn in the recipe section on page 327. It's so easy to make, and you can avoid all of these health pitfalls. Make it in advance and throw it in a reusable bag for the office or movie theater.

---

food in glass jars. Two great brands are Good Boy Organics Yellow Barn Biodynamic and Bionaturæ. As for canned beans, forget about them. Buy organic dried beans and cook them yourself. You can avoid BPA and save money, too.

6. HIGH-FRUCTOSE CORN SYRUP (HFCS)

I gripe about this additive all the time. HFCS is a chemical derivative of corn syrup. It's found in foods too numerous to count. A few examples: bread, sodas, flavored yogurt, crackers, and cookies. A review published in the *International Journal of Obesity* in 2008 noted that the rise in obesity in the last thirty-five years has paralleled the rising use of HFCS, which made its debut on the food scene just before 1970. HFCS makes you fat largely by impacting two hormones, insulin and leptin. When you ingest HFCS, insulin skyrockets, and insulin promotes fat storage. Not only does this sweetener make your insulin level surge, it also wreaks havoc on the hormone leptin, the body's appetite regulator. HFCS suppresses your response to leptin, and you get so hungry you want to eat everything in sight. The result: Your body gets very adept at hoarding fat.

Another concern about HFCS is cited in a study by the American Chemical Society on carbonated soft drinks. Rutgers University Professor of Food Science Chi-Tang Ho, PhD, conducted chemical tests on eleven different carbonated soft drinks containing HFCS. He found "astonishingly high" levels of reactive carbonyls in those beverages. These undesirable compounds associated with "unbound" fructose and glucose molecules are believed to cause tissue damage. By contrast, reactive carbonyls are not present in table sugar, whose fructose and glucose components are "bound" and chemically stable.

The Food Babe Way: Read package labels for high-fructose corn syrup. It's in more products than you might imagine. Later on, I'll show you how to spot other hidden sources of sugar and how to choose products with nonrefined sugars such as fruit, dates, coconut sugar, maple syrup, and honey.

7. ARTIFICIAL SWEETENERS

If you think drinking diet soda is the way to lose weight, think again. Artificial sweeteners, from aspartame to saccharin and everything in between, are bad news for weight control. They can be found in diet foods, beverages, candy, desserts, and many other processed foods. Look for aspartame, neotame, saccharin, sucralose, erythritol, acesulfame potassium, and acesulfame K on the label. You can also find them under the brand names NutraSweet, Sweet'N Low, Equal, and Splenda.

Artificial sweeteners may do more harm than good—for three reasons. First, some of these sweeteners, such as acesulfame potassium and aspartame, may slow down your metabolism. Second, artificial sweeteners actually train people to crave sweets. Third, the presence of artificial sweeteners in a product doesn't automatically mean natural high-calorie sweeteners aren't present, too. Some food manufacturers use both.

What about the overall safety of artificial sweeteners? This has been a topic of hot debate for decades. Some studies say they're safe, others say they're not. All I know is that I haven't seen little pink, yellow, or blue packets of sweeteners growing on trees, so I avoid the stuff.

The Food Babe Way: Use low-cal options such as pure stevia leaf powder or liquid, but in moderation.

8. PRESERVATIVES

As you stroll down the aisles of the grocery store, start thinking about the shelves of boxed, canned, jarred, and packaged foods as caskets holding dead food. It's all embalmed with preservatives that will make you feel dead, too.

Among the worst of these preservatives are nitrates, used in meats to prevent bacteria growth and maintain color. Toxic to the brain, nitrates are linked to Alzheimer's disease and many types of cancer. I see no reason to eat chemically preserved cured and smoked meat.

Then there are the preservatives BHA and BHT, both banned all over the globe but still allowed in the United States. BHA and BHT are petroleum derivatives used to preserve fats and oils. They have produced cancers in rats, mice, and hamsters. The International Agency for Research on Cancer and the US National Toxicology Program classify the preservative BHA as "reasonably anticipated to be a human carcinogen"—but as I mentioned in the previous chapter, the FDA still allows it.

Studies found that rats fed the FDA's maximum limit for the endocrine-disrupting preservative propyl paraben in food had decreased sperm counts.

Another controversial preservative is propylene glycol, used as a thickening agent to absorb water. Large oral doses in animals have caused central nervous system depression and kidney damage.

Then there's propyl gallate, used to keep oils in processed food fresh. It can cause stomach or skin irritation in sensitive people.

A source of many preservatives is fast food. Watch out for dimethyl-polysiloxane in particular, a type of silicone with antifoaming properties that is used in cosmetics and a variety of other goods like Silly Putty. You'll find it in Chick-fil-A chicken sandwiches, McDonald's French fries, KFC mashed potatoes and biscuits, Taco Bell cinnamon twists, Five Guys French fries, Domino's breadsticks, and on and on.

The Food Babe Way: Choose foods that are fresh or do not contain preservatives. There's no reason to embalm your body before you're dead.

9. TRANS FATS

Most people recognize the term "trans fat" because these nasty fats have made headlines. Minute amounts of trans fats occur naturally in red meats and full-fat dairy products, but most come from a man-made process called hydrogenation that morphs vegetable oil into solid fat. Trans fats help processed food stay solid at room temperature and lengthen shelf life.

But the processed kind of trans fats can be deadly, even in trace amounts. According to a 2012 study published in *Annals of Internal Medicine,* a mere forty-calorie-per-day increase in trans fat, maybe from a store-bought cookie or two, can up your risk of heart disease by 23 percent! In fact, the Centers for Disease Control and Prevention (CDC) has attributed up to 7,000 deaths and over 20,000 heart attacks to the substance. Trans fats are suspected of doing other damage, too. They may raise blood sugar, hurt your immunity, make your fat cells bigger, and create more of them.

For fun, I looked into the history of these deadly fats. They were created back in the early 1900s by a chemist who wanted to find a cheap substitute for candle wax. He discovered that boiling cottonseed oil and then cooling it would cause it to harden into blocks of fat that you could burn as candles. Seeing dollar signs, Procter & Gamble bought the patent and began producing cheap food fat. Yuck.

The Food Babe Way: Trans fats are easy to hunt down. Look for "partially hydrogenated" on the ingredient labels of foods like crackers, cookies, pies, and other bakery items; dough; and snack foods. Don't believe the "No Trans Fat" label on some food packages; there still could be some lurking inside because of an FDA loophole. Always check the ingredient list.

I'll introduce you to foods that have nonthreatening oils in them like coconut oil, sesame oil, olive oil, hempseed oil, and red palm fruit oil. So don't worry. You can have your fat and eat it, too. A footnote: Trans fats are being gradually phased out of foods, thank goodness!

10. ARTIFICIAL AND NATURAL FLAVORS

Warning: This section contains material that may be upsetting to those who are about to eat a meal.

Added flavoring can come artificially from cheap toxic ingredients like petroleum or can be made from anything in nature — including animal parts!

Readers of my blog know that the next time you lick vanilla ice cream from a cone, there's a chance you'll be swirling secretions from a beaver's anal glands around in your mouth. This one rates really high on my upchuck meter.

Called castoreum, this secretion is used as a "natural flavor" not only in vanilla ice cream but also in strawberry oatmeal and raspberry-flavored products.

If you chew gum, you may also be chewing lanolin, an oily secretion found in sheep's wool that is used to soften some gums. What nutritional value do you think these disgusting additives have for your body?

None! They exist just to get you to buy something fake or that shouldn't be food, rather than a real alternative.

What about "natural flavors"? They're anything but. Natural flavor can legally contain naturally occurring glutamate by-products that act like MSG, which is a known excitotoxin. Excitotoxins make food irresistible to eat but can cause stroke, Alzheimer's disease, Parkinson's disease, obesity, migraines, fatigue, and depression.

The natural and artificial flavoring chemicals in our foods are contributing to what David Kessler, former head of the FDA, calls a "food carnival" in your mouth. They trick your mind into wanting more and more. The big food companies are hijacking our taste buds one by one and lining their corporate pockets at the same time, as we buy more products with these addicting synthesized flavors in them.

The Food Babe Way: The word "natural" on a label is virtually bogus. It doesn't equate with "good." Read labels. If they list artificial or natural flavors, put those foods back on the shelf. You have a choice. You can let the food companies and flavor factories conduct chemical warfare on you. Or you can treat them like the enemy and stop buying their products. Instead, choose organic and other products that do not use added flavoring.

11. FOOD DYES

Artificial food dyes are created synthetically and/or derived from petroleum, a known carcinogen, or even insect parts. (And ironically, the ones made from insect parts might be less bad for you than the ones made from oil.) If you eat pickles, snack bars, ice cream, candy, jam, maraschino cherries, or cake regularly throughout your life, you'll probably eat up to one pound of red dye over your lifetime.

We tend to eat with our eyes as well as our mouths, and food manufacturers capitalize on this. Dyed foods trick you by making processed food more appealing. Artificial food dyes are linked to hyperactivity in children, asthma, allergies, and skin issues. They are banned in certain countries and require a warning label in Europe. Color me worried!

The Food Babe Way: Check labels! The worst offenders are Yellow

#5 or tartrazine (E102) and Yellow #6 (E110), both of which may be contaminated with the human carcinogen benzidine. Other harmful dyes are Citrus Red #2 (E121), Red #3 (E127), Red #40 (E129), Blue #1 (E133), and Blue #2 (E132). Also, watch out for "caramel coloring," which can be artificially derived. These artificial dyes are found in sodas, candies, and baked goods, and are even used to dye some fruit, such as cherries and fruit cocktails. There are plenty of foods made without artificial dyes, and you'll learn about them here.

12. DOUGH CONDITIONERS

There's a reason most commercially baked bread keeps so well for so long: dough conditioners. These chemicals are added to bread dough to strengthen its texture, extend shelf life, and reduce processing time.

One of the ingredients in dough conditioners is the amino acid L-cysteine. It's made from either human hair or duck feathers. Appetizing, huh?

A dough conditioner lets companies pass off chemically processed cheap food as "freshly baked" because it creates perfect, evenly spaced air pockets within the dough, improving the texture after the dough comes out of large industrial processing machines. Several dough conditioners have been linked to cancer, allergies, and asthma. Read the ingredient lists of fast-food products, and you'll discover that dough conditioners are in practically every bun, piece of bread, muffin, biscuit, roll, and tortilla.

The Food Babe Way: I choose or make freshly baked breads. For convenience, try sprouted bread like Food For Life's Ezekiel bread, which is found in the freezer section of most health food stores. And always check the ingredient list of store-bought baked goods. Look for "dough conditioners" or specific names like azodicarbonamide (the yoga mat chemical), DATEM, potassium bromate, monoglycerides, and diglycerides.

13. CARRAGEENAN

I bring up carrageenan again because you'll read in various articles and online that this seaweed-derived additive is safe. To which I say: BS!

This additive is an inflammatory agent found in a bunch of products from desserts to toothpaste. Carrageenan is used as a thickener, stabilizer, and/or emulsifier (a substance that keeps liquids from separating). Unfortunately, it is allowed in some organic foods, such as nondairy milk, even though it has been linked to gastrointestinal problems ranging from irritable bowel syndrome to colon cancer. The organic watchdog group the Cornucopia Institute has called for an outright ban on the use of carrageenan in all food products.

The Food Babe Way: Carrageenan is listed on the labels of some dairy and nut milks, yogurt, cheese, cottage cheese, sour cream, cream cheese, whipping cream, ice cream, and processed deli meats, among other foods. Because this additive is so suspect, I prefer to make my own nut milks, ice cream, yogurt, and other foods whenever possible, or choose products that do not contain carrageenan on the ingredient list.

14. MONOSODIUM GLUTAMATE (MSG)

This "flavor enhancer" is found in fast foods and many processed foods. It heightens the flavor of food by exciting neurons in the brain when eaten. This sounds like a good idea for spicing up bland foods, but MSG has a long rap sheet. Let me tally up its offenses for you: If you're one of the people who are allergic to this common ingredient, it could lead to skin rashes, itching, nausea, vomiting, headaches, asthma, heart arrhythmias, depression, and even seizures.

MSG is also linked to obesity. A 2008 study from researchers at the University of North Carolina looked at the diets of 752 men and women living in three villages in north and south China. Most of the people ate a natural foods–type diet, but about 80 percent added MSG to their cooking. After adjusting for factors like smoking and physical activity, they found those who used MSG were almost three times as likely to be overweight as those who used none. Experts think MSG makes food taste so good that we help ourselves to too much. Food companies engineer their food to make a flavor irresistible and memorable so you eat more.

No thanks. I stick to nutritious foods that are flavorful on their own, without MSG.

The Food Babe Way: MSG is listed as monosodium glutamate on labels and is found in restaurant foods, chips, dips, frozen dinners, salad dressings, and soups. Some companies trick the consumer and say "No added MSG" on the label; however, MSG is a master of disguise. Hidden MSG (free glutamic acid) can be found under certain common names, which I've listed below.

Deceptive Nicknames for MSG

Glutamic acid	Whey protein
Glutamate	Whey protein concentrate
Monopotassium glutamate	Whey protein isolate
Calcium glutamate	Soy protein
Monoammonium glutamate	Soy protein concentrate
Magnesium glutamate	Soy protein isolate
Natrium glutamate	Anything "protein"
Anything "hydrolyzed"	Anything "protein fortified"
Any "hydrolyzed protein"	Soy sauce
Calcium caseinate	Soy sauce extract
Sodium caseinate	Protease
Yeast extract	Anything "enzyme modified"
Torula yeast	Anything containing "enzymes"
Yeast food	Anything "fermented"
Yeast nutrient	Vetsin
Autolyzed yeast	Ajinomoto
Gelatin	Umami
Textured protein	

---

15. HEAVY METALS AND NEUROTOXINS

How would you like a nice big helping of aluminum, lead, mercury, or arsenic for dinner? Sounds crazy, I know. But you could be filling your body with heavy metals without knowing it. So how do they turn up in our bodies? The answer is through pesticide-sprayed food, farmed fish, and food packaging material.

The problem is that your body can't easily eliminate heavy metals or break them down. They get stored in places like fat tissue and eventually make their way through your bloodstream and invade your brain, lungs, heart, eyes, stomach, liver, and sexual organs. Heavy metals are particularly toxic to your brain cells, where they can cause memory loss, migraines, and premature brain aging.

The Food Babe Way: It's difficult to avoid exposure to heavy metals, so I recommend choosing the following plant foods known to detox your system and help strip the body of these poisons:

- Cilantro, otherwise known as coriander or Chinese parsley, which helps remove mercury, aluminum, and lead from the body by crossing the blood-brain barrier to work its removal magic.
- Cruciferous vegetables, such as broccoli, kale, and cabbage, and others such as dandelion. These veggies contain antioxidants that increase the production of detoxifying enzymes in the body.
- Sulfur-rich foods, such as onions and garlic. These help your body eliminate heavy metals.

I also advise that you limit fish to once or twice a week and go to seafoodwatch.org to choose fish with low levels of mercury.

FOOD BABE ALERT:
YOUR BRAIN ON METALS AND TOXINS

We're getting dumber and dumber. The total IQ of Americans has dropped 41 million points, according to Dr. David Bellinger, writing in a 2012 paper published by the National Institutes of Health. A 2014 study published in *The Lancet Neurology* named certain everyday chemicals as responsible not only for the drop in IQ but also for autism spectrum disorder and ADHD. The experts have pointed to a collection of brain-damaging chemicals called neurotoxins as causes of these and other brain problems.

(Continued)

Neurotoxin	Sources	Effects on the Brain and Body
Arsenic	Pesticide that has been found in rice; brown rice syrup and products containing this syrup (cereal and energy bars, toddler formula, and high-energy foods for athletes); apple juice; and grape juice	Long-term exposure to arsenic at low levels has been linked to skin and lung cancers and cardiovascular disease. It may contribute to problems in pregnancy, such as miscarriage and low birth weight, and may cause problems in breathing and brain development in infants.
Chlorpyrifos	Pesticide sprayed on grains, citrus, grapes, broccoli, and almonds	Damages the nervous system and impairs brain development in fetuses and children.
DDT/DDE (a DDT metabolite)	Though banned in the US, DDT/DDE can be passed to us through imported food exposed to them.	Linked to Alzheimer's disease.
Ethanol	Alcoholic beverages	Causes depression and slows down areas of the central nervous system responsible for heart rate and breathing, as well as motor control.
Fluoride	Tap water	In high doses, lowers IQ and harms brain development in children.
Lead	Rice imported into the US	In young children, can diminish learning ability and intellectual development. In adults, increases blood pressure and causes cardiovascular disease.
Manganese	Tap water, stainless steel, and soda cans	May cause learning and coordination disabilities, behavioral changes, and a condition that resembles Parkinson's disease.
Mercury	Larger fish that eat others— tuna, swordfish, and shark	Linked to cancers and reproductive abnormalities, headaches, irritability, fatigue, depression, and poor concentration.
Polychlorinated biphenyls (PCBs)	Though banned, these chemicals are found in farmed salmon and oily parts of other fish	Interfere with verbal learning and memory in children, as well as fetal brain development.

LET'S EAT AN AMAZING ARRAY OF FOOD

I realize I've just lobbed a hand grenade into your pantry and fridge. You're probably wondering: Jeez, is there anything left to eat? Lettuce, anyone? I'm going to show you an amazing array of foods you can eat, from meats to veggies to pastas to desserts. Nothing is off-limits unless you know, by reading ingredient labels and consulting the information here, that it's loaded with chemicals.

There's so much you can do to help yourself and your family. I'm going to put you, rather than the food companies, in control of what you eat. My program does not require crazy-drastic changes in how you eat or how you live your life. You'll start by making one change a day. That may sound like super–slow motion, but trust me, one new change every day for twenty-one days will make a huge difference in your life. All you have to do is clean up your diet and be more conscious of not putting unnecessary chemicals in your mouth.

Yes, you'll toss out the bad sugars, the trans fats, the processed foods, the artificial sweeteners, the gross additives and dyes, and the boxed garbage. You'll eat real food, like wild salmon, grass-fed meats, avocados, organic pesticide-free fruits and veggies, nuts, olive oil and coconut oil, and much more. You'll stop your metabolism from being poisoned by toxic chemicals. Your body will start functioning again like the perfect machine it was created to be.

I know you've picked up this book for many reasons, and I'm sure one of them is that you'd like to lose weight. In all honesty, your body can never be lean unless it is clean of fattening toxins. But if you nourish it with healthy, delicious food, you can achieve the shape you have always wanted — without ever feeling hungry or deprived.

This is what I want to talk to you about next — ridding yourself of chemical calories so you can drop pounds, feel more energetic, and get back on the road to health.

CHAPTER 3

CUT OUT THE CHEMICAL CALORIES

IT'S HARD FOR ME to believe that I was once thirty pounds overweight. First as a teenager, then later as a professional management consultant in my twenties, I was fat, tired, and stressed. Always. All I did was work, work, work. If I had a spare half hour, I'd grab some fast food. If not, I'd reach for the closest sugar-packed snack I could find to fend off the hunger shakes.

I didn't want to continue to live in this unhealthy body that stared back at me from the mirror. So I read. I studied everything I could get my hands on to figure out what was going on with me.

I eventually dropped refined sugars and most meats. I avoided processed foods like the poison they are. I fed my body fresh organic foods — fruits, veggies, grains, good fats, and other whole foods — and made time to nourish my body back to health.

The one thing I did not do was go on a "diet." I just became more aware of the things I ate and stuck to what made sense.

I started losing those pounds and gaining more and more energy — although I really wasn't making heroic efforts to get thinner. I got back to an attractive normal weight, and I've stayed there — even by eating up to 2,000 calories a day, normally a lot for a woman with my frame.

What had changed?

I was eating clean, toxin-free food, and that made all the difference.

THE RISE OF THE OBESOGENS

Everyone knows Americans are fat and getting fatter. Some startling statistics:

- More than 65 percent of Americans are overweight, and 33 percent are obese.
- 32 percent of children are either obese or overweight.
- It's projected that in ten years, 43 percent of Americans will be obese.
- After the nasty habit of smoking, obesity is America's biggest cause of premature death, and is linked to 70 percent of heart disease and 80 percent of diabetes cases.

Why are we blimping up?

Well, it's not just from eating too many cookies. There's more to it than that. Now we know that the chemicals in our food are making us not only sick but fat, too, no matter how faithfully we diet.

These chemicals are called obesogens, a term coined by Bruce Blumberg of the University of California, Irvine, for certain chemicals that trigger our bodies to store fat even though we might be restricting calories.

The theory that obesogens in our food and environment could be making us fat has been gathering steam ever since researcher Paula F. Baillie-Hamilton published an article in the *Journal of Alternative and Complementary Medicine* in 2002, presenting strong evidence that chemical exposure caused weight gain in experimental animals. Since then, researchers have gathered even more evidence that chemicals may make us fat, too.

"Over the past ten years, and especially the past five years, there's been a flurry of new data," said Kristina Thayer, director of the Office of Health Assessment and Translation at the National Toxicology Program (NTP), in an article in *Environmental Health Perspectives* by Wendee Holtcamp. "There are many studies in both humans and animals. The NTP found real biological plausibility."

Robert H. Lustig, an obesity researcher and professor of clinical pediatrics at the University of California, San Francisco, notes in the book he edited *Obesity Before Birth: Maternal and Prenatal Influences on the Offspring* that different obesogens work differently in the body. Some plump up the number of fat cells, others expand the size of fat cells, and still others influence appetite, fullness, and how well the body burns calories. But the bottom line is that these chemicals certainly have a negative effect on our weight. They get into your body through food and screw up hormone production and metabolism. When you eat crappy chemicals, your body becomes a fat, toxic waste dump.

FOOD BABE ALERT: THE FATTENING CHEMICALS		
Some Common Obesogens	Source	How They May Cause Weight Gain
Atrazine	Pesticide	Increases body fat in kids
BPA	Plastic containers	Programs fat cells to incorporate more fat, so fat cells become very large
Estradiol	Synthetic estrogen given to dairy cows to increase milk production; may be in nonorganic milk	Interferes with the body's normal fat storage and fat formation mechanisms
Fructose (high-fructose corn syrup)	Processed foods, soda	Is metabolized in the body like a fat
Genistein	A natural chemical in soy foods	Mimics the action of estrogen, a fat-forming hormone
Monosodium glutamate (MSG)	Many processed foods and Asian dishes	Flavors food to make it more appealing and addictive; consumers wind up eating more calories than they need
Phthalates	Food packaging	Increases waist circumference in men and creates problems handling insulin, a fat-forming hormone
Tributyltin (TBT)	Fish and shellfish	Triggers genes that cause the growth of fat cells

WHY I WAS FAT AND SICK

I'm sure that in my formerly unattractive and unhealthy days, I was eating every obesogen on the planet. Obesogens were packing fat on me without my permission!

Just recently, I decided to analyze my diet as a teenager to see what kinds of chemicals and obesogens I was ingesting. It was shocking. Here's my analysis of a typical day of eating. I was eating all of the Sickening 15 every single day (the offending chemicals and obesogens are highlighted in bold):

Breakfast

Florida lemonade: Water, lemon juice, **sugar,** grapefruit juice pulp. (27 grams of sugar!)

Apple Cinnamon Nutri-Grain Bar: Crust: whole grain oats, **enriched flour** (wheat flour, niacin, reduced iron, vitamin B1 [thiamin mononitrate], vitamin B2 [riboflavin], folic acid, whole wheat flour, **soybean and/or canola oil, soluble corn fiber, sugar, dextrose, fructose,** calcium carbonate, whey, wheat bran, salt, **cellulose,** potassium bicarbonate, **natural and artificial flavor,** cinnamon, **mono- and diglycerides, soy lecithin,** wheat gluten, niacinamide, vitamin A palmitate, **carrageenan,** zinc oxide, reduced iron, guar gum, vitamin B6 (pyridoxine hydrochloride), vitamin B1 (thiamine hydrochloride), vitamin B2 (riboflavin). Filling: **invert sugar, corn syrup,** apple puree concentrate, glycerin, **sugar, modified corn starch,** sodium alginate, malic acid, **methylcellulose,** dicalcium phosphate, cinnamon, **citric acid, caramel color.** (12 grams of sugar!)

Lunch

Buddig Turkey Meat: Turkey, **mechanically separated turkey,** turkey broth, salt, less than 2% of: **modified food starch,** potassium lactate, **dextrose, sodium phosphate, carrageenan,** sodium diacetate, **sodium erythorbate, sodium nitrite,** honey, **natural flavoring.** (I was eating WHITE SLIME—leftover turkey scraps—and nitrates almost every day in high school!)

Nature's Own Whitewheat Bread: **Unbleached enriched flour** (wheat flour, malted barley flour, niacin, reduced iron, thiamine mononitrate, riboflavin, folic acid), water, **sugar,** wheat gluten, fiber (contains one or more of the following: **soy,** oat, **cottonseed,** or cellulose), yeast, contains 2% or less of each of the following: calcium sulfate, **soy flour,** salt, **soybean oil,** cultured wheat flour, calcium carbonate, **dough conditioners** (contains one or more of the following: **sodium stearoyl lactylate, calcium stearoyl lactylate, monoglycerides and/or diglycerides, distilled monoglycerides, calcium peroxide, calcium iodate, DATEM, ethoxylated mono- and diglycerides, enzymes,** ascorbic acid), vinegar, guar gum, **citric acid, monocalcium phosphate,** sodium citrate, **soy lecithin,** niacin, iron (ferrous sulfate), thiamine hydrochloride, riboflavin, folic acid, ammonium sulfate, natamycin (to retard spoilage).

Fruit Roll-Up: Pears from concentrate, **corn syrup, dried corn syrup, sugar, partially hydrogenated cottonseed oil, citric acid,** sodium citrate, **acetylated mono- and diglycerides,** pectin, malic acid, **natural flavor,** vitamin C (ascorbic acid), **color (Red 40, Yellows 5 & 6, Blue 1).**

Doritos: **Corn,** vegetable oil (sunflower, **canola, and/or corn oil), maltodextrin (made from corn),** salt, **whey, monosodium glutamate, buttermilk, romano cheese (cow's milk, cheese cultures, salt, enzymes), cheddar cheese (milk, cheese cultures, salt, enzymes),** onion powder, **natural and artificial flavor, dextrose,** tomato powder, **artificial color (including Yellow 6, Yellow 6 Lake, Yellow 5 Lake, Yellow 5, Red 40 Lake),** spices, sodium caseinate, **lactose,** lactic acid, **citric acid, sugar,** garlic powder, red and green bell pepper powder, **skim milk, disodium inosinate, and disodium guanylate.** Contains milk ingredients.

Dinner

Lasagna noodles: Semolina, **durum flour,** niacin. (Processed flour!)

Ragú sauce: Tomato puree (water, tomato paste), diced tomatoes in tomato juice, **sugar, vegetable oil (corn and/or cottonseed and/or canola),** salt, onion powder, spices (basil, oregano, spice), dehydrated garlic, **citric acid,** dehydrated parsley, and **flavoring.** (Inflammatory oils!)

Polly-O ricotta: **Pasteurized milk, whey, milkfat,** salt, vinegar, guar gum, **carrageenan, xanthan gum.** (Possible hormones plus antibiotics!)

Kraft shredded mozzarella: **Low-moisture part-skim mozzarella cheese (pasteurized part-skim milk, cheese culture,** salt, enzymes), **cream cheese powder (milkfat, nonfat milk, milk, sodium phosphate,** salt, carob bean gum, **cheese culture); cellulose powder** added to prevent caking; natamycin (a natural mold inhibitor). Contains: milk. Cellulose powder is wood pulp! (Possible hormones plus antibiotics!)

My Typical Snacks

Fruit—various kinds, but I loved apples: Thank goodness my mom would cut fruits that she got from the farmers' market or local grocery store when I got home from school; we didn't buy organic, so this means a nice dose of pesticides.

Fruit, however, was never my main snack. I ate snack cakes and Cheetos, mostly—all foods loaded with chemicals, trans fats, oils, sugar, MSG, artificial flavorings, acids, and all sorts of questionable ingredients.

This was my daily diet when I was a teenager. My skin looked horrible, and I was chubby and felt terrible and sick. I rest my case: I was a chemical stockpile of obesogens.

THE DIET DILEMMA

More than 80 million of us are dieting, yet without a lot of success. What is it about diets that don't work? Any diet book will tell you to eat right and exercise, but what does that really mean? I've seen people "eat right" by eating unlimited amounts of red meat and fat, and I've seen people "work out" daily for more than four hours, exhausting their body and pushing themselves too far.

I decided to search for some answers. My search was inspired not by any diet book, but rather by an eye-opening article in *The Atlantic* titled: "Science Compared Every Diet, and the Winner Is Real Food." The article summarized an independent study, published in the *Annual Review of Public Health* in 2014, that reviewed every major diet and concluded, "A diet of minimally processed foods close to nature, predominantly plants, is decisively associated with health promotion and disease prevention."

I was pumped just reading the full study. It supported and validated what I had been doing and preaching for years: A natural, plant-based diet is the secret to staying in shape, feeling vital, and being healthy. Other diets just don't cut it long-term, and one reason is that they induce you to eat a lot of chemical calories and lock you into habits that kill your ability to maintain your weight. At the end of each section below, I've listed the chemicals that you might eat on a particular diet, and I've boldfaced the worst offenders. Take a look.

1. THE LOW-CALORIE DIET

What it is: A low-calorie diet is based primarily on cutting up to 500 calories a day or more. It operates on the theory that "a calorie is a calorie."

Why I think it's flawed: All calories are not equal. For example, you can choose to eat a 100-calorie flavored yogurt cup, or an apple, also 100 calories. However, when you look at the ingredient list on most yogurts, you'll find that it contains artificial sweeteners—sucralose and acesulfame potassium (Ace-K). Both of these ingredients work against you by making you crave more. There may be other unhealthy ingredients in the yogurt, too, whereas an apple is a natural, high-fiber food. The low-calorie diet is also difficult to stick to, and many people end up gaining back weight after they go off it.

The chemicals you might eat on this diet:

Diet Pepsi—Carbonated water, **caramel color, aspartame, phosphoric acid, potassium benzoate** (preserves freshness), caffeine, **citric acid, natural flavor, acesulfame potassium.**

Yoplait 100-calorie Greek yogurt—Vanilla-pasteurized grade A nonfat milk, **sugar.** Contains 2% or less of: **cornstarch, potassium sorbate** (added to maintain freshness), **natural flavor,** yogurt cultures (L. bulgaricus, S. thermophilus), **sucralose, acesulfame potassium,** vitamin A acetate, vitamin D3.

Weight Watchers Smart Ones Chicken Enchilada—Chicken Enchilada (filling consists of white meat chicken, dark meat chicken, water, salt, **isolated soy protein, modified cornstarch,** and **sodium phosphate**); water, enchilada seasoning (**modified cornstarch,** emulsifiers [**modified cornstarch, corn maltodextrin, soy lecithin, sodium stearoyl lactylate, xanthan gum,** guar gum], **masa corn flour,** nonfat milk, dehydrated onion, salt, garlic powder, chicken fat, cultured whey, spices, whey, **artificial flavor [corn maltodextrin, modified cornstarch, partially hydrogenated cottonseed/soybean oil, citric acid, calcium disodium EDTA, BHA],** dehydrated chicken broth, **natural smoke**

flavor, **corn maltodextrin**], green chili flavor [salt, **autolyzed yeast extract,** dehydrated green bell peppers, **corn maltodextrin,** spices, **natural flavor**], dehydrated jalapeño peppers, **citric acid,** chicken flavor [**hydrolyzed corn, soy,** and wheat gluten protein, **autolyzed yeast extract,** dehydrated chicken broth, chicken fat, thiamine hydrochloride, **corn syrup solids**], dehydrated cilantro, green chiles (green chile peppers, **citric acid**), **modified cornstarch, cornstarch, methyl cellulose,** egg white powder, **xanthan gum,** guar gum], tortilla [**white corn flour,** water, **modified food starch, mono- & diglycerides,** salt, **xanthan gum,** guar gum, lime]), sauce (water, light sour cream [cultured skim milk and cream, **modified cornstarch,** gelatin, **disodium phosphate,** guar gum, **carrageenan,** locust bean gum], green chiles [green chile peppers, **citric acid**], nonfat milk, onions, jalapeños [jalapeño peppers, citric acid], **modified cornstarch,** cream, **enriched wheat flour.**

Gatorade G2 Low Calorie Sport Drinks Grape—water, **sucrose syrup, high-fructose corn syrup (glucose-fructose syrup),** citric acid, sodium citrate, salt, **natural and artificial flavors, monopotassium phosphate, sucralose, acesulfame potassium, red 40, blue 1.**

2. THE LOW-FAT DIET

What it is: This type of diet counts fat grams and keeps fat intake at 20 percent (or less) of your daily calories. The diet is often followed to reduce heart disease, but also to lose weight.

Why I think it's flawed: A low-fat diet focuses on the percentage of fat in your food, and not on anything else that you may be eating. It also sanctions replacing full-fat versions of a food with a fat-free counterpart—such as fat-free salad dressing. The problem with these fat-free alternatives is that they are nothing more than processed garbage full of sugar, starches, and gums. Consequently, you'll be eating a lot of unhealthy carbs such as sugar and white flour, which can wreak havoc on your insulin levels, increase your diabetes risk, and ironically, increase your chances of a heart attack. The low-fat diet has proven unsuccessful in helping people lose weight. We need a certain amount of fat in our diets, anyway. It helps us absorb vitamins A, D, K, and E. Unsaturated fats from nuts, olive oil, sesame oil, and avocados prevent heart disease. Coconut oil helps lower cholesterol and reduce abdominal fat.

The chemicals you might eat on this diet:

Lean Cuisine Apple Cranberry Chicken—Blanched whole wheat orzo pasta (water, whole durum wheat flour), cooked white meat chicken (white meat chicken, water, modified tapioca starch, chicken flavor (dried chicken broth, chicken powder, **natural flavor**), **carrageenan,** whey protein concentrate, **soybean oil, corn syrup solids, sodium phosphate,** salt), water, carrots, green beans, wheat berries, apple juice concentrate, dried cranberries (cranberries, sugar, sunflower oil), apples (apples, **citric acid,** salt, water), 2% or less of butter (cream, salt), **modified cornstarch,** chicken broth, orange juice concentrate, apple cider vinegar, sugar, **soybean oil,** sea salt, ginger puree (ginger, water, **citric acid**), **yeast extract,** spices, lemon juice concentrate, **citric acid.**

Skinny Cow Low Fat Vanilla Ice Cream Sandwich—Skim milk, wafer (**bleached wheat flour, isomalt*, malitol*, caramel color, sorbitol*,** palm oil, cocoa, **corn flour, modified cornstarch,** salt, baking soda, **natural flavor, soy lecithin**), **maltodextrin, polydextrose, sorbitol*,** cream, stabilizer (**mono- and diglycerides, cellulose gel, cellulose gum, carrageenan**), **sucralose (Splenda brand),** vitamin A palmitate, **acesulfame potassium, natural flavor, artificial flavor.** *Sensitive individuals may experience a laxative effect from excess consumption of this ingredient.

Nestlé Nesquick Low Fat Chocolate Lowfat Milk with Vitamin A Palmitate and Vitamin D3 Added—Sugar, less than 2% of cocoa processed with alkali, calcium carbonate, **cellulose gel, natural and artificial flavors,** salt, **carrageenan, cellulose gum.** Contains: milk ingredient.

Special K Low-Fat Granola with Honey—Whole grain oats, sugar, **corn syrup,** oat bran, rice, contains 2% or less of honey, **modified cornstarch, soy grits,** molasses, soluble wheat fiber, **natural flavor, corn flour,** acacia gum, salt, **soy protein isolate,** oat fiber, evaporated cane juice, **malt flavoring, BHT for freshness.** Vitamins and minerals:

niacinamide, reduced iron, vitamin B6 (pyridoxine hydrochloride), vitamin B1 (thiamin hydrochloride), vitamin B2 (riboflavin), vitamin A palmitate, folic acid, vitamin D, vitamin B12. Contains soy and wheat ingredients.

3. THE LOW-CARB DIET

What it is: This type of diet is fairly high in protein and fat and very low in carbs. It focuses on controlling insulin levels to lose weight and prevent diabetes — both worthy goals.

Why I think it's flawed: You eat large amounts of high-fat meat and cheese on this diet. The meats may be heavily processed with nitrates (bacon) or be from hormone- and antibiotic-injected cows. Also, the reduction in carbs means you'll be eating fewer fruits and vegetables, resulting in nutrient deficiencies. This is why vitamin and mineral supplements are often recommended on these diets.

The chemicals you might eat on this diet:

Atkins Sesame Chicken Stir-Fry—Grilled seasoned chicken strips (Chicken breast meat, water, less than 2% lemon juice concentrate, vinegar, salt), water, broccoli, green beans, red bell pepper, **canola oil, soy sauce** (water, wheat, **soybeans,** salt, alcohol, vinegar, lactic acid), contain less than 2% of the following: chicken stock, toasted sesame oil, garlic puree, chicken fat, ginger puree (ginger, water), raisin juice concentrate, **modified food starch,** wok oil flavor (safflower oil, sesame seed oil, rice bran oil, **natural flavors**), toasted sesame seeds, apple cider vinegar, **caramel color, soy lecithin, xanthan gum, disodium inosinate, disodium guanylate,** spices, **sucralose.**

Atkins Advantage Dark Chocolate Almond Bar—Roasted almonds, toasted coconut, dark chocolate flavored coating (palm kernel oil, **maltitol,** milk protein concentrate, cocoa [processed with alkali], **dextrose, soy lecithin,** vanilla extract), **polydextrose, maltitol syrup,** water, sunflower oil, salt, **natural flavor, sucralose.** Contains almonds, coconut, soy, and milk. This product is manufactured in a facility that uses eggs, wheat, seeds, peanuts, and tree nuts.

4. THE PALEO DIET

What it is: Based on a "caveman" style of eating, this diet recommends eating lots of proteins and fewer carbs while restricting dairy foods and beans. Although vegetables, fruits, nuts, and seeds are allowed, the emphasis is on meat and fats.

Why I think it's flawed: In truth, the meat you eat on this diet is not at all like the meat of our caveman ancestors. Theirs wasn't factory-farmed, pumped full of antibiotics and hormones. You would need to have access to pastured-raised, organic meat all the time for this diet to work, and that's just not realistic if you plan to ever leave your home or travel. What's more, you aren't allowed to eat grains, beans, or legumes—which can be important sources of fiber and nutrients. Advocates of Paleo diets claim that legumes contain "antinutrients." One is lectin, a protein that binds to cell membranes and supposedly destroys tissue. The flaw in this reasoning is that this reaction happens mostly in animals, not humans.

I can't believe that a diet would tell you to eat no beans. There is irrefutable evidence that beans reduce the risk of cancer and enhance longevity. Plus, because they're full of fiber, they help you lose weight, as all natural fiber-rich foods do.

Another antinutrient is phytic acid, a compound that prevents the body from absorbing minerals such as calcium, magnesium, and iron. Legumes are only moderately high in phytic acid. Does that mean you should stop eating them? No! Just eat a variety of plant foods, and you'll moderate how much phytic acid you eat.

What's more, unless you eat an abundance of vegetables, these diets are also low in health-giving probiotics and can be acid-forming. An acidic diet can cause cancer cells to thrive. Also, animal protein stimulates the growth factor IGF-1, a naturally occurring protein produced by the liver. Similar to insulin, high levels of IGF-1 may accelerate aging and growth of cancer cells later in life. Protein-rich plant foods like seeds, nuts, beans, and dark leafy greens do not raise IGF-1.

Unlimited helpings of meat, oil, eggs, and fish could get you slim but not healthy in the long run. Also, if everyone ate a Paleo diet, we'd run out of meat. Paleo seems like a great idea, but it's not sustainable, unless you make vegetables the main component.

The chemicals you might eat on this diet: Hormones, GMOs, antibiotics fed to livestock, pesticides, carrageenan, synthetic vitamins, and natural flavors.

Almond Breeze Original Unsweetened Almond Milk—Almond milk (filtered water, almonds), calcium carbonate, sea salt, potassium citrate, **carrageenan,** sunflower lecithin, **natural flavor, vitamin A palmitate, vitamin D2, and D-alpha-tocopherol (natural vitamin E).**

5. THE RAW FOODS DIET

What it is: This regimen is a plant-based diet of unprocessed raw foods (vegetables, fruits, sprouted grains, nuts). This is also known as the living food diet—as the theory of this diet is to keep food as alive as possible.

Why I think it's flawed: The raw foods diet has a lot going for it, and I recommend that you eat raw fruits and veggies frequently—at least 50 percent of the time. This sort of diet also eliminates your exposure to most of the Sickening 15. But a 100 percent raw diet is difficult to maintain. It's so limited in food choices, and excludes some healthy superfoods such as cooked quinoa, beans, and sweet potatoes. While most veggies are best eaten raw, the nutritional content of some foods, particularly carrots and tomatoes, actually increases when cooked. Also, this kind of diet can be dangerously deficient in nutrients such as calcium, iron, vitamin B12, vitamin D, and omega-3 fatty acids.

The chemicals you might eat on this diet:

Pesticides found in fruits and vegetables.
Raw agave nectar (a form of refined sugar).
Carrageenan used as a stabilizer and thickener in some raw desserts.

6. THE GLUTEN-FREE DIET

What it is: This diet completely eliminates foods that contain gluten, a protein in wheat, barley, and rye. A gluten-free diet is medically necessary for people with celiac disease (1 percent of the population) or who have an allergy to gluten. Other people try this diet because they might be intolerant of gluten. It is possible that gluten causes digestive problems and other disorders, or that the diet will help them lose weight. The reason these diets don't work for people who want to lose weight is because an entire ingredient is eliminated, making you choose lesser-quality ingredients to replace it and consuming processed foods just because they are "gluten free."

Why I think it's flawed: My biggest beef with the gluten-free diet is that it encourages the use of processed foods such as refined sugar, white rice, soda, and oil. The popularity of the gluten-free diet has given rise to an industry of gluten-free convenience foods that contain suspicious additives, added sugar, and ingredients such as insulin-raising, nutrient-empty potato starch and tapioca starch. Brown rice is often substituted in gluten-free breads, pastas, and cakes, but it can be contaminated with arsenic. You can go gluten-free without exposure to these ingredients. If you have a sensitivity to gluten, choose naturally gluten-free food such as quinoa, nuts, seeds, fruits, and vegetables.

The chemicals you might eat on this diet:

Pillsbury Gluten Free Thin Crust Pizza Dough — Water, **modified tapioca starch,** whole sorghum flour, whole millet flour, **rice flour, fructose,** egg white, brown sugar, **soybean oil.** Contains 2 percent or less of: salt, extra virgin olive oil, **hydrogenated soybean oil, xanthan gum,** leavening (**sodium aluminum phosphate,** baking soda), guar gum, **natural and artificial flavor,** yeast, **yeast extract.**

Udi's Gluten Free Whole Grain Bread — Udi's Best Blend (tapioca and potato starch, brown rice and teff flour, modified tapioca starch), water, non-GMO vegetable oil (**canola,** sunflower, or safflower oil), egg whites, **evaporated cane juice,** tapioca **maltodextrin,** tapioca syrup, yeast, flaxseed, **xanthan gum,** salt, baking powder (**sodium acid pyrophosphate,** sodium bicarbonate, **cornstarch, monocalcium phosphate**), **cultured corn syrup solids** (natural mold inhibitor), dry molasses, enzymes.

Gluten Free Honey Nut Chex Cereal — **Cornmeal, sugar, whole grain corn,** honey, salt, barley malt extract, brown sugar molasses, rice bran and/or **canola oil, color added, natural and artificial flavor, natural almond flavor.**

Glutino Gluten Free Covered Pretzel Fudge — Fudge coating (**sugar,** palm kernel oil, nonfat dry milk solids, cocoa powder, **soy lecithin,** salt, **natural flavor**), pretzel (**corn starch,** potato starch, rice flour, **soluble corn fiber,** palm oil, **sugar,** salt, **cellulose gum, soy lecithin, yeast extract,** sodium bicarbonate, **sodium acid pyrophosphate, citric acid**).

7. THE VEGAN DIET

What it is: Vegans eat a strict plant-based diet that excludes anything that has come from an animal (meat, eggs, dairy, even honey). This diet is typically adopted for ethical reasons, rather than for its health benefits or to lose weight.

Why I think it's flawed: The vegan diet generally does not take into account whether the food is organic or non-GMO. Vegans are at risk for developing a vitamin B12 deficiency. B12 can only be sourced from animal products, so supplementation is necessary. Vegans often rely heavily on processed meat substitutes and an abundance of soy products that can mess with hormones and could be GMO-derived. There are definitely right and wrong ways to be vegan, but as a generalized plan to lose weight, the vegan diet has many pitfalls, unless you follow the principles outlined in the chapters ahead.

The chemicals you might eat on this diet:

Beyond Meat, Beyond Beef Feisty Crumbles — Water, non-GMO pea protein isolate, **non-GMO expeller-pressed canola oil,** spices, beef flavor (**yeast extract,** maltodextrin, **natural flavoring,** salt, sunflower oil, onion powder), chicory root fiber, rice flour, tomato powder, caramel color (natural), **sugar,** contains 0.5% or less of: calcium sulfate, potassium chloride, lime juice concentrate, **citric acid,** onion extract, chili pepper extract, garlic extract, paprika extract.

Daiya Cheddar Style Shreds—Filtered water, tapioca and/or arrowroot flours, **non-GMO expeller-pressed canola** and/or non-GMO expeller-pressed safflower oil, coconut oil, pea protein, salt, inactive yeast, **vegan natural flavors,** vegetable glycerin, **xanthan gum, citric acid** (for flavor), annatto, **titanium dioxide** (a naturally occurring mineral).

Original Vegan Boca Burgers—Water, **soy protein concentrate,** wheat gluten, contains less than 2% of **methylcellulose,** salt, **caramel color,** dried onions, **yeast extract,** sesame oil, **hydrolyzed wheat protein, natural and artificial flavor (non-meat), disodium guanylate, disodium inosinate.**

8. THE PESCETARIAN DIET

What it is: A pescetarian eats fish but excludes all other animal proteins.

Why I think it's flawed: This diet does not fully emphasize the dangers of processed foods. Plus, you can still eat farmed salmon that's been fed antibiotics, GMOs, and dyes.

The chemicals you might eat on this diet:

Farmed salmon—Antibiotics, GMOs, and dyes, often contaminated with PCBs. Shark, swordfish, king mackerel, tilefish, and tuna have higher amounts of mercury.

Trans-Ocean Crab Classic Flake Style Imitation Crab (commonly used in California rolls)—Alaska pollock, water, egg whites, wheat starch, **sugar, cornstarch, sorbitol,** contains 2% or less of the following: king crab meat, **natural and artificial flavor,** extracts of crab, oyster, scallop, lobster, and fish (salmon, anchovy, bonito, cutlassfish), refined fish oil* (anchovy, sardine), rice wine (rice, water, koji, yeast, salt), sea salt, modified tapioca starch, **carrageenan,** yam flour, **hydrolyzed soy, corn,** and wheat proteins, potassium chloride, **disodium inosinate and guanylate, sodium pyrophosphate, carmine,** paprika, color added. *Adds a trivial amount of fat. Contains pollock, salmon, anchovy, bonito, cutlassfish, sardine, crab, lobster, soy, egg, wheat.

9. THE DETOX DIET

What it is: A detox diet promotes the elimination of toxins in the body—a process that is indeed important—through the use of fiber, juices, vegetables, and herbs. On some detox diets, fasting is recommended.

Why I think it's flawed: My major criticism of most types of detox diets is that they fail to prepare your body beforehand and do not give you long-lasting advice on how to eat afterward. For a diet to be effective, it needs staying power; it needs to be something you can do for the rest of your life. I'm all in favor of occasional juice cleanses, but you need a plan before and after that makes sense to follow in the long-term. A detox diet tends to be short-term and can set you up for harmful yo-yo dieting. It usually eliminates several ingredients and foods that could be healthy long-term. Fasting is not always healthy, especially for people with diabetes or heart disease. If you are eating the right foods from the get-go, your body will always be naturally detoxing. *The Food Babe Way* will show you how.

The chemicals you might eat on this diet: Pesticides sprayed on nonorganic produce and additives in juices. Supplements are often suggested that may contain synthetic or chemically processed ingredients.

10. THE MEDITERRANEAN DIET

What it is: This diet is based on a pattern of eating followed in Mediterranean countries, such as Greece and Italy. Foods emphasized include fruits, vegetables, grains (including refined grains—white flour!), nuts, seeds, and beans. The main sources of fat are olive oil, cheese, and yogurt. You're allowed to eat some red meat and drink wine—all in moderation. A study published by the *New England Journal of Medicine* revealed that a Mediterranean-type diet, with its emphasis on olive oil, nuts, and red wine, could reduce the risk of stroke by up to 30 percent.

Why I think it's flawed: The Mediterranean way of eating is fairly well balanced, and it discourages processed foods. My issue with this diet is that it generally doesn't emphasize where the food comes from, whether it's organic, or whether it contains GMOs. You eat a lot of grains on this diet, so if you have problems with gluten, you'd have to find substitutes. Refined white bread and pasta are like sugar, so you don't want to consume them on a regular basis. Here's a big uh-oh, too: If you eat too much olive oil, cheese, nuts, and wine on this diet, you'll pack on pounds.

The chemicals you might eat on this diet:

> Added sulfites in wine
> Fake olive oil with added GMO oil fillers
> Pesticides
> Antibiotics and GMOs in conventional yogurt and cheese
> Refined white pasta and white bread

EAT REAL FOOD, AKA THE FOOD BABE WAY

Maybe the whole diet thing hasn't worked out for you. Maybe you eat well for a few days or a few hours but then find yourself face-first in a gallon of ice cream or stuffing yourself with cookies. Or maybe you're doing your best to live a healthy, active life, but you just keep riding the rollercoaster of dieting for years on end.

Isn't it time to quit your back-and-forth battle with food? As I explained earlier in this chapter: Losing weight and getting healthy don't have as much to do with calories or fat grams or carb counting as you've been led to believe.

The secret is to break free from food additives and obesogens that are getting in your body's way as it tries to burn fat and keep you healthy. You can do this by eating 100 percent pure, toxin-free, real food. You won't have to worry about sugar, artery-clogging fats, calories, carbs, or chemicals—all the stuff that comes from poisoned, processed foods. If you follow the recommendations in this book, your weight—and your health—will take care of themselves.

HERE'S HOW IT WORKS...

The Food Babe Way is a twenty-one-day program designed to launch you into better health and a new, thinner, fitter body. It's designed for high-speed healing and slimming. It requires forming some new habits and breaking some old ones. And it is something you can do easily and successfully.

Psychologists say it takes twenty-one days to form good habits, and holistic nutritionists say it takes twenty-one days to change the chemistry of the body. This program is designed around those two premises. Each day, I'll give you a new habit to practice, or an unhealthy pattern to give up (like eating fast food), along with a meal. Everyone wants menu planning and weight control to be brainless. Always thinking about what to eat next can be overwhelming, so I have done everything for you, from the menus to the recipes. Day by day, you're going to gradually replace fatty, sugary, chemical-laden food with wholesome, nutrient-intact, organic food. This program will not only keep you on track; it will help you lose weight if you need to and/or maintain the healthy lifestyle you may have already built.

You won't have to count anything or obsess over calories or carbs, either. You just have to read labels, change some food-buying and food-prep practices, and enjoy food the way it was meant to be—natural and whole.

Everyone can eat the Food Babe Way, I'm convinced. The only reason I've been able to maintain my ideal weight for over ten years now and feel amazing is because of my habits, food choices, and routine. And now I want to share that with you.

Once you get started, expect to feel revitalized even after the first day. And after the second day, expect your digestion to improve practically overnight and your energy levels to zoom. I promise! Keep going, and you'll start feeling the tune-up of a lifetime, regaining lost horsepower within a day. Your body will be humming along like a sports car, complete with a new paint job. Watch out, though: You may find that you need to be quite humble when people start to compliment you on how fit, attractive, sexy, and vibrant you have become.

Let me ask you: Do you like the lifestyle you've set for yourself and your family? If not, it is never too late to change, and it takes only twenty-one days.

Day 1 starts now.

PART II

21 DAYS OF GOOD FOOD AND GOOD HABITS

CHAPTER 4

WEEK 1 — FLUID ASSETS FOR FOOD BABES

WELCOME TO WEEK 1! The goal this week is to clean up your body, ridding it of the toxins and antinutrients the food industry has been putting in our food. The easiest and quickest way to do that is by putting the right fluids in your body. The fluids will flush out toxins, hydrate your body, and help your system metabolize fat more efficiently. Best of all, you'll start feeling lighter and more energetic after the very first day. After I gave up horrendous sodas and sugary juices for pure, clean fluids, my skin, my energy, my weight, and my entire body changed for good.

Whatever you put in your mouth affects your body, so be sure to also start my 21-Day Food Babe Way Eating Plan, which begins on page 281. It will help you control your eating habits, and it will also show you how to eat wisely and well. By continuing the plan, which will quickly become second nature, you'll naturally start losing weight and keeping it off. The Food Babe Way Eating Plan is not a diet, but a way of living. Follow it closely and expect your body, and your life, to change.

Day 1 — Cleanse Daily with My Morning Lemon Water Ritual

MOST OF US WOULD love to be thinner, more energetic, and healthier, but we make the excuse that our busy lives deny us the time or the energy to accomplish this. Good news: It's possible to get fitter and healthier without making radical changes to your life. And the first step in that direction is ultraeasy: Drink a cup of warm lemon water with cayenne pepper as soon as you get up in the morning.

I know from personal experience that adopting this daily habit has amazing health benefits. Once upon a time, I had cravings for sugary foods like granola bars or muffins as soon as I got up in the morning. But those cravings vanished after I began this habit. Now I crave whole and satisfying foods instead. Starting my day with a healthy action sets me up for success for the rest of the day and is a reminder that my health comes first.

You'll get some amazing benefits from this one little habit.

First, even though lemon juice is acidic, its low-sugar and high-alkaline mineral content has an alkalizing effect. Our bodies have different levels of acidity and alkalinity, and one of the keys to good health is learning to strike the right balance between the two. Some parts of your body are naturally a little more acidic, such as your stomach with its digestive juices, but too much acidity can be very harmful. When your diet is high in acidic foods—such as white bread, soda, processed and fast foods, and, to a lesser extent, meat and eggs—your body starts siphoning off minerals such as calcium to neutralize the acid, decreasing the body's ability to absorb important nutrients, to produce energy, and to repair and detoxify itself. An acidic system can increase your risk of many degenerative diseases, from arthritis to heart disease to cancer.

To help your body function at its peak, it's best to maintain a balance that errs on the side of alkalinity. In this state, normal chemical reactions can take place in cells and tissues, such as metabolism, immune cell protection, proper blood flow, and weight regulation. You can take control of your acid-alkaline balance and increase alkalinity through the foods you eat. Alkaline foods include fresh fruit, vegetables, and certain nuts and whole grains such as almonds and quinoa.

The second reason to start your day with lemon-cayenne water is that this wonderful morning ritual stimulates your liver, which is the main detoxing organ in the body. The liver has hundreds of vital functions that support health. I won't list them all, as it would take up too many pages, but here are a few liver benefits that are relevant to staying healthy: healthier skin, clearer eyes, better attitude, and more balanced weight. The liver is at its most active in the morning, and the lemon helps speed up the elimination of toxins. Don't be surprised if you have to go to the bathroom quickly; this indicates the habit is working.

Third, lemon water increases your fat burn by improving your digestion. If your digestive system is not working up to par, it's nearly impossible to shed pounds or keep your weight in check. Faulty digestion can prevent your body from absorbing the nutrients it needs to burn fat. Drinking warm lemon water stimulates saliva and sends a signal to the body to get digestion rolling.

Fourth, there are important health-building nutrients in lemons. One is vitamin C. This amazing vitamin fights cell damage and chronic inflammation, strengthens your immune defenses, and accelerates wound healing. Before starting this habit, I was sick all the time. But drinking lemon juice, spiced up with cayenne pepper, every morning has helped prevent me from getting colds and the flu and has kept me going strong.

Another nutritious component of lemon juice is limonin. It helps prevent cancer, strengthens blood vessel linings, elevates beneficial enzymes in the liver, and reduces artery-clogging cholesterol.

Why do I add the cayenne? Here are a few of the scientifically proven benefits of this miracle spice:

- It burns your body fat by boosting your metabolism (any hot, spicy food does this).
- It increases energy expenditure and feelings of satiety.

- It fights food cravings.
- It enhances blood circulation.
- It is high in vitamins A, C, and B complex; calcium; and potassium.
- It has a healing effect on your digestive system.

If you don't like the lemon water and cayenne drink, I've got an alternative for you: Try apple cider vinegar in a cup of warm water. This powerhouse vinegar has been used for centuries as a natural remedy to cure allergies (including those to pets, foods, and the environment), sinus infections, acne, high cholesterol, flu, chronic fatigue, candida, acid reflux, sore throats, contact dermatitis, arthritis, and gout.

Besides that, apple cider vinegar can burn some serious booty. Widely used for weight control, it helps break down fat in the body and can boost your metabolism. It also lowers glucose levels and reduces insulin spikes that can lead to weight gain.

If this option appeals to you, start today! Remember to buy the good stuff. Bragg makes a great version that is organic, raw, and unfiltered.

Sound good? Then follow my lead, and you'll be able to do this successfully every single day.

THE FOOD BABE WAY

START THE NIGHT BEFORE

Every night, I fill my electric teakettle with filtered water, and I take one lemon from the fridge and place it on the counter, along with the cayenne pepper bottle and a cup filled halfway with water. As soon as I get up in the morning, I put on my robe and walk into the kitchen to turn the electric kettle on. I then go into the bathroom, and by the time I finish putting in my contact lenses and splashing my face with water, the electric kettle has finished heating up my water.

Next, I pour the hot water into the glass half full of room-temperature water. I want the water to be warm, not hot. Why? Warm water is close to your body's own temperature, and you'll be able to process it — and the nutrients in the drink—better; water that's too hot can kill off beneficial live enzymes in the lemon. You want these alive, not dead, because they strengthen the enzymes in your liver to break down fat. Next, using a lemon squeezer (to get as much juice as possible), I squeeze half of the lemon on top, sprinkle with cayenne pepper (for extra detoxifying and metabolism boosting), and drink. (Again, if you don't like lemon or cayenne, apple cider vinegar is a great substitute, or try lime.)

SIP AND SOOTHE

I sip this mixture with a glass straw so that my teeth aren't exposed to the acid. I drink at least twelve ounces, followed by another eight ounces of water, before I eat or drink anything else. I've done this every morning for several years. I even bring lemons with me when I'm out of town. I just toss them in my suitcase and ask my hotel for an electric kettle upon arrival. If they don't have one, I'll request hot water in the morning. There have been a few times when I've been out of town without access to lemons or limes and thus haven't been able to follow my morning ritual. On those days, I've noticed an immediate difference in how I feel and look—I tend to be drained and more sluggish.

This ritual is just too easy not to do—so drink up and start each day with this healthy habit.

> **FOOD BABE ALERT:**
> **STARBUCKS SABOTAGE**

Starting the new lemon water habit may mean weaning yourself off your morning Starbucks. I understand the allure; Starbucks makes more than 80,000 different kinds of drinks, but hear me out: You're paying a premium for these drinks—and for coffee that's riddled with potential toxins.

At most locations, Starbucks doesn't serve organic coffee or organic milk; they serve nonorganic coffee made from beans doused with pesticides, and milk from cows fed GMOs and given antibiotics. If you drink

(Continued)

Starbucks on a daily basis, you're exposing yourself to pesticides, GMOs, and antibiotics every day.

Starbucks gets some of its beans from developing nations, where chemical spraying is less regulated. You could be drinking toxins that are banned in the United States but not elsewhere. One of these is the pesticide chlorpyrifos, which has been linked to birth defects and is highly toxic to wildlife.

And you can forget about decaf. Most conventional decaffeinated coffees are made by soaking the beans in a chemical called ethyl acetate, which is used in nail polish and glues, and a carcinogen called methylene chloride, which Starbucks uses.

The fancy drinks at Starbucks can really pack on the pounds, too (there are sixty grams of sugar in one Grande White Chocolate Mocha Frappuccino). The syrups and potions they use to make some of their signature drinks also may contain artificial flavors made from petroleum, carcinogenic caramel coloring, and many preservatives.

I personally love coffee. But I always brew organic coffee at home, and that's a great habit to start now as well.

CHECKLIST

Today:

✓ I did my morning lemon water ritual.

Day 2 — Be a Lean, Green Drinking Machine

STARTING TODAY, DRINK A green drink every day.

By green drink, I mean a smoothie or a juice made mostly from kale, romaine, spinach, and other leafy veggies.

I know what you're thinking: That sounds repulsive. But listen, greens are among the healthiest foods you can eat—and you can make them very yummy. A green drink is the best fast food available and a superb way to add more veggies to your diet. And once you start to pump your body with greens, you'll start craving them.

Not convinced? Here are three reasons why this daily habit is vital to your ultimate health.

1. YOU'RE MAKING SURE YOU GET YOUR SIX (OR MORE) DAILY SERVINGS.

Nutritionists say we should eat six to eight servings of veggies and fruits a day for good health. Calorie for calorie, greens hold the most concentrated nutrition of any food. They protect against all types of cancer; work wonders on your bones, arteries, and blood pressure; help keep you thin and fit; and more. Greens can also decrease chronic, health-damaging inflammation, boot out toxins, and even improve your digestion.

But six to eight servings a day is tough to do. For most Americans, a vegetable serving is as small as a piece of lettuce and a slice of tomato on a sandwich—and that might be it for the whole day. (When I was little, I went days without seeing anything green—I can't help thinking this contributed to my poor health as a child.) If you blend or juice your fruits and veggies, though, getting all you need is a cinch. Consider this: A twelve-ounce glass of fresh vegetable juice supplies a whole day's worth of servings.

I like to drink fresh green vegetable juice on an empty stomach, usually ten minutes after my lemon water habit. Drinking a tall glass of juiced kale, spinach, or collards (mixed with other vegetables) is a good way to get some of the nutrients that you might not ordinarily eat at breakfast. After all, who's going to sit down and eat a bowl or two of kale in the morning? It's much more satisfying to drink vegetable juice.

When I juice, I use a wide range of vegetables, giving my body the variety of vitamins and minerals it needs to repair damaged cells, prevent disease, and look and feel younger.

2. YOU'RE COMPENSATING FOR DEPLETED SOIL.

Pesticides, genetically modified seeds, and conventional farming practices have depleted important vitamins and minerals from our soil. A stalk of today's broccoli, for example, doesn't yield the same amount of nutrition as broccoli did twenty years ago.

Studies published within the past fifteen years indicate that much of our produce is low in phytonutrients, which are natural disease-fighting chemicals in fruits and vegetables. These chemicals have the power to reduce four of the scariest diseases in our modern lives: cancer, heart disease, diabetes, and dementia. Up until about fifty years ago, our fruits and veggies were abundant in phytonutrients. But over time, modern farming practices began inadvertently stripping away these protective nutrients.

Consequently, we need to overcompensate by eating as many whole plant foods as possible. Enjoying a daily green drink is one easy way to do that.

3. YOU'RE DETOXING NATURALLY.

Many diseases are triggered by poisons in the body that come from polluted foods. Consuming green drinks is the quickest and easiest natural way I've found to detox from these poisons. Chlorophyll, which is what makes a leaf green, is a key factor. This pigment helps plants absorb light energy for use in photosynthesis and growth, and it is essential to all life on earth.

Though nutrition experts have known about the power of

chlorophyll for quite some time, not much scientific research has been done on it until recently. An exciting study published in *PLOS ONE* in 2011 showed that chlorophyll supplements, along with yogurt and cruciferous veggies like broccoli, cleared up DNA damage in colon tissue. DNA damage leads to cancer, so this combination of foods appears to lower the risk of developing colon cancer.

Another impressive chlorophyll study, published in *Appetite* in 2013, had to do with chlorophyll and weight control. Chlorophyll is found inside plants in saclike membranes called thylakoids, which help the plant absorb sunlight. This study found that thylakoids given in a supplemental form suppressed hunger and prevented further weight gain in a group of overweight women. No wonder I feel full and satisfied after enjoying a green drink.

I like to blend chlorophyll-rich foods like spinach, kale, and collards with fruit, which adds a dash of sweetness, cuts down on any bitterness that might come from the greens, and gives me extra fiber to regulate my blood sugar.

I've found, too, that this type of blend alleviates cravings because it provides a burst of nutrition — one that's not usually present in the typical American diet. When your body doesn't get what it needs, nutritionally speaking, cravings kick in. And if you give in to those cravings, you're back on the road to gaining weight.

I hope you are now pumped to incorporate green drinks into your diet every day.

THE FOOD BABE WAY

Getting your daily greens doesn't have to be complicated. Here are three easy ways to "go green."

HAVE A SHOT OF WHEATGRASS

The simplest is to knock back a shot of wheatgrass juice — but let me warn you! It's going to be strong in taste, so it's not for the faint of heart. Wheatgrass, however, is one of the best sources of living chlorophyll available. In the 1970s, Ann Wigmore popularized the use of fresh-squeezed wheatgrass juice to treat cancer patients who had been written off as "incurable" after conventional cancer treatment. In a miraculous turn of events, Wigmore saved her own gangrenous legs from amputation with her wheatgrass treatments and eventually competed in the Boston Marathon.

Consuming a mere ounce of wheatgrass is the nutritional equivalent of eating two pounds of dark green leafy vegetables, making it an easy way to ramp up your daily vegetable intake. You can buy premixed wheatgrass juice or wheatgrass powder, which you can blend with water or any type of organic fruit or vegetable juice. I've listed more benefits of wheatgrass and chlorophyll on my website, foodbabe.com.

BLEND YOUR GREENS

The second way to go green is to make a green smoothie. This method is the first one I tried when introducing more greens into my diet. I like to blend greens into a smoothie because this preserves the beneficial fiber of the greens. The fiber gives me something to chew on. Juice (and smoothies) are food and should be chewed. It's important to swish around the juice or smoothie in your mouth or move your jaw up and down for a couple of seconds before swallowing it to release your saliva, which contains digestive enzymes that are crucial in delivering key nutrients to your cells.

I take a handful of kale and throw it right in my blender along with frozen fruit—usually berries, and some good fat and protein (like chia and hempseeds). I used to take this smoothie along with me to work in a glass container and sip on it slowly throughout the morning for my breakfast, and everyone would ask what I was drinking. It's an unconventional approach to breakfast, but one that makes me feel amazing before a long day of work and gives me long-lasting energy to make it through the day. Whenever I travel out of town, I ask the hotel kitchen to make me green smoothies. Most hotels have greens, fruit, and a blender available, so it's a rather simple request—you just need to ask!

Depending on the kinds of fruits or vegetables you toss into your smoothie, you'll get a healthy, hefty dose of vitamins, minerals, live enzymes, and phytonutrients. All of these nutrients boost your antioxidant intake and enhance your body's natural detoxification process.

In the recipe section (Chapter 8), you'll find instructions for making My Basic Green Smoothie and other green drinks.

Recommended Blenders

Blender	Features	Cost
Vitamix	A self-cleaning machine that lets you chop, blend, cream, puree, and more.	Up to $600
Blendtec	A powerful blender that can easily crush ice, make hot soup, blend nut butters, grind seeds, puree fruit, and much more. Excellent for making green and other smoothies.	Up to $500
NutriBullet	An all-in-one blender featuring a convenient flip-top lid and to-go cups and lids (BPA-free plastic). It has a one-speed setting for ease of use.	Up to $150
Ninja	A blender that can be used for juicing, food processing, frozen blending, and dough mixing.	Up to $200

JUICE IT

The third way to get your daily fill of green is by juicing greens. I love this method. After I learned how to juice a few years ago, my body weight stabilized, and I've been able to fit easily into everything in my closet since then. This is important, because I love my wardrobe and don't want to grow out of it! If you're trying to drop pounds but you've got hard-to-control food cravings, it might be because your body is deficient in some essential vitamins and minerals. Drinking juice replenishes those elements and zaps your cravings so you can lose weight.

Juicing your greens (and other produce) delivers as many nutrients to your body as possible—a real jolt of concentrated nutrition. When juice is separated from the fiber of fruits and vegetables, it is easier for your body to absorb all of the nutrients, giving you an instant boost of energy. Consuming the abundance of live enzymes, vitamins, and minerals in juice is like drinking a natural version of Red Bull. There's nothing wrong with a little organic coffee in the morning, but I was able to break my dependence on caffeine after I started having fresh juice daily.

Want to look more beautiful? Drink juice. After I started putting carrots in my green juice on occasion, my eyelashes started to grow longer and my eyes became brighter within just a couple of weeks. Feeling the extra energy boost is one thing, but seeing the results in the mirror can be quite dramatic and can make you a firm believer in the powers of drinking juice.

I use fresh juices in two ways: either as a daily snack or as my daily green drink. You can find several delicious juice recipes in the recipe chapter. And for more information on juicing, check out the juicing guide on my website, foodbabe.com.

To get going, all you need is a good juicer (see my recommendations on page 93) and a batch of organically grown fruits and vegetables. Now you can go crazy with produce and juice every fruit or veggie in sight!

I Did It the Food Babe Way

I suffer from rheumatoid arthritis and osteoporosis, although I stay active. One Saturday, I went for a bike ride. The next day, I woke up with a very swollen, angry, hot knee. I whipped up Hari Shake (see the recipe on page 292) and began drinking it periodically over a two-day period. Guess what? The swelling subsided, and the pain is minimal. I am amazed!

—Wanda

Drink green juice on an empty stomach. Recently, a blogger friend of mine tried juicing for the first time, and after finishing her first juice, she complained that it gave her heartburn. I asked her if she drank her juice on an empty stomach, and she said, "No, I had it after breakfast."

Fresh juice should be consumed only on an empty stomach. The benefit of drinking juice is diminished if you don't, and it can end up giving you digestive issues like what my friend experienced. Drinking juice on an empty stomach allows the vitamins and minerals in the juice to go straight to your bloodstream. Having fiber or a meal already in your stomach prevents your body from quickly absorbing the nutrients from the juice. A good rule of thumb is to wait at least two hours after a meal to drink a green juice and to wait twenty minutes after drinking a green juice to consume a meal.

Drink your green juice right away. As soon as fresh green juice is exposed to air, its live enzymes begin to degrade, decreasing the nutritional content. There's a difference in how I feel after drinking fresh juice versus an older juice. The live enzymes of a fresh juice give me immediate energy, whereas older juice just doesn't give me the same kick. For this reason, unless you have a slow masticating juicer, twin-gear, or Norwalk press juicer, I recommend that you always drink your juice fresh, within fifteen minutes of making it. This is especially important if you make your juice without a juicer, using just a blender and strainer. For juice made in a slow or twin-gear juicer, store it in an airtight container (filled to the top with no air gap) for up to thirty-six hours; with a press juicer, you can store it up to seventy-two hours. If you decide to store your juice, remember to keep it refrigerated until you drink it. This is also important to keep in mind when you buy premade, raw, unpasteurized juice because as soon as the juice becomes warm, harmful bacteria can begin to grow. Always keep your juice in a cooler if you're traveling. If you notice that your favorite juice bar keeps juices longer than seventy-two hours, make sure they are using high-pressure pasteurization technology (as Suja juices and BluePrintCleanse do). Otherwise, they are selling you lower-quality and nutritionally degraded juice.

Limit sweet fruits and vegetables in your green juice. Sweet fruits and vegetables like watermelon, apples, pears, and carrots are nutritious

(Continued)

when consumed whole, but juice too many of them and you're suddenly feeding your body too much sugar and fructose. A high-sugar juice can affect insulin levels pretty dramatically, causing cravings and weight gain. This is why I recommend limiting the sugary fruits and vegetables in your green juice to a maximum of one piece per serving. Adding one green apple, or a lemon or lime, for example, is a great option for sweetness and does not spike insulin levels the way other fruits do. (One note: If you're trying to get your children to switch over to green juice, you can start by adding two fruits per serving and then slowly decrease this over time as they become accustomed to the taste.)

Try different greens. Rotate the types of greens you use in your juice each week to prevent the buildup of oxalic acid (which can affect the thyroid gland) and provide a balance of vitamins and minerals for your body. For a real jolt of nutrition, juice frequently with the following greens, rated by Whole Foods as the top ten most nutrient-dense green vegetables:

1. Mustard/turnip/collard greens
2. Kale
3. Watercress
4. Bok choy/baby bok choy
5. Spinach
6. Broccoli rabe
7. Chinese/Napa cabbage
8. Brussels sprouts
9. Swiss chard
10. Arugula

Enjoy juice as a snack, not a meal. Juice isn't a meal replacement—it's a meal enhancer or snack. Since fresh juice is nature's vitamin pill, you'll want to consume it like a supplement: within twenty minutes before a complete meal. Additionally, drinking juice before a meal reduces carb and sweet cravings and changes your taste buds so that you'll begin to desire plant-based foods versus heavy or processed foods.

Clean your juicer thoroughly. Life is busy, and it's easy to procrastinate when it comes to cleaning your juicer. But I can tell you from personal experience that cleaning your juicer (at least rinsing it off) will save you and your knuckles a lot of scrubbing later. If I know time is going to be tight, I'll often throw all the parts of the juicer in the sink and let them soak with water and a little dish soap. That way, when I get around to cleaning the juicer later, it will be much easier. I also save time in the morning by washing the vegetables the night before, which eliminates this step the next day and allows me more time to clean the juicer right after using it. I've got my juicing routine down to twenty minutes when using a two-step press juicer, which is time well spent. And when I use a centrifuge or another type of juicer, my timing is usually around fifteen minutes from start to cleanup.

Recommended Juicers

Juicer	Type	Cost
Slow Juicer (Breville, Hurom, or Omega)	A masticating juicer that grinds the vegetables against a filter, rather than working as a centrifuge (this is one of my favorites).	Up to $400
Green Star Juicer	A masticating juicer.	Up to $500
Norwalk Juicer	A juicer with a *vortex triturating head* for complete cutting and grinding and a *hydraulic press* that extracts the nutrients from the pulp provided by the *triturator*.	Up to $2,500
Breville Juicer	A stainless steel centrifuge juicer that spins vegetables until they separate into juice and pulp.	Up to $300
Jack LaLanne Juicer	A centrifuge juicer. It's lower in price than most centrifuge juicers because it is made of white plastic. It may stain easily and be harder to clean.	Up to $150

WHAT ABOUT STORE-BOUGHT JUICES?

There's nothing like making fresh raw vegetable or fruit juice at home with your own juicer. But juicing takes time, energy, and a commitment to the routine. The availability and variety of store-bought juice concoctions have soared in recent years. This exploding market tempts us with its convenience, unreliable marketing, and pseudohealthy buzzwords. Here's the scoop on how to understand juice labels at the grocery store and choose the best store-bought juices for you and your family.

"100% juice" doesn't mean anything: Food companies are allowed

to say "100% juice" on the label even when their juice contains additives, flavorings, or preservatives.

"Concentrate" is just a fancy name for syrup: Juice concentrates are made from fruits and vegetables that are heated down to syrup and then have water added back in. The concentration process involves both the addition and subtraction of chemicals and natural plant by-products in order to condense the juice. During concentration, fruits and vegetables lose flavor. This is why companies then have to put "flavoring" back in to give the juice a fresh taste.

"Not from concentrate" could mean flavored: According to the book *Squeezed: What You Don't Know about Orange Juice,* by Alissa Hamilton, companies store orange juice in giant tanks and extract the oxygen from them. This preserves the liquid and prevents it from spoiling for up to a year. However, this storage system causes the orange juice to lose all of its flavor. So the industry uses "flavor packs" to reflavor the juice.

GMOs: Many juice companies use citric acid to extend the shelf life of their product. You would think citric acid comes from citrus, like lemons, oranges, and limes, but it doesn't. Most food manufacturers use genetically engineered corn and sugar beets to create citric acid, by synthetically fermenting the glucose from these crops in a laboratory. And some juice companies go as far as adding sugar (which could be from GMO sugar beets), high-fructose corn syrup (from GMO corn), and other ingredients that could contain GMOs.

Synthetic ingredients: The sneakiest ingredients lurking in juice come in the form of synthetics made in a laboratory. These include Fibersol-2 (a proprietary synthetic digestion-resistant fiber), fructooligosaccharides (synthetic fibers and sweeteners), and inulin (an artificial and invisible fiber that's added to foods to increase fiber content). Avoid synthetic ingredients in your diet, because they're usually made from petroleum, coal, and GMOs, none of which provide any nutrients.

Pasteurization: This process kills raw enzymes, minerals, and vitamins, which means it kills off our reasons for drinking juice in the first place. Heat kills the bad stuff and the good stuff, making the juice pretty much worthless. Juice companies sometimes even replenish the lost vitamin content with synthetic vitamins because there is barely any nutrition left after processing. Furthermore, most companies create vitamins through chemical manipulation and synthesis, not from actual fruits and vegetables.

CHOOSE THE BEST STORE-BOUGHT JUICE

Now that I've exposed commercial juices, you must be wondering if there are any store-bought juices that are nutritious. I created the following chart to help you navigate the juice aisles more confidently and choose the best store-bought juice. Thankfully, there are lots of good options!

How to Choose the Best Store-Bought Juice

Best: Fresh Raw Organic		
Suja juice	Organic Avenue	TurmericALIVE
Suja Elements	Luna's Living Kitchen	Blue Print
Juice Press	Viva Raw	Evolution Fresh (some)

Better: 100% Organic, Not from Concentrate		
Uncle Matt's Organic	Lakewood	Odwalla (some)
365 Everyday Value	Bolthouse Farms	Trader Joe's (some)

Questionable: Organic, but from Concentrate or with Additives	
Santa Cruz Organic	Purity
Honest Kids	

Worst: Nonorganic, Pasteurized		
V8	Simply Orange	Mott's
Naked Juice	Tropicana	Del Monte
Zico	Ocean Spray	Welch's
POM Wonderful	Minute Maid	

CHECKLIST

Today:

    ✓ I did my morning lemon water ritual.

    ✓ I enjoyed a green drink.

Day 3 — Stop Drinking with Your Meals

LET'S DO A QUICK checkup: Do you have any of these symptoms?

- ✓ Indigestion
- ✓ Heartburn
- ✓ Irritability
- ✓ Bloating
- ✓ Fatigue
- ✓ Headaches
- ✓ Food cravings
- ✓ Difficulty losing weight
- ✓ Depression

If you checked one or more of these, you might have one bad habit that is contributing to these symptoms. You won't believe the likely culprit: the habit of drinking fluids with your meals. Never mind the fact that everybody does this; unfortunately, it runs roughshod over digestion and triggers nasty symptoms like these.

For most of my life, I'd wake up, have breakfast, and then immediately feel bloated, uncomfortable, and sick to my stomach. Some mornings, I didn't feel well enough to go to school—I didn't even want to go out the door. In the summers, I couldn't even put on my bathing suit or zip up my jeans. I would feel sluggish all day long. I took all the standard advice, such as drinking lots of water, eating plenty of fiber, and sipping ginger ale, but nothing worked. I think I knew, subconsciously, that something was going on.

While still working as a management consultant, I began to delve into Ayurvedic medicine. Originating in India, Ayurveda is an ancient healing system based on lifestyle and diet. Adherents to Ayurveda practice meditation and yoga, use herbs to treat illness, and follow a diet customized to their constitution.

While studying Ayurvedic practices, I took my first trip to India. Other than the splendor of the scenery, I observed something fascinating about the culture: In restaurants, water was rarely served with meals, and when it was, the water was at room temperature. If you asked for ice, you'd be lucky to get a single cube. Usually, the only liquid you'd have with meals would be warm ginger tea, to enhance digestion.

This habit is so unlike the experience we have at American restaurants, where we swallow our food and slam back ice water, several soda refills, and maybe some beers.

After that trip, I got into the habit of not drinking fluids with my meals, with the occasional exception of warm ginger tea. I paid attention to the food I was eating. I slowed down my eating and thoroughly chewed my food. Overall, I began to eat more mindfully. And when I did, I started feeling full faster; I was no longer overeating. I began to feel the energy from my food go to work in my body.

In one short week, my stomach symptoms eased. The bloating and feelings of heaviness disappeared, and there was no more bubble gut. My food gave me so much more satisfaction, and I suddenly had more energy.

During late-night work sessions or when we were out of town and eating at restaurants, my coworkers noticed my new habit. "What are you doing?" they asked. "Without water to wash it down, won't you choke on your food?"

At the same time, they noticed my newfound energy and alertness. I made believers out of people. Though this habit might sound crazy, it is key to healthy digestion, satiety, and overall vibrant health.

Stop This Sticky Habit Today

A lot of people think chewing gum aids digestion. It does not; chewing food does. The process of digestion begins in the mouth, where saliva starts breaking down food. If you chew gum, you tax your saliva glands and digestive enzymes, and you won't have enough enzymes to properly digest real food as you age.

(Continued)

Chewing gum can also make you feel bloated. When you chew gum, you swallow excess air, leading to abdominal pain and bloating. What's more, chewing gum sends your body physical signals that you're about to eat food. In response, your body releases enzymes and acids, but without the food they're supposed to digest. The net effect is more bloating and an overproduction of stomach acid.

Gum is also made with synthetic rubbers and contains additives such as texture modifiers, plasticizers, softeners, fillers, and emulsifiers to give specific properties to the gum. Many popular brands contain artificial sugars linked to cancer, artificial food dyes made from petroleum, and preservatives banned in other countries. If you're chewing gum, you're chewing chemicals you shouldn't be putting in your mouth.

Stop this sticky habit and you'll look and feel better right away.

Check out the worst offending brands on foodbabe.com.

GUT FEELINGS

Drinking liquids with your meals interferes with the production of spit, or saliva, the substance you swish around in your mouth. Saliva is your friend. It helps break down food in the mouth. It helps us swallow food. It protects tooth enamel.

The salivary glands in your mouth churn out saliva to the tune of about four cups a day. Over your lifetime, these glands will produce 10,000 gallons of saliva, enough to fill a backyard swimming pool. As long as you chew your foods thoroughly, you'll create saliva, which lets you eat comfortably without lots of liquids. Let your saliva naturally help you swallow your food.

Drinking fluids with meals also dilutes digestive enzymes (which diminish with age) and stomach acids, making digestion incomplete, and that will delay your poop train. As a consequence, you'll have trouble losing weight, getting rid of toxins, and feeling like a happy, energetic person. With bad digestion, toxins can build up in your digestive organs. This can inhibit the body's ability to break down fat. It also causes insatiable cravings and interferes with your body's ability to register hunger or fullness.

You don't want to mess with these enzymes, acids, and saliva, so avoid drinking fluids with your meals. Start this habit today.

POP QUIZ: WHAT IS THE HEALTHIEST-SOUNDING BUT *WORST* LIQUID TO DRINK WITH MEALS?

Answer: cold water. (Cold soda is just as bad!)

After several studies were published a few years ago demonstrating that consuming cold water increases your metabolism, you could literally hear the ice plopping into glasses across the country. People thought: "Wow, if I just drink cold water all day, I can lose weight!" Well, this bit of wisdom is a double-edged sword. True, drinking cold water does speed up your metabolism (about four extra calories for every eight ounces of water). It does so by using energy to heat up the cold water to body temperature.

But here's the problem: If you drink cold water with your meal, energy required for digestion is diverted. That's not good. While eating, you want all of your energy directed at breaking down food so your body can easily assimilate the nutrients and eliminate waste and toxins.

Be careful at restaurants. The wait staff is trained to bring huge glasses of ice-cold water to your table. I see people at restaurants getting refill after refill of cold liquids while gulping down huge amounts of inadequately chewed foods. These are very bad habits, and your digestion will hate you for it.

THE FOOD BABE WAY

When should you drink fluids? Here are my recommendations:

DRINK WATER OR OTHER LIQUIDS TWENTY MINUTES BEFORE MEALS

That way, the beverage won't interfere with digestion—and you'll knock off pounds. This advice seems unconventional, given our current habits as a society; but try it, and you'll see that it actually works.

According to one study, people who drank two glasses of water before eating their meals lost about fifteen pounds over a three-month period, compared to the eleven pounds lost by a non-water-drinking group following the same low-calorie diet. Why the difference? Researchers suggested that water reduced the dieters' calorie intake either by swelling their stomachs and making them feel more full, or by making it less likely that they would revert to drinking sugary drinks with their meals.

DRINK FLUIDS AFTER A MEAL

The next-best time to drink fluids is after your meal, but you should wait at least thirty minutes and up to an hour. This allows your food to be adequately digested without complicating matters for your tummy and intestines.

Don't overthink this habit. Just slowly go from drinking with meals to drinking between meals. Mindful drinking (and eating) will have a positive impact on the way you feel.

IF YOU MUST DRINK WITH YOUR MEALS, SIP ON A WARM BEVERAGE

Good options include herbal tea or warm water with lemon. Because the temperature is closer to your body's normal heat, warm water will ease digestion rather than disrupt it. Ginger is my favorite type of tea to drink with or after meals because it naturally and gently moves food from the upper part of the digestive tract into the lower. The wait staffs at my favorite restaurants know to bring me a cup of ginger tea right after I'm seated — no ice water.

At home I just cut up a few pieces of fresh gingerroot and pour hot water over them. On the go, I always carry ginger tea bags with me. Yogi tea, Numi, and Traditional Medicinals are my favorite digestive teas.

BE CAREFUL ABOUT STEEPING PESTICIDES

Tea is something I drink every single day. It's sacred at my house, and I have a whole drawer devoted to it. I drink it because it is amazing for

your health. There are so many varieties of tea that can improve digestion and metabolism and even prevent certain diseases.

But what I'm about to share with you rocked my world when I first
heard it, and I've never been able to look at tea in the same way again.

Did you know that most tea is not washed before it is put into bags?
That means if the tea was sprayed with cancer-causing pesticides, those
pesticides go right into your cup.

Many popular tea brands get away with using the ingredient "natural flavors" to make us think we're buying better, cleaner ingredients;
however, companies are just covering up the inferior taste and low quality of their tea. Fortunately, there are brands that are putting the kibosh
on the use of "natural flavors" and are instead using only real ingredients. I was happy to learn that Ahmed Rahim, CEO of Numi Tea, is
just as disgusted by this ingredient as I am. He told me, "You can break
down anything that is found in nature and if it ends up tasting like the
flavor you wish to use, you can add it to any product and call it 'natural
flavor' on the ingredient label. It could come from a stone in the ground
and you'd never know." This is why I put a product down and run far, far
away when I see the words "natural flavor" listed on a label. I want to
know what I am eating! Don't you?

WATCH THAT TEA BAG

A recent article in *The Atlantic* discussed the "silky sachet" and "luxuri-
ous mesh bags" that hold loose-leaf teas (like in the brand Tea Forté).
Terms like "silky sachets" and "corn-based biodegradable tea bags" mis-
lead customers into believing a product is more natural and sustainable
than it really is. It turns out that these modern-day bags, which are
meant to showcase the tea leaves, are made of plastics such as polylactic
acid (PLA) or polyethylene terephthalate (PET). *The Atlantic* pointed
out that researchers have found that PET leaches estrogen-mimicking
pollutants into water. Although the actual tea bag is not an ingredient
like teas and herbs, it is still an element you put into boiling water and
may leave traces of harmful ingredients in the tea you drink.

The bottom line: Avoid drinking liquids with your meals, and time your fluid intake so that it works with your digestion, not against it. Stick to approved teas rich in truly natural ingredients, and drink plenty of clean water (at the appropriate times) to help your body flush toxins.

CHECKLIST

Today:
- ✓ I did my morning lemon water ritual.
- ✓ I enjoyed a green drink.
- ✓ I stopped drinking fluids with my meals.

Day 4 — Be Aware of What's in Your Water

SPEAKING OF WATER AND fluids: It's great if you're in the habit of drinking the recommended eight glasses of water a day, but the important question is whether or not you are drinking "clean" water.

Many of the doctors and scientists I've had the chance to speak with about what's happening to our food supply say that what's happening to our water as a result could be even more disastrous. Our tap water is laced with toxins, including pesticide runoff, pharmaceutical residues, and hormone impersonators.

In 2010, the Environmental Working Group, a nonpartisan, nonprofit organization, reported that tap water from forty-five states contained more than 300 contaminants! You'll be shocked at what some of those contaminants were: radon, a radioactive gas; Freon, a refrigerant pumped into air conditioners; the weed killer metolachlor; and acetone, the liquid used to remove nail polish.

The Environmental Protection Agency even admits that there's so much perchlorate in drinking water that it needs to be more tightly regulated. Perchlorate is an ingredient in rocket fuel. Yes, rocket fuel. We're all looking for that extra pick-me-up in the morning, but personally I would rather stick to my green smoothie. (For other toxins in drinking water, see the chart on page 108.)

> ### FOOD BABE ALERT:
> ### FUROR OVER FLUORIDE
>
> Every time you have a sip of water from the tap, cook a meal with tap water, or take a bath or shower, you're exposing yourself to fluoride. It has been added to our drinking water for decades, put there to ward off tooth cavities from childhood on. But fluoride is essentially a toxic waste product fed to us through our taps.
>
> *(Continued)*

The fluoride in our drinking water can be a stealth source of arsenic contamination. Arsenic is a powerful carcinogen that promotes the risk of several types of cancer, and it gets into the water supply by way of fluoride. The most common form of fluoride is hexafluorosilicic acid, which is the type frequently contaminated with arsenic.

There's mounting evidence that fluoride itself poses grave health risks to infants and children—including reductions in IQ. Further, arsenic exposure may cause lasting damage to the developing brains and endocrine and immune systems of fetuses, toddlers, and infants.

Amazingly, the debate over the dangers of fluoride has raged on for more than sixty years. Yet study after study confirms that fluoride is a dangerous poison that accumulates in your body, and that ultimately it isn't even very effective at preventing dental decay.

Are you starting to get the picture? I, for one, am glad the government is watchdogging our water supply, but we can't rely on others to protect our health. We've got to take control of it ourselves.

THE FOOD BABE WAY

Stop drinking water straight out of your tap. Tap water is poisoned with a variety of toxins (again, I refer you to the chart). Some recommendations to help you:

FILTER YOUR WATER

The easiest way to ensure you are getting safe water without contaminants is to filter your tap water directly under your kitchen sink. Simple carbon filters that mount on your faucets or come in a pitcher can reduce contaminants, while more costly reverse osmosis filters can filter out fluoride, arsenic, and chromium. These will not, however, filter out perchlorate and nitrates.

Personally, I recommend getting at least a two-stage water filter. It takes a plumber or a crafty helper a short time to install one, but it is totally worth it. You can learn more about water filters from the Environmental Working Group at www.ewg.org/report/ewgs-water-filter-buying-guide.

CHANGE YOUR WATER BOTTLE

When you go out, drink water out of reusable stainless steel or glass water bottles. Fill them at home and take them with you when you're on the go. My favorite water bottles are:

Klean Kanteen (www.kleankanteen.com)
Thinksport (www.gothinksport.com)
bkr (www.mybkr.com)
Life Factory (www.lifefactory.com)

FILTER YOUR SHOWER WATER

Harmful chemicals can enter your body through opened skin pores while you're showering, which is why I have a water filter on my shower head, too. At first, I wasn't sure whether filtering my shower water was worth it, until an experience at my hairdresser's salon settled the question.

I've been going to the same hairdresser, Megan, for more than ten years. She knows my hair, inside and out. A few years ago, I had taken a six-month hiatus from getting my hair cut, because I wanted to grow it a little longer. After the six months were over, I went in to see her. She began to comb her fingers through my hair to see what needed to be done.

"What are you doing to your hair?" she asked.

I was a little alarmed. "What's wrong?"

"Nothing! It is so much thicker. It feels like a whole new head of hair!"

At first, I couldn't pinpoint exactly what had changed. I was still eating a nutritious, additive-free diet and living a healthy lifestyle.

Then I put two and two together. A water filter company had contacted me, asking me to try out a shower filter. Given that your body is over 60 percent water, that your skin is your largest organ, and that you expose yourself to nearly twenty-five gallons of water on average when you shower, bathing with clean water is crucial for a healthy body.

After receiving the shower filter, I opened the box and immediately thought, "Is the filter going to affect the water pressure? Do I really want to install this? What am I doing?" All I could think about was the fact that my hair was going to take longer to shampoo and condition.

After my husband installed it (it took about two minutes), I turned on the faucet, and much to my surprise, the water pressure was so good that I didn't miss my old shower head at all.

After showering in filtered water for several months, I could see noticeable differences in my hair and skin. There were barely any stray hairs left in the drain. Very little hair fell out when I blow-dried my hair (my bathroom floor used to be covered!). My hair had luster and was never dry. I needed to use less shampoo and conditioner. After I got out of the shower at home, I needed fewer oils and moisturizers on my skin. None of these results constitute a scientific study, but they made a miraculous change for me personally. And the real magic was happening in ways I couldn't even see — namely, the reduction of the daily toxins I was being exposed to, which could accumulate and cause disease and aging in my body over time.

Unfiltered shower water contains potentially hazardous chemicals, of which chlorine is the most common. It can cause dry skin and hair, itchiness, and eye irritation. It is also linked to cancer, asthma, and allergies.

I'm a believer in shower filters and will continue to use one. This lesson taught me that what I put on my skin is just as important as what I put in my body.

SAY NO TO BOTTLED WATER — AS MUCH AS POSSIBLE!

Break the bottled water habit. First of all, many bottled waters are just tap water in disguise. But second, plastic water bottles may contain BPA (bisphenol A) and other obesogens that increase the size of fat cells. These chemicals leach from the bottle into the water. I always carry a stainless steel or glass container of water around with me — to the gym, in the car, to meetings, and even to some restaurants! Once you start drinking your delicious filtered water at home, you'll never want to drink anything else. You will start to taste the chlorine and other impurities from other water sources. But this is a good reminder to always carry your water with you. The only time I get bottled water is when I'm in a foreign country or traveling somewhere where I don't have access to filtered water in a glass bottle. If I can hit a Whole Foods while I'm traveling, I'll always buy Mountain Valley Spring Water from Hot Springs, Arkansas, which is sold in a big green glass bottle. Sometimes I'll have a case of it delivered to my hotel so that I have it on a long business trip. It makes a major difference in the way I feel.

STOP REHYDRATING WITH SPORTS DRINKS

Sports drinks are little more than sugar-laden soft drinks packed with a cocktail of additives, preservatives, tooth-eroding acids, and colorings. Some used to contain brominated vegetable oil, or BVO—which is banned in many countries because it is a fire retardant. BVO can cause headaches and exhaustion, and can take a serious toxic toll on your body.

Fortunately, Coca-Cola announced in 2014 that it would drop this controversial ingredient from its Powerade sports drink, after a similar move made by PepsiCo's Gatorade in 2013. These positive actions were taken after a Mississippi teenager, Sarah Kavanagh, targeted both products in Change.org petitions. Her Powerade petition had more than 59,000 online supporters, while the Gatorade petition had more than 200,000.

It's ironic, but if a sports drink is very sugary (more than 8 percent added sugar—as most are), the beverage will dehydrate you. These sugary beverages draw water out of cells and dump it into the stomach to dilute the drink before digestion.

You can find a lot of research validating the benefits of sports drinks, but that could be because much of this research is funded by sports drink entities, such as the Gatorade Sports Science Institute. The marketing hype around sports drinks makes them sound attractive, but they provide virtually no benefits when compared to plain, pure water for the average person.

For moderate workouts under an hour, water is all you need for rehydration. Instead of filling up on sports drinks, a healthful postworkout snack such as a banana is a better choice to replenish minerals and nutrients lost in sweat. One of my favorite rehydrators is coconut water. But you have to be careful and read labels because a lot of coconut waters on the market contain added sugar or added flavorings. My advice is to purchase coconut water produced by Harmless Harvest. Its product is not made from concentrate, and it is not heated, so it retains nutrients; it also does not contain added flavors or sugars.

Another effective rehydrator is green juice that includes celery juice. The celery juice replaces lost electrolytes, rehydrates the body with its rich minerals, and is a much better alternative to the synthetic ingredients in most sports drinks.

STAY INFORMED

Get in touch with your local water company. Legally, they must issue an annual report that lists all the contaminants found in your water supply, disclose the quality of your water, and reveal the source of your local water. They can mail you a copy, or you should be able to find it online at www.epa.gov/safewater/ccr/whereyoulive.html.

Having access to clean and unpolluted water is vital to your health. You can eat the best organic food on the planet, but if you're drinking water that is full of toxins, that effort could be compromised. Water needs to be clean and free of toxins and harmful microbes to keep you at your best.

Contaminants in Tap Water	
Toxins	Potential Adverse Health Effects
Aluminum	May cause cognitive decline in the elderly.
Arsenic	May contribute to cancer, organ failure, reproductive problems, and other diseases.
Chlorine	May increase cancer risk.
Chromium	Causes allergic dermatitis (skin reactions) and may increase cancer risk.
Fluoride	In excessive amounts, may cause bone fractures in adults and developmental problems in children; may increase cancer risk.

Gas, oil	May damage kidneys, liver, or other organs.
Lead	Can cause learning, neurological, and behavioral problems in children.
Microbes (bacteria and viruses)	Linked to upset stomach, diarrhea, and more serious illnesses.
Nitrates	Associated with birth defects and miscarriages.
Perchlorate	Can decrease production of thyroid hormones, which are important for normal metabolism and good mental function.
Pesticides	May damage kidneys, liver, or other organs.
Prescription drugs	May increase cancer risk, cause organ damage, and promote the development of antibiotic-resistant bacteria.

CHECKLIST

Today:

✓ I did my morning lemon water ritual.

✓ I enjoyed a green drink.

✓ I stopped drinking fluids with my meals.

✓ I drank, and bathed in, pure, clean, filtered water.

Day 5 — Ease Back on
Dairy Foods

Many popular diets demonize dairy foods and insist that you cut them out altogether, forever.

I disagree. I don't think you have to give up dairy to live a healthy lifestyle. But I do believe that we need to eat less of it. The reason? Most dairy foods are laced with hormones and chemicals.

EAT LESS DAIRY, ENJOY IT MORE

I didn't need to search far to learn how to include dairy nutritiously in my diet; I just listened to the stories of my parents. For thousands of years, my ancestors in India had one cow that they shared with the rest of the villagers. Traditionally in India, the cow is allowed to give its milk to its calf first, and what remains is used for human consumption. This leaves a very small amount to use throughout the week for cooking (and it's not in gallon-size containers that can stay fresh for weeks).

From that single cow, my ancestors made yogurt, cheeses, and other dairy products, but they used those foods as condiments for their meals, eating very little.

They did eat a small amount of dairy every day, however. And they were able to do this without negative health consequences because the milk they received from the cow was pure, raw milk. It was not poisoned with pesticides, chemicals from genetically modified crops, antibiotics, growth hormones, or toxins from feedlots, where livestock is fed before slaughter. The milk was unpasteurized and completely free of chemical processing, making it a healthy nutritional addition to a strict vegetarian diet.

ADULTERATED DAIRY

By contrast, on typical farms in the United States, calves are slaughtered shortly after birth for their meat; this creates a great deal of pain and suffering for the mama cow, causing her to secrete massive amounts of stress toxins that are released into her milk. These toxins are then passed down to us, along with all the other unknown antibiotics, growth hormones, and chemicals the industry uses to produce the milk. This didn't happen in India where my parents are from because the cow is sacred and the majority of Indians don't eat beef.

Milk is pasteurized to control bacterial growth. Pasteurization, however, destroys many vitamins found in raw milk. A 2011 study published in the *Journal of Food Protection* reported that pasteurization decreases vitamin E, and several B vitamins, including B1, B2, B12, and folate. The heat also destroys enzymes your body needs for proper digestion. One of these is phosphatase. Without this enzyme, the calcium lingers in your bloodstream and can accumulate in your arteries. As a result, your arteries get stiff and it's more difficult for them to pump blood. Stiff arteries give rise to hypertension (high blood pressure), chest pain, and heart failure.

Calcium can also build up in plaque, the cholesterol-filled pouches lining the interior of arteries. This process constricts the arteries and potentially chokes off blood supply to the heart and other vital organs. Should a plaque rupture, you'd be at risk of a heart attack or stroke.

The pasteurization process is why America is still one of the top nations suffering from bone-related illnesses—even though we are one of the top three dairy consumers in the world—and why our rates of heart disease continue to rise.

Drinking cow's milk may also contribute to various types of cancers. This is because cow's milk is pumped full of synthetic hormones that end up in your glass. Consider some evidence:

- **Prostate cancer.** Researchers writing in 2012 in *Nutrition & Metabolism* noted that prostate cancer is "the most common dairy-promoted cancer in men of Western societies."

- **Breast cancer.** Researchers writing in a 1997 issue of *Medical Hypotheses* noted: "Dairy products contain both hormones and growth factors, in addition to fat and various chemical contaminants, that have been implicated in the proliferation of human breast cancer cells."
- **Other cancers.** Calves are routinely injected with a hormone called IGF-1, the protein I mentioned earlier that in excess levels can promote aging and tumor development. It is used to spur fast growth in the animals. From a 2011 study in the *Proceedings of the Nutrition Society*, researchers point out that "even within well-nourished western populations, men and women with relatively high intakes of protein from dairy products have higher blood levels of IGF-1. These observations have led to the hypothesis that high intakes of protein from dairy products may increase the risk for some cancers by increasing the endogenous production of IGF-1." IGF-1 is resistant to pasteurization.

The Indian customs illustrate how we should use dairy today: Eat it in limited quantities and use it as a condiment. That's what I do.

THE FOOD BABE WAY

You don't have to give up milk and dairy products for the rest of your life. Simply dial down your dairy consumption. The Food Babe Way is not about deprivation or denial. I can't imagine never eating ice cream again, or sour cream on top of a taco, or cheese on pizza.

Fortunately, if you're a milk and dairy lover, you have more options than ever — options that will help you develop today's habit for life.

CONSIDER RAW MILK

Most of my family immigrated to the United States from India, where they had access to raw milk. In raw milk, all the natural minerals are intact and easily absorbed by the body. Raw milk also contains several types of naturally occurring probiotics that help populate your digestive system with beneficial bacteria. Of course, you must refrigerate it and use it before it spoils. Raw milk keeps seven to ten days in the fridge.

Unfortunately, buying raw milk is illegal in the following states: Delaware, Iowa, Louisiana, Maryland, Montana, New Jersey, Nevada, and West Virginia. It is legal only for pet food in Florida, Georgia, and North Carolina. Raw milk laws vary from state to state. In many states, you can buy raw milk only from a farmer. A good source for information on where you can buy raw milk is www.farmtoconsumer.org.

It is unfortunate that the government can impose bans that override our rights as consumers to decide what we want to eat and drink, especially when they cut out something that is healthier than the alternative.

It saddens me that my relatives in certain states can't get raw milk, with all its nutrition, the way they could in their childhood. Indian immigrants and other immigrants from raw-milk-producing countries are being duped by the US dairy industry and don't even know it. I'd really like to see my family recipes passed down from generation to generation, but I am not sure we can do this safely for our future children and grandchildren unless we can all get access to real raw milk.

INTRODUCE GOAT CHEESE INTO YOUR DIET

I love goat cheese and like to use it in salads, spreads, and any recipe that calls for regular cheese. From a health standpoint, using goat cheese makes sense. Because goat's milk contains smaller fat molecules than cow's milk, it's easier to digest and absorb. Therefore, many people who have trouble eating other dairy products can more easily tolerate and enjoy goat cheese.

Goat cheese contains only 80 calories and 6 grams of fat per ounce. Compare this to cow's milk cheese, at 110 calories and 10 grams of fat per ounce. Goat cheese is lower in cholesterol, too, and it's full of essential nutrients such as vitamin A, vitamin K, phosphorus, and various B vitamins.

FALL IN LOVE WITH NONDAIRY MILKS

The popular alternatives these days are milk substitutes such as almond, coconut, and hempseed milks. They're low in calories and fat. They're hormone- and lactose-free and thus better for health and digestion.

MAKE YOUR OWN NONDAIRY MILK

My favorite solution for milk lovers is to make your own nondairy milk. In most cases, it's just a matter of soaking raw, unsalted nuts or seeds in water, then blending and straining the mixture through a cheesecloth. Take almond milk, for example. Simply soak raw almonds in water at a 1:4 ratio overnight. Then blend and strain. It's that easy. Even easier is my Homemade Organic Cashew Milk (see page 295 in the recipes chapter, Chapter 8). You don't have to strain the nuts from the pulp, and the result is a rich, creamy milk that's slightly sweet on its own.

Here are some guidelines on making milks from other nuts and seeds:

Nuts	Soaking Time
Almonds	8 to 12 hours
Brazil nuts	Not necessary
Cashews	2 to 3 hours
Hazelnuts	12 hours
Macadamias	Not necessary
Pecans	4 to 6 hours
Pistachios	Not necessary
Walnuts	4 hours
Seeds	Soaking Time
Flax	8 hours
Hemp	Not necessary
Sesame	8 hours
Sunflower	2 hours

I recommend some store-bought alternatives—but with some reservations. Not long ago, I learned from the Cornucopia Institute, a public information group that backs locally produced and organic food, that many nondairy milks, even if certified as organic, contain carrageenan, an additive derived from red algae. Carrageenan is not something you want to put in your body on a regular basis, as a collection of scientific studies links it with immunity problems, gastrointestinal inflammation, and cancer.

I felt tricked after hearing this. I assumed that once a product was certified organic, it was perfectly safe to drink. I suggest that you check the ingredients on any box or carton of nondairy milks to ensure that it is carrageenan-free. Also if the nondairy milk is not organic, you can expect some other synthetic ingredients you should probably avoid.

To help you, here are some organic milk substitutes that don't have carrageenan:

- Natural Value organic coconut milk
- So Delicious culinary coconut milk (regular and light versions)
- Native Forest coconut milk
- Thai Kitchen organic coconut milk
- Pacific Hemp Original
- Whole Foods 365 Everyday Value almond milk
- Tree of Life almond milk

CHOOSE ORGANIC DAIRY MILKS

Don't like the taste of almond milk or its nondairy buddies? Here's some good news: British scientists analyzed milk from organically farmed animals and conventionally farmed animals. What they found really opened my eyes: The organic milk had 67 percent more antioxidants and vitamins than conventional milk, as well as 60 percent more conjugated linoleic acid, or CLA, a beneficial fat that may shrink tumors. The reason for these astounding nutritional benefits is simple: Organically raised cows often feed on fresh grass and clover. Also, their milk is produced without antibiotics, synthetic hormones, and harmful pesticides.

Here we come to one of the most processed food products on the planet: frozen yogurt. When a company feeds people chemicals instead of pure food, they make a lot of money. And frozen yogurt makers are raking in the dough.

Even when frozen yogurt restaurants market their products with buzzwords like "natural" and "healthy," these places are often still serving heavily processed dairy products with harmful additives that could affect your health. My previously favorite frozen yogurt establishment has a slogan on the wall in their stores that says "I'm homemade, organic, and delicious." That sign should state: "I'm homemade in a factory with artificial trans fat, GMOs, and petroleum-ridden blue food coloring!" This is what I found when I researched what was in my favorite flavor of frozen yogurt. I'd been eating this stuff every time I passed it at the mall, completely misled about what I was actually putting in my body.

Depending on the product, frozen yogurt might contain processed sugars, sugar alcohols, emulsifiers, stabilizers, carrageenan, natural and artificial flavors, dyes and colorings (many of which are potential carcinogens), artificial sweeteners, growth hormones and antibiotics, and genetically engineered corn syrup.

What's a frozen yogurt lover like me to do? The answer is to buy good organic vanilla frozen yogurt from the freezer section of a natural food store. Top it with a few organic chocolate chips, and it will taste just like one of those high-calorie chocolate chip cookie ice cream sandwiches you can get at the gas station. To go even healthier, you can purchase plain frozen yogurt with no added flavorings and add a nonsugary item like chopped nuts. Be cautious about which toppings you decide to add, and remember to keep your portion size under control when you order frozen yogurt, and especially when you serve yourself at dispensers.

A popular Indian proverb reminds us, "A harvest of peace grows from seeds of contentment." Likewise, I think if we can be content with eating less dairy, we'll be pleasantly surprised to find ourselves growing healthier and more peaceful as a result of following today's habit.

CHECKLIST

Today:

✓ I did my morning lemon water ritual.

✓ I enjoyed a green drink.

✓ I stopped drinking fluids with my meals.

✓ I drank, and bathed in, pure, clean, filtered water.

✓ I ate less dairy and made healthier dairy choices.

Day 6 — No More Big Gulps!

YOU ARE WHAT YOU drink, too. If you're a soda drinker, you're ingesting a lot of bad chemicals that are screwing with your weight, your health, and your life. Read on for the scary details—and how to stop this horrible habit.

SCARY SUGARS

Take a teaspoon of sugar and dump it on your kitchen table. Do this ten times. What do you have?

Yes, you've got a mess, and no, I'm not cleaning it up for you. But you also have the amount of sugar found in one twelve-ounce can of soda.

Obviously, if you're hooked on soda, you're swilling down a huge amount of sugar and calories (around 140 calories in each can). A sugary habit like that is the doorway to poor nutrition, weight gain, type 2 diabetes, and other health complications.

Most soda companies sweeten their beverages with high-fructose corn syrup (HFCS), one of the Sickening 15 I covered in Chapter 2. HFCS is becoming increasingly unpopular these days—so unpopular that Pepsi decided in March 2014 to put sugar in its colas instead of HFCS. To my mind, this is not a solution. For one thing, replacing HFCS with another type of sugar will have little effect on obesity and diabetes. Ultimately, it's like replacing a cigarette with a cigar.

COLOR ME CANCER?

To food companies and their customers, color is everything. It gives a food product glitz, appeal, and the expectation of delicious taste. With more products emerging in different hues, color continues to be one of the most crucial aspects of food. At the same time, it's becoming one of the most controversial, especially in sodas.

Sodas use "caramel coloring" to give them that dark, delicious look. Not to be confused with real caramel, caramel color is the single most used food coloring in the world. It is created by heating ammonia and sulfites under high pressure — a process that produces a cancerous substance called 4-methylimidazole (4-MEI). Although there are no FDA limits on the amount of 4-MEI that can be present in soft drinks, a federal study in 2007 concluded that 4-MEI caused cancer in mice, and in 2011 the International Agency for Research on Cancer determined that the chemical is "possibly carcinogenic" to humans.

If you're a soda drinker, please be aware that your favorite soft drink may contain high levels of 4-MEI. In January 2014, *Consumer Reports* had a long list of soft drinks tested for 4-MEI: Pepsi, Diet Pepsi, Pepsi One, Malta Goya, Sprite, Diet Coke, Coca-Cola, Coke Zero, Dr Pepper, Diet Snap, Brisk Iced Tea, and A&W Root Beer. Under California's Proposition 65 law, any food or beverage that contains more than 29 micrograms of 4-MEI per day must carry a health warning label. *Consumer Reports'* tests showed that each of the twelve-ounce samples of Pepsi One and Malta Goya had more than 29 micrograms per bottle. Neither carries a warning.

Pepsi responded by stating: "We believe their conclusion is factually incorrect and reflects a serious misunderstanding of Proposition 65's requirements." Pepsi also said it was working to reduce 4-MEI levels in its products.

Regular Pepsi, which was obtained in New York State, contained as much as 174 micrograms. A second test showed levels at 32 micrograms. Also purchased in New York, Pepsi One ranged from 39.5 micrograms to 195.3. Malta Goya had the highest levels, averaging from 307.5 micrograms to 352.5 micrograms.

These findings concern me. We are being unnecessarily exposed to a potential carcinogen just because companies want their beverages to look brown. Ask yourself: How small a dose of poison are you willing to consume on a regular basis?

THE BUZZ OVER CAFFEINE

The reason why so many sodas, particularly the low-calorie versions, contain caffeine is that the manufacturers want you to get hooked on them. Caffeine is addicting because it stimulates you, and you keep coming back for the buzz. The sugar in sodas is addicting, too, so you've got a double whammy keeping you on this stuff.

Soda may have as much as 71 milligrams of caffeine per twelve ounces. Caffeine in energy drinks often ranges from 160 milligrams to 500 milligrams a serving. That's way too high. Caffeine forces your adrenal glands to work harder, causing lack of energy and exhaustion in the long term. What happens when you're constantly exhausted? You stop moving and exercising, and you're likely to pack on pounds. Caffeine also depletes the body of vitamin C and leaches minerals like magnesium and calcium from your bones.

To me, the most alarming caffeine-loaded products on the market are those made by Monster Beverage Corporation. Its energy drinks have been referenced in the deaths of several people, according to reports submitted to the FDA. Despite this issue, Monster drinks are still on the market.

Excess doses of caffeine can increase heart rate and drive up blood pressure significantly. For someone who has an underlying heart condition, these side effects can be fatal. In one of these deaths, an autopsy concluded that the victim died of an irregular heart rhythm ("cardiac arrhythmia" due to caffeine toxicity after consuming two twenty-four-ounce energy drinks in twenty-four hours).

GMOs IN SOFT DRINKS

Many soft drinks may be laced with GMOs. That's because corn-based products such as sorbitol, fructose, aspartame, maltodextrin, and citric acid are hidden within these drinks.

The American Academy of Environmental Medicine (AAEM) reported, "There is more than a casual association between GM foods and adverse health effects....The strength of association and consistency between GM foods and disease is confirmed in several animal studies." AAEM also stated that GMOs prevent the body from using insulin properly, and faulty insulin regulation leads to diabetes and obesity. Based on this research, we should definitely follow GMO-free diets for weight and blood sugar control—and that means no soft drinks.

PUSHING PRESERVATIVES

Unbeknownst to the average person, the preservatives in soft drinks can be harmful. For example, sodium benzoate is a preservative found in many soft drinks that when combined with the ascorbic acid (vitamin C) in the drinks produces benzene, a known carcinogen.

Preservatives in sodas, particularly phosphoric acid, also acidify your body. Jameth Sheridan, Doctor of Holistic Medicine, states that it takes thirty-six glasses of water to realkalize your body after drinking just one diet soda. Thirty-six glasses!

I Did It the Food Babe Way

You really saved my life!! I am a single mother of three, who works three jobs and tries to eat "healthy." I drank a couple of pots of coffee, however, and at least one twelve-pack of Diet Coke daily (I was truly a soda addict). I developed severe acid reflux and was in great pain. After reading your website, I quit drinking pop, coffee, and caffeinated tea. I started eating organic foods.

The result: No longer do I have acid reflux. I have more energy than ever. And I just feel like I'm getting healthier from the inside out. You have been such an inspiration.

—Dawne

FOUNTAIN OF CHEMICALS?

When I drank soft drinks as a teenager, I always wondered why fountain drinks tasted better. My friends and I would go on and on about how fountain drinks were the best, and then we'd hit up the local gas station to get our fix. Thank God those days are over. Giving up soda was the first habit I adopted on my journey toward healthy, organic living. Almost immediately after I stopped drinking soda, I began to see changes in my skin. It was no longer dull-looking, dry, and pocked with eczema. Instead, it became glowing and vibrant.

During my investigative work, I found out that fountain drinks have a totally different formula than their bottled or canned counterparts found on store shelves. One of the scary ingredients in fountain drinks is dimethylpolysiloxane. This additive is commonly used in vinegary-smelling silicone caulks, adhesives, and aquarium sealants; as a component in silicone grease and other silicone-based lubricants; and in defoaming agents, mold release agents, damping fluids, heat transfer fluids, polishes, cosmetics, and hair conditioners. It is also the major component in Silly Putty.

The food industry doesn't want you to know about the differences between formulas for fountain drinks and drinks in cans and bottles. How many more lawsuits might they face if people knew that their sodas contained the main ingredient in Silly Putty?

Digging a little deeper, I found out that fountain drinks can be contaminated with dangerous bacteria. In 2010, researchers at Virginia Western Community College in Roanoke analyzed ninety beverages of three types (sugared sodas, diet sodas, and water) from thirty commercial soda fountains for microbial contamination. Coliform bacteria, including E. coli, were detected in nearly half of the beverages. Coliform is found in the poop of all warm-blooded animals and humans. Seventeen percent of the beverages contained other pathogens. Among them: klebsiella, responsible for an often-fatal form of pneumonia; staphylococcus, which can cause food poisoning and other serious infections; and candida, a fungus that may cause fatigue, headache, poor memory, and weight gain. Just thinking about this makes my body hurt!

ARTIFICIAL SWEETENERS MAKE YOU FAT AND SICK

As for diet sodas, don't fool yourself into thinking you've been "good" by drinking this stuff. A January 2012 study reported in the *American Journal of Clinical Nutrition* suggested that a daily diet soda habit (at least one per day) could hurt your circulatory system and increase the possibility of vascular events such as stroke and heart attack.

This was the first study that ever probed a connection between diet sodas and heart health, and researchers aren't clear on why these beverages might be tied to heart attack and stroke. They speculate that it might be because daily diet soda drinkers tend to be heavier and already have heart risk factors such as high blood pressure, diabetes, and unhealthy cholesterol levels.

If you're trying to lose weight, drinking diet sodas is not the solution, either. The artificial sweeteners they contain have been proven to stimulate your appetite, increase carbohydrate cravings, and promote fat storage and weight gain. Researchers from the University of Texas at Houston discovered that drinking diet sodas will expand your waist (translation: bigger belly), which is a risk factor for type 2 diabetes.

When you eat something sweet—even when it has no calories— your brain is tricked into wanting more calories because your body is not getting enough energy (i.e., calories) to be satisfied. So you keep craving sweets, eating sweets, and gaining weight.

Furthermore, there are more dangerous side effects from artificial sweeteners—especially aspartame, which is considered one of the most dangerous substances allowed in our food supply. Since 1980, more than 10,000 complaints have been filed with the FDA about this substance; it was never proven safe before it was approved for use in our food supply. In one study, the researchers found that aspartame raised blood sugar in diabetes-prone mice. Besides diabetes, aspartame is linked to autoimmune disorders, depression (which can also cause you to eat more), birth defects, and several forms of cancer.

Another suspect sweetener is erythritol, a sugar alcohol found in Vitaminwater Zero. The body does not easily digest sugar alcohols, and as a result, they can cause diarrhea, headache, and other intestinal disorders in some people.

You might see a widely used beverage sweetener such as acesulfame potassium, or Ace-K, in many popular "diet" drinks. According to the Center for Science in the Public Interest (CSPI), this product is anything but safe. CSPI reported that safety tests of Ace-K conducted in the 1970s were faulty. Specifically, two rat studies suggested that the additive might cause cancer, but these studies were never addressed by the FDA before it approved the sweetener for use in soft drinks. Large doses of acetoacetamide (a breakdown product of this sugar) have been shown to affect the thyroid in rats, rabbits, and dogs. As you might know, the thyroid gland regulates the endocrine system, which is responsible for a healthy metabolism.

Need Extra Incentive to Ditch the Diet Soda?

I was so addicted to soft drinks that I drank soda five times a day. I rarely drank anything else. My friends would say, "Just drink water." But replacing soda with water? Impossible! I LOVED soda.

My weight climbed to 190 pounds—40 pounds higher than I should be for my height and frame. I was so fat that my shirts stretched apart at the buttons so far that you could see my BFB (that's short for Big Fat Belly). My ballooning weight was a "smack in the face" that forced me to take action. I knew that the soft drinks were making me fatter. I had to do something.

Whenever I felt thirsty, I realized I'd open my refrigerator and mindlessly grab a can of soda. That's the behavior I wanted to interrupt. For starters, I decided to put a roadblock between me and my refrigerator. A scale! I made the rule, "Before I open the refrigerator, I must weigh myself." Any weight gain was another "smack in the face" to keep me from drinking soda.

Being familiar with psychology, I knew that I couldn't just stop or start doing a bad habit; I had to replace it with something. I replaced soda with sparkling, lemon-flavored water.

All of this worked. I dropped ten pounds right away, without increasing my workouts or changing what I was eating. All I did was stop drinking five soft drinks a day. Now I have a sparkling water habit... and a shirt that fits.

Let's break down why this works and how you can use it to hack your behaviors.

First, smack yourself in the face. Not literally, but you need a trigger to remind yourself that you want to make a change. For me, the smack was my weight.

Second, create a rule to interrupt your usual behavior. My rule was to weigh myself before opening the refrigerator.

And finally, replace your behavior with a better behavior.

Follow that three-step strategy and bam! You're set.

—Derek Halpern, founder of socialtriggers.com

THE FIZZ OVER BVO

BVO stands for brominated vegetable oil, an additive that has been used to make soft drinks since the 1930s and has GRAS ("generally recognized as safe") status. BVO is found in some citrus-flavored soft drinks and sports drinks.

Banned in the European Union, BVO has been found to increase triglycerides and cholesterol. In high amounts, it can damage the liver, testicles, thyroid, heart, and kidneys, as well as cause skin ulcers called bromoderma. It is also used in flame retardants.

THE FOOD BABE WAY

I prefer drinking plain, filtered water over liquid with sugar, artificial sweeteners, preservatives, artificial flavors, Silly Putty, bacteria, and brominated vegetable oil. Don't you? Here are my suggestions for kicking this habit:

BE AWARE OF YOUR HABIT

For starters, look at the back of the can and see how many chemicals you are drinking—that alone should steer you in another direction. Then be honest about how many sodas you drink in a week. Add them up by keeping a food diary for seven days. For sticker shock, use a calculator to add up how many calories and sugar grams you're guzzling in that period. Your soda is not only costing you your health, it's also costing you money. Prices of soft drinks vary, but if you drink two twelve-ounce cans of soda daily, you spend about $2 a day or more, or $730 a year.

EASE OFF SODA

Can't go cold turkey? Try cutting back by a fourth the first week, half the second week, and so on until you can quit your soda habit for good.

MAKE SUBSTITUTIONS

Drink lots of clean, filtered water instead of soda. Purchase a refillable water bottle and keep it with you at home, at work, and in your car.

Plus, find other fizz. Miss the refreshment and mouth feel of sodas? Don't worry: I have you covered with a quick switch to a few of my favorite healthy and refreshing soda alternatives:

- GT's Enlightened Organic Raw Kombucha
- Sparkling water
- Sparkling water + lime juice + organic cranberry juice
- Water + cucumbers + strawberries
- Sparkling water + lemon juice + fresh-pressed organic juice
- Zukay probiotic drinks
- 100% raw coconut water
- Cold brewed organic tea

Remember that soda is loaded with calories, sugar, and chemicals—all hazardous to your health. I don't want you to be the first person whose obituary lists the cause of death as complications from soda consumption. Can your soda habit today!

CHECKLIST

Today:

- ✓ I did my morning lemon water ritual.
- ✓ I enjoyed a green drink.
- ✓ I stopped drinking fluids with my meals.
- ✓ I drank, and bathed in, pure, clean, filtered water.
- ✓ I ate less dairy and made healthier dairy choices.
- ✓ I stopped drinking all sodas.

Day 7 — Love Your Liver

I'M FREQUENTLY ASKED, "WHAT about alcohol? Can I still enjoy a drink or two while following an organic lifestyle?"

The short answer is yes. But I have two caveats: First, if you're trying to get thin and fit, it's best to lay off alcohol. Second, you've got to know how to choose the best organic wines, beers, and spirits, because the alcohol industry often uses harmful chemicals to make its products.

For today's habit: Go alcohol-free to lose weight, and if you do imbibe, learn all you can about organic choices and the controversial chemicals the alcohol industry uses.

FAT BURNING AND ALCOHOL

Alcohol affects your liver, one of the hardest-working organs in your body. One of the liver's primary jobs is to skim environmental toxins from your body. If it is overtaxed with alcohol, the normal process of toxin removal becomes extremely diminished and can result in rapid aging, loss of libido, and disease.

The liver is also your major fat-burning organ, so if you treat it well, it will work to full capacity and you'll eliminate maximum fat. Your liver normally burns fat for energy, but when you drink alcohol, your body "switches fuel" and burns up the booze instead of fat. In one study, volunteers were given two ninety-calorie vodka and lemonades. For several hours afterward, their fat-burning rate dropped by a whopping 73 percent.

Alcohol also weakens your willpower by shutting down mechanisms in the brain responsible for self-restraint—which is why you reach for forbidden fatty and sugary foods. Studies show that people who have a predinner tipple eat far more calories than those who have a soft drink.

The morning after, you might wake up with a hangover and try to eat your way out of it. Hangover hunger is caused by a slump in blood sugar, brought on by too much booze. Your body wants fast-fix carbs, as these give you an instant sugar hit. If you give in, those sugary calories just turn into body fat.

Finally, booze dehydrates you. Alcohol is a diuretic, which means it makes you pass more fluid than you take in. Dehydration makes your metabolism drop, meaning you burn fewer calories than usual.

To drink or not to drink while on a diet? It's clear that alcohol will tax your fat-burning ability, so it's best to kick it out of your diet if you want to get slim and fit and feel great.

BEER: BREWING CHEMICALS

I got curious about the chemicals in alcohol because my husband loves beer. I wanted to know exactly what was in his favorite brews, so I started some intensive research to find out. I questioned several beer companies. And the information I unearthed was shocking.

Under normal circumstances, beer is essentially a brew of only four ingredients: water, hops, malt, and yeast. However, beer makers add many other ingredients to clarify, stabilize, preserve, and enhance the color and flavor of beer. I discovered that there is a long list of additives the government has approved for use in beer:

- Caramel coloring, classified as III or IV, made from ammonia, and considered a carcinogen. This coloring agent is heated with ammonia and contains two toxins, 2-methylimidazole and 4-methylimidazole. In 2007, studies by the US National Toxicology Program revealed that both chemicals cause cancer in lab animals.
- Calcium disodium EDTA, an additive made from formaldehyde, sodium cyanide, and ethylenediamine.
- Many different types of sulfites and antimicrobial preservatives, which have been linked to allergies and asthma.
- Natural flavors, which can come from anything, including a beaver's anal gland.

- High-fructose corn syrup, a sweetener linked to obesity.
- GMO sugars, such as dextrose and corn syrup.
- Artificial food dyes and artificial flavors made from petroleum.
- Animal-based clarifiers, including isinglass (dried fish swim bladder), gelatin (from skin, connective tissue, and bones), and casein (found in milk).
- Foam control (used for head retention), which is achieved through the addition of glyceryl monostearate, propylene glycol, and pepsin, all potentially derived from animals, or propylene glycol alginate, which is derived from seaweed.
- BPA (bisphenol A), a component in many can liners that may leach into the beer. BPA can mimic the female hormone estrogen and may affect sperm count and other organ functions.
- Carrageenan, which is linked to inflammation in the digestive system and to irritable bowel syndrome (IBS) and is considered a carcinogen in some circumstances.

During my initial investigation, I couldn't get a single mainstream beer company to share the full list of ingredients contained in their beer. But I did get some of them to fess up to the use of these ingredients in writing. I've summarized this information in the chart on the next page.

The alcohol industry has lobbied for years against efforts to require ingredient labeling because they don't want you to know what you're drinking. So in June 2014, I turned up the heat on the beer industry. I launched a nationwide petition, asking two of America's most popular beer companies — Anheuser-Busch and MillerCoors — to disclose their beer ingredients and publish them online. Nearly every other food and beverage provider is legally required to make this information available — yet these two companies, which collectively sell more than $70 billion in beer each year, have not. Ingredient labeling on food products and non-alcoholic beverages is required by the Food and Drug Administration, but the same requirement does not apply to beer, wine, or liquor. As a result, we know more about what's in a bottle of Windex than in one of the world's most popular drinks.

In less than a day, my petition received over 40,000 signatures, plus millions of page views online and in mainstream media.

After this media firestorm, Anheuser-Busch reached out to me to announce they would disclose the ingredients on their website.

An Anheuser-Busch representative wrote:

"We are working to list our beer ingredients on our website, just as you would see for other food and non-alcohol beverage producers. We are beginning immediately, having incorporated this information earlier today on www.tapintoyourbeer.com for our flagship brands Budweiser and Bud Light, and will be listing this for our other brands in the coming days."

After Anheuser-Busch's response, MillerCoors responded by listing some ingredients on their Facebook page and website, but they have not officially agreed to list all ingredients yet.

I was thrilled with Anheuser-Busch's quick response. This petition is further proof that making your voice heard can change the policies of a multibillion-dollar company overnight. MillerCoors needs to step up to the plate and agree to make all their ingredients public, and so should EVERY other beer company. Below is a chart that shows what additives are in the beers that have had their ingredients disclosed. Please note, this is just a sampling of the products on the market—there are many more whose ingredients we don't know anything about at all.

Additives	Beers
Caramel coloring	Newcastle Stella Artois REDD'S Apple Ale Leffe Johnny Appleseed Cider Bud Light Lime Straw-Ber-Rita Bud Light Lime Apple-Ahhh-Rita Bud Light Lime Lime-A-Rita
Added colors	Stella Artois Cidre Sparks Bud Light Lime Straw-Ber-Rita Bud Light Lime Mang-O-Rita Bud Light Lime Raz-Ber-Rita

(Continued)

Additives	Beers
Corn (may be GMO)	Shock Top Twisted Pretzel Wheat Bass Pale Ale Busch Non-Alcoholic Michelob Golden Draft O'Douls Leffe Stella Artois Blue Moon (via email)
Corn syrup (may be GMO)	Coors Corona Foster's Miller Light Pabst Blue Ribbon Red Stripe Redbridge Blue Moon (via email)
Corn syrup, dextrose syrup, or rice syrup (may be GMO)	Bud Ice Bud Light Platinum Select 55 (Budweiser) Select (Budweiser) Busch Busch Ice Busch Light Busch Signature Copper Lager Rolling Rock Hurricane King Cobra Natural Natty Daddy Michelob ULTRA Lime Cactus Bud Light Lime Straw-Ber-Rita Bud Light Lime Apple-Ahhh-Rita Bud Light Lime Lime-A-Rita Bud Light Lime Mang-O-Rita Bud Light Lime Raz-Ber-Rita
Caramelized sugar syrup	Bud Light Platinum
High-fructose corn syrup (may be GMO)	Bud Light Lime Michelob ULTRA Lime Cactus Bud Light Lime Straw-Ber-Rita Bud Light Lime Apple-Ahhh-Rita Bud Light Lime Lime-A-Rita Bud Light Lime Mang-O-Rita Bud Light Lime Raz-Ber-Rita O'Douls O'Douls Amber Busch Non-Alcoholic
Isinglass from fish swim bladders	Guinness Nelson Organic (some varieties) St. Peter's Organic Ale

Additives	Beers
Carrageenan (Irish Moss)	Sierra Nevada North Coast Brewing Co. Deschutes Fish Tail Organic Brooklyn Brewery Mill Street Original Organic Eel River Organic Fuller's Honey Dew Organic Bridgeport Brewing
Propylene glycol alginate	Corona
Hop extract	Bud Light Lime Bud Light Platinum Bud Ice Rolling Rock Select 55 (Budweiser) Busch Ice Busch Light Busch Signature Copper Lager Hurricane King Cobra Landshark Lager Michelob Golden Draft Michelob ULTRA Lime Cactus Natural Natty Daddy Bud Light Lime Straw-Ber-Rita Bud Light Lime Apple-Ahhh-Rita Bud Light Lime Lime-A-Rita Bud Light Lime Mang-O-Rita Bud Light Lime Raz-Ber-Rita
Natural flavor and/or artificial flavor	Shock Top Honey Bourbon Cask Wheat Shock Top Twisted Pretzel Wheat Bud Light Lime Michelob ULTRA Lime Cactus Bud Light Lime Straw-Ber-Rita Bud Light Lime Apple-Ahhh-Rita Bud Light Lime Lime-A-Rita Bud Light Lime Mang-O-Rita Bud Light Lime Raz-Ber-Rita Johnny Appleseed Cider Michelob ULTRA Light Cider Stella Artois Cidre REDD's Apple Ale
Sulfites	Johnny Appleseed Cider Michelob ULTRA Light Cider

(Continued)

Additives	Beers
Malic acid (may be GMO)	Michelob ULTRA Lime Cactus Bud Light Lime Straw-Ber-Rita Bud Light Lime Apple-Ahhh-Rita Bud Light Lime Raz-Ber-Rita Michelob ULTRA Light Cider Stella Artois Cidre Johnny Appleseed Cider
Sucrose (sugar) (may be GMO)	Shock Top Twisted Pretzel Wheat Stella Artois Cidre Johnny Appleseed Cider
Sucralose (Splenda) (artificial sweetener)	Bud Light Lime Straw-Ber-Rita Bud Light Lime Mang-O-Rita Bud Light Lime Raz-Ber-Rita
Sodium citrate (may be GMO)	Stella Artois Cidre Bud Light Lime Straw-Ber-Rita Bud Light Lime Apple-Ahhh-Rita Bud Light Lime Lime-A-Rita Bud Light Lime Mang-O-Rita
Ascorbic acid (synthetic vitamin C) (may be GMO)	Corona

WHAT'S WRONG WITH WINE?

If you think beer has a lot of additives, that's nothing compared to what you'll find in wine. I'd always thought of wine as a natural product, since it's made from grapes. Sadly, the truth is not quite so simple. In researching this issue, I found my way to the US Government Printing Office website, which listed "materials authorized for the treatment of wine and juice." There are nearly fifty ingredients on the list, and in my opinion, many of them may be harmful. I've summarized some of the usual suspects below.

- Acacia (gum arabic). This additive is used to clarify and stabilize wine, but it is also linked to mild-to-severe asthma attacks and rashes.
- Acetaldehyde. Used to stabilize the color of wine and juice, acetaldehyde can cause severe headaches in some people.
- Aluminosilicates (hydrated) such as bentonite (Wyoming clay) and kaolin. Both are natural minerals found in the earth's crust, but they can irritate the lungs and eyes.

- Animal by-products such as egg white powder, milk products, beef gelatin, and sturgeon-derived isinglass (fish bladder). The additives make certain wines inappropriate for vegans and vegetarians.
- Heavy metals. These include mainly vanadium, copper, and manganese. Manganese can accumulate in the brain and has been linked to Parkinson's disease. And don't forget that heavy metals are one of the Sickening 15.
- Oak chips or particles, uncharred and untreated. These increase the tannin levels in wine, and many people are highly sensitive to tannins.
- Pesticides, sprayed onto grapes. Another of my Sickening 15, pesticides are linked to many illnesses, including cancer. I was shocked to learn that wine growers treating grapes with chemicals have to wear hazmat-style clothing and breathing devices to protect themselves while spraying their grapes!
- Polyvinylpolypyrrolidone (PVPP), a chemical used to clarify wine. It reduces levels of quercetin in wine, a disease-fighting phytochemical.
- Sugar. In a process called chaptalization, cane sugar is added to grape juice to increase the alcohol in the finished wine. Added sugar is of course troublesome, since it negatively affects levels of glucose and blood fats in your system. Please note: Adding cane sugar is not legal in California, Argentina, Australia, southern France, or South Africa, so producers use sugar-rich grape concentrate to simulate the same results.
- Sulfites. These chemicals can be dangerous to people suffering from asthma because they can trigger an asthmatic attack; such episodes have caused the deaths of ten to twenty people in the last three years, according to the Center for Science in the Public Interest.
- Sulfur dioxide. This gas produces headaches, migraines, asthma, eczema, and other skin problems.
- Tribromophenol. This chemical lurks in wooden wine barrels, wooden wine racks, and the crates used to transport the grapes.

It's basically a fire retardant—and it's very toxic. If you put a tiny amount into a large aquarium, the fish will die.

- Yeasts (genetically modified). We know from a large and growing body of research that GMO products can be toxic, allergenic, and far less nutritious than their natural counterparts.

BE CHOOSY ABOUT BOOZING

Now we come to distilled liquor, namely, vodka, whiskey, gin, Scotch, tequila, and liqueurs. If you thought wine and beer had a lot of additives, hold on to your martini glass: Distilled liquors are rife with chemicals. On a government website that lists every ingredient in booze, (www.ttb.gov/ssd/limited_ingredients.shtml), I counted more than sixty additives, plus several suspect food colorings.

When it comes to liquor, it's also important to watch out for GMOs. Did you know, for example, that Jack Daniel's whiskey and Smirnoff vodka are made primarily from corn?

In the list below, I'm calling out some of the nastiest chemicals you may find in your favorites.

- Benzoic acid/sodium benzoate. These additives deter the growth of microorganisms in acidic foods. In sensitive people, they can cause hives, asthma, or other allergic reactions. One product that's really loaded with this additive is Skinnygirl Margarita, marketed as a low-calorie cocktail and designed to appeal to dieters who still want to imbibe.
- BHA. I've mentioned this food preservative throughout the book; it's highly toxic and may cause cancer.
- BHT. This is another food preservative I gripe about frequently. It can build up in your fat tissue and has been known to cause cancer in lab animals.
- Brominated vegetable oil (BVO). Here we are again with BVO, a chemical that keeps oils in suspension in foods. Ingesting BVO

leaves residues in body fat, as well as fat in the brain, liver, and other organs.

- Caffeine. As I've mentioned, caffeine is addictive. Even the FDA warns of the dangers of added caffeine in alcoholic beverages, which may cause people drinking them to become more intoxicated than they realize. Some vodkas may be infused with caffeine, and many mixed drinks such as rum and Coke give you a jolt of caffeine (from the soda).

- Propylene glycol. This clear, colorless liquid is often used in antifreeze as well as in processed foods. Not cleared for general food use in Europe, propylene glycol may cause organ damage and harm to the central nervous system after prolonged or repeated exposure. Fireball Whisky was recently pulled from shelves in Europe because the amount of propylene glycol was out of compliance with European standards.

- Sorbitol. In large amounts, this sugar alcohol exerts a laxative effect and may even cause diarrhea.

- Sucrose and other refined sugars. Excessive amounts of these sweeteners boost blood sugar levels and affect triglycerides (fat) and LDL ("bad") cholesterol levels in blood, and may thereby increase the risk of heart disease. Malibu rum and Kahlúa don't use high-fructose corn syrup in other countries, but they do in their products sold in the United States — it's the worst kind of sugar, one of my Sickening 15.

COLORINGS

Ever wonder what makes Bailey's Irish Cream so deliciously brown, or blue curaçao so tropically blue? It's all the coloring agents. Below is a list of coloring agents that may be used in beverage products — with their possible side effects.

- Annatto extract. Made from the seeds of a tropical shrub, annatto causes hives in susceptible people.

- Caramel coloring. Guilty parties using caramel coloring include Jack Daniel's Tennessee Honey Whiskey, Captain Morgan Spiced Rum, Bailey's Irish Cream, and Kahlúa.
- Carmine (cochineal extract).
- FD&C Blue #1.
- FD&C Blue #2. Although animal studies have found some evidence that this dye causes brain cancer in male rats, the FDA insists it is safe.
- FD&C Green #3. A 1981 study hinted that this dye caused bladder and testicular tumors in male rats, but the FDA concluded that it was not carcinogenic after doing tests of its own. Fortunately, this suspect dye is not widely used.
- FD&C Red #3. There is strong proof that this dye causes thyroid tumors in rats. It has mostly been used to color the maraschino cherries floating in your Manhattan or old-fashioned. Lobbying by the cherry industry in the 1980s prevented the dye from being banned outright. Though still used, Red #3 has been largely replaced by Red #40.
- FD&C Red #40.
- FD&C Yellow #5.
- FD&C Yellow #6. Animal tests indicate that this dye causes tumors of the adrenal gland and kidney. It can also be contaminated with the carcinogens benzidine and 4-aminobiphenyl.

THE FOOD BABE WAY

MAKE BETTER BEER CHOICES

If you enjoy an occasional beer and wish to maintain your healthy life-style, reach for one without GMOs and additives. Here are some good choices:

- Additive-free mainstream beers. A few popular brews exist that don't have chemicals and GMOs. These include Heineken and

Amstel Light. You can find a list of additional clean beers at foodbabe.com/cleanbeer.

- German beers. The Germans are very serious about the purity of their beers. They follow a purity law called the *Reinheitsgebot* that requires all German beers to be produced only with the core ingredients water, hops, yeast, and malted barley or wheat. Advocates of German beers insist that they taste cleaner, and some even claim they don't suffer from hangovers as a result.
- Certified organic beers. By law, these beers cannot include GMOs or other harmful additives. Organic beers also support environmentally friendly practices, reduce the amount of pesticides and toxins in our air, and support organic farmers — which is a huge plus. Samuel Smith's Brewery makes several delicious organic varieties.
- Craft and microbrew beers. My husband now buys his beer from local craft breweries and microbreweries. These companies will give you a list of the ingredients they use. Be aware, though, that big beer makers are slowly closing in on craft beers and buying them up one by one. Anheuser-Busch did this with Rolling Rock and Goose Island Beer Company. Make sure your favorite craft beer and microbrew are still independently owned and controlled before taking a sip.

In the end, if you decide to drink beer, drink it infrequently and quiz the beer companies for the truth. Find a beer that you can trust and stick with it.

CHOOSE ORGANIC WINE

Organic wine is produced from organically grown grapes and is officially certified in accordance with the USDA's guidelines for organic products. For a wine to be certified organic, no synthetic pesticides can have been used for three years before harvest.

If the wine is labeled organic, not only are the grapes organic, but the wine-making process is also certified organic. This means that the entire process—crushing the grapes, fermenting the wine, bottling, and other procedures like cleaning—must meet USDA standards.

I recommend you start choosing organic wine. My favorites are Cabernet Sauvignon from Frey Vineyards and the organic biodynamic wines from Robert Sinskey Vineyards in the Napa Valley.

Look for sulfite-free wines, too. The label will state "sulfite-free," "no sulfites added," or "NSA."

Avoid GMO wines. A genetically modified yeast called ML01 has been approved for use in the United States as well as Canada and South Africa. Since there is no law requiring lists of ingredients on wine labels, GMOs may be present in conventionally made wine in America. Reportedly used on a limited scale, the GM yeast essentially flies under the radar with consumers and advocacy groups kept in the dark. Other wine-making countries such as Australia and New Zealand require ingredients including yeast to be listed on the label. As far as I'm concerned, if a wine producer, or a food company for that matter, won't disclose this information to you, it's best to steer clear of their products. USDA certified organic wines and biodynamic wines cannot be made with GMO yeast. According to organicconsumers.org in 2007, the following wine producers do not use GMO yeast:

Atlas Peak Vineyards

Beaulieu Vineyard

Buena Vista Carneros

Chappellet Winery

Charles Krug Winery

Clos Du Val Wine Company

Clos Pegase Winery

Duckhorn Vineyards

Far Niente

Flora Springs

Grgich Hills Winery

Groth Vineyards

Heitz Wine Cellars

Joseph Phelps Vineyards

Madonna Estate

Markham Winery

Merryvale

Quintessa

Robert Mondavi

Rothschild/Mondavi (Opus One)

Rubicon Estate Winery

Shafer Vineyards

Silver Oak

Spring Mountain Vineyard

Sterling Vineyards

Trefethen Vineyards

Tres Sabores

V. Sattui Winery

William Hill Estate

BE DISCERNING WITH DISTILLED LIQUOR

If distilled liquor is your alcoholic beverage of choice, the cleanest drink you can enjoy is tequila. I'm not talking about a margarita, which is full of sugar and calories, but pure tequila served on the rocks with a wedge of lime. This is exactly what I order when I want a cocktail, and it is a good choice (as long as you don't drink too many of them and end up dancing on the bar!).

You can also choose distilled liquor that is labeled organic. Let's say you like gin. If you order or purchase organic gin, that means that the juniper berries, coriander, angelica root, and other ingredients used to make it have all been grown according to USDA organic requirements. Some products will be labeled as "made with" organic ingredients. This means that at least 70 percent of the agents in the liquor must be certified organic.

Finally, I'd stay away from liqueurs — those after-dinner-type drinks that are so syrupy sweet. They are laced with all kinds of flavorings that do your body no good at all.

Be aware, too, that the health benefit claims about alcohol that might make drinking it seem like a good idea are a little suspect, considering alcohol can be addictive and capable of inflicting organ damage. Many studies say a beer or a glass of wine a day is healthy for you, but a lot of people don't stop at just one.

I feel that the decision to drink alcohol is a personal one. I enjoy wine, champagne, and tequila every now and then. When I do, I make the best choices I can. Having or not having alcohol is not a judgment call that any of us should make for others, unless excessive drinking is ruining someone's health, family, and personal life. The important thing is to be educated about alcohol, what's in it, how much should be consumed, and whether you feel it's something you want to have in your lifestyle.

CHECKLIST

Today:

✓ I did my morning lemon water ritual.

✓ I enjoyed a green drink.

✓ I stopped drinking fluids with my meals.

✓ I drank, and bathed in, pure, clean, filtered water.

✓ I ate less dairy and made healthier dairy choices.

✓ I stopped drinking all sodas.

✓ I loved my liver by paying attention to alcohol consumption.

CHAPTER 5

WEEK 2 — FOOD HABITS FOR FOOD BABES

CONGRATULATIONS! YOU'VE MADE IT to Week 2.

Before we start the second week, take some time to reflect on how you feel after developing those first seven good habits. Fix yourself a cup of herbal tea and sit in a quiet place. Now ask yourself:

- Do I feel lighter and more energetic?
- Has my skin improved?
- Have any pesky health conditions subsided or disappeared — allergies, skin flare-ups, tummy cramps, sluggishness, or others?
- Has my sleep improved?
- Do I feel less bloated?
- Have my cravings dissipated?
- Have I seen other positive effects?

Week 1 was about cleansing your body of potential troublemakers. We concentrated on fluids to help your body eliminate toxins and support a healthy digestive system.

In Week 2, we're going to take it up a notch by learning to support your body with the nutrition it needs: good proteins, raw fruits and veggies, beneficial fats, fiber-rich grains, and some "superhero" foods. I'll also show you how to get away from the biggest health offenders around: fast food and refined sugar.

Food, including healthy beverages, is the best source of vitamins, minerals, phytochemicals, and other healthful components. You'll now discover what it feels like to treat your body to clean food. And take it from me: It's going to feel amazing.

Day 8 — Pass on Fast Food

FAST FOOD IS MASS-PRODUCED, mass-processed, and designed to be slapped together quickly. Virtually nothing is prepared on-site and nothing is really fresh, so the food is generally devoid of vitamins, minerals, and other nutritional value, and it's encased in packaging that may expose us to harmful chemicals.

I've seen a lot of things that have made me angry over the years, from "100% whole grain" snacks full of toxic processed chemicals to food marketed to children that's full of artificial sweeteners. But fast foods, and the chemicals in them, really ruffle my feathers! We must stop the epidemic of fast food. We must stop the obesity and the unnecessary degenerative diseases that are caused by fast foods. We must stop kids from eating and craving this junk. Today is the day to make that commitment: Give up fast food!

Getting off fast food is not going to be easy, if you're used to eating it. Beyond the dangerous processing and packaging, fast food is also formulated and manufactured to be addictive, a fact proven by various scientific studies. A 2007 report titled "The Link Between Fast Food and the Obesity Epidemic," published in the journal *Health Matrix,* stated: "Fat, sugar, and cholesterol [found in fast food] have addictive qualities similar to the drug nicotine."

I don't need science to tell me this. I know from personal experience, and once again, it has to do with Chick-fil-A. Long before I became the Food Babe, I was addicted to eating at Chick-fil-A. I remember the first time I tasted their food. It was at the mall when I was very young, and the restaurant used to pass out the free samples of hot, fresh pieces of newly fried chicken on little toothpicks. It was free, so of course my parents let me try it. The smell alone was intoxicating, not to mention the taste. My addiction to Chick-fil-A continued throughout my childhood and into my college years, when I ate their food nearly every day. Even though I haven't had Chick-fil-A food in more than a decade now, I still know what a Chick-fil-A sandwich smells and tastes like—that's because they engineer it so you won't ever forget it.

Much later, during a visit to Chick-fil-A headquarters, I noted that the fast-food company prided itself on its "healthy" menu items, one of which was oatmeal. Though not organic, their oatmeal was pushed as having no artificial flavors or additives. I got to sneak behind the scenes to watch store employees prepare this oatmeal, and I couldn't believe my eyes.

The oatmeal is not prepared on-site; instead, it's shipped to the restaurants already cooked and stored in plastic bags. Sometimes it's put in the freezer until needed. After you order oatmeal, an employee boils the bag containing the oatmeal, rips open the bag, and serves it to you, steaming hot, in yet another plastic container.

During this entire process, plastic may have leached into your food—a typical fast-food practice that could have disastrous long-term health consequences. You now may be ingesting chemicals without your knowledge or permission. And we also don't know what's in the water that's being used to boil the oatmeal.

If you eat fast food, you can be exposed to chemicals known as perfluoroalkyl acids (PFAAs). These acids are found in the wrappers that encase your cheeseburger and other fast foods. They are also present in microwave popcorn bags, dust, tap water, stain-resistant carpets, waterproof fabrics, and a host of other household products.

PFAAs can migrate from the wrappers into our food. According to research from the University of Toronto, we can ingest these chemicals, which then get into our blood.

Elevated levels of these chemicals in the blood are worrisome and potentially dangerous to humans. Specific types of these chemicals, perfluorooctanoic acid (PFOA) and perfluorooctanesulfonate (PFOS), have been associated with changes in sex hormones and cholesterol levels, according to the Agency for Toxic Substances and Disease Registry (an agency of the US Department of Health and Human Services).

Think about this the next time you're tempted to pick up some fast food. The way fast food is prepared and packaged can be unhealthy.

There just might also be plastic cooked into your food. Yes, you read that correctly—plastic.

THE MSG ISSUE

Among the most addicting additives dumped into fast food is MSG, one of my Sickening 15 ingredients, and it's especially rampant in one of my favorite foods—pizza. In 2011 Congress voted to declare pizza sauce a vegetable in the school lunch program. But there's a lot going on behind closed doors that nobody wants us to know or talk about, and it all starts with the ingredients.

After I started researching fast-food pizza ingredients, one thing became abundantly clear: Fast-food pizza chains didn't like the questions I was asking. I found a couple of ingredient lists online and began calling the top pizza chains to find out more. But when I called most pizza restaurants and asked questions, they blatantly refused to share ingredient lists, and their customer service reps were oblivious to what their ingredients were. For example, Papa John's does not post its ingredients online even though their competitors Pizza Hut and Domino's do. Little Caesars, California Pizza Kitchen (CPK), and Mellow Mushroom have all refused to answer my questions about their ingredients. I was told by Mellow Mushroom's corporate offices that they will comply only with government regulations, which merely require them to publish an allergen list and nothing more. Little Caesars told me that if I was concerned about what was in their food, I *"just shouldn't eat there."* Ha—don't worry, I won't!

Why are these ingredients so hard to find? Why do some companies refuse to share their ingredients? What is it that they don't want us to know? Could it be large amounts of MSG?

Some restaurants don't want to get a bad rap by putting MSG on their ingredient or allergen statements, so they found another way to secretly add this potent flavor enhancer to your food, without the average customer's realizing it. They are using an FDA loophole to sneak processed free glutamic acid into your food, which has the same effect as

MSG—and they are doing it all without warning you. Other forms of glutamic acid in fast food include:

- Autolyzed yeast extract (hidden MSG)
- Textured or hydrolyzed proteins (hidden MSG and GMO)
- Hydrolyzed corn (hidden MSG and GMO)
- Modified starches (hidden MSG and possible GMO)
- Natural flavors (possible hidden MSG)
- Disodium inosinate or disodium guanylate (MSG enhancers)

These forms of MSG allow fast-food chains to have "clean labels" that can lead you to believe their products contain no MSG—when they actually contain its equivalent!

Remember, MSG tricks your brain into believing that what you're eating tastes so great, you want more of it. Your taste buds sense that there is more protein in the food than there really is—which is great for food manufacturers who want to save money by using less meat. And repeat business keeps the pockets of these businesses lined with cash.

MORE UNHOLY ADDITIVES

Fast food consists mostly of high-calorie, low-nutrition meals that are laden with cheap sugars, fat, and excessive salt. Most people know this. But what most people don't know is that fast food contains other very nasty additives.

If you make your own pizza at home, you'll need Ezekiel sprouted wheat tortillas, organic pizza sauce, veggies, and organic cheese. If you buy a pizza from a fast-food outlet, it may be made with any or all of the following: artificial colors, partially hydrogenated oils, cellulose (wood pulp), GMO soybean oil, BHT/BHA (butylated hydroxytoluene/butylated hydroxyanisole, used in embalming fluid and fuel jets), sodium nitrite, enriched flour, caramel coloring, BPA, modified food starch cellulose (powdered wood pulp), aluminum, high-fructose corn syrup, carrageenan, propylene glycol, sodium citrate, citric acid, sodium aluminum phosphate, lactic acid, sorbic acid, natamycin (mold inhibitor), and corn maltodextrin.

There is not enough space to list and explain every additive here, so for now I'll highlight some of the most offensive ingredients. Some of those ingredients you wouldn't feed to your pets. Some you could use to light a fire or caulk up a leaky sink.

Did you know that Wendy's chili contains silicon dioxide (found in sand) or that McDonald's apple pie contains L-cysteine (derived from poultry feathers)? Are you aware that Jack in the Box puts cellulose (the same ingredient that is in sawdust) in many of its cheeses, sauces, and shakes? Or that Wendy's puts dimethylpolysiloxane (used in Silly Putty) in its Natural-Cut Fries? These are not ingredients you'd find sitting next to the sweet potatoes and asparagus in the produce department. If you check the fast-food companies' ingredient lists posted online, you'll see that these chemical names are all there in black and white.

I'd like to bring up, once again, one of the scariest additives: azodicarbonamide (the yoga mat chemical), which is often used in foamed plastics but is also used to bleach flour and condition dough. You'll find it in many fast-food burger buns and sub sandwich buns (even whole wheat varieties). This ingredient is banned as a food additive in the United Kingdom, Europe, and Australia. If you get caught using it in Singapore, you can get up to fifteen years in prison and be fined $450,000. The UK has recognized azodicarbonamide as a potential cause of asthma if inhaled, and advises against its use in people who have sensitivity to food dyes and other common food allergies, because it can worsen the symptoms. Another study reviewed by the Center for Science in the Public Interest found that when azodicarbonamide is heated, it forms a carcinogen!

If a server is slapping processed meat on that azodicarbonamide-containing sandwich bun (and it's likely they are), you're also going to be ingesting nitrates. The consumption of nitrates is serious: In the body, nitrates morph into nitrosamines, which have been proven to increase the risk of disease dramatically.

The World Cancer Research Fund recommended that people avoid processed meat (with high concentrations of nitrates) because it poses a "convincing" risk for bowel cancer. The Fund based their conclusion on a large, independent scientific review conducted in 2007 and confirmed in 2011. Studies have shown it may only take 1.8 ounces of high-nitrate processed meat daily to increase the likelihood of cancer by 50 percent, the likelihood of heart disease by 42 percent, and the likelihood of diabetes by 19 percent.

Speaking of fast-food meat, maybe you've heard of pink slime, which is leftover beef scraps. After being treated with ammonia to kill bacteria, the meat is run through a centrifuge and then added to ground beef to bulk up the meat and reduce the fat content. Eww!

These disgusting substances are considered "safe" additives. Companies put these ingredients into their products and then dare to call it food.

I should also point out that fast-food joints often use foods that have been sprayed with pesticides. A good example is the Russet Burbank potato, used by McDonald's to make hash browns and French fries. Fellow food activist and author Michael Pollan has reported that the fast-food giant insists on using these potatoes, even though they are extremely sensitive to Irish potato blight and difficult to grow. These potatoes tend to be afflicted with net necrosis, a viral infection that causes spots and lines on the potatoes. McDonald's won't buy blemished potatoes, and the only way to prevent net necrosis is to spray potatoes with a pesticide called methamidophos. This pesticide is so toxic, writes Pollan, "that the farmers who grow these potatoes in Idaho won't venture outside and into their fields for five days after they spray."

Methamidophos is typically sprayed on potato fields from the air by crop dusters, which means it can drift and affect unsuspecting people in nearby areas. Exposure to methamidophos in the air can cause immediate coughing, gagging, and vomiting. And after Russet Burbank potatoes are harvested, they have to be stored in giant, atmosphere-controlled sheds the size of football stadiums for six weeks so that they gas off all the pesticides and chemicals. Now, doesn't that sound appetizing?

It's time to get back to the basics and only eat food that is clean and chemical-free.

WHY DO WE BUY FAST FOOD?

To move toward a healthier diet, we need to consider why we buy fast food. And one of the main reasons we buy fast food is because it's cheap! Unfortunately, it's cheap because it's not real food. And if you eat cheap, your health will gravely suffer. You are what you eat, so don't be fast, easy, and cheap.

My dad has always liked fast food because it's cheap, and that's why he fed us at fast-food restaurants when we were kids. He just doesn't believe in spending a lot of money on food. Growing up in India, he was brought up to believe that food's sole purpose was to keep you alive, and you never wasted food. Buying food cheap was the only way to get it. After moving to the United States, he subsisted mostly on fast food because it was a good buy.

Sadly, this reasoning meant that my dad never paid attention to the nutritional value of good food. Over time, he developed type 2 diabetes. Right before I started my blog, he got very ill and had to be rushed to the hospital. He spent days in the hospital with doctors and nurses poking and prodding him, trying to figure out what was wrong. He didn't feel well and he couldn't concentrate. A couple of months later, he had a prostate specific antigen (PSA) test. His PSA was high, and the doctors confirmed that he had prostate cancer. It was stressful and saddening news, particularly because my mother-in-law had died just a year earlier from ovarian cancer. It was an overwhelming time for my family and me. I adore my dad, and I don't know what I'd do without him.

Fortunately, the disease is in its earliest stage. My dad found a doctor in Charlotte who advises "active surveillance": watching the situation, repeating the PSA test every three months, and following up with the doctor. My dad has also been advised to avoid red meat and dairy — two contributors to prostate cancer in men.

I'm afraid that a lifetime of eating fast food has severely and irrevocably hurt my dad's health. It infuriates me that our food system, pushing cheap, additive-filled food, is so full of poison. I do not want to be part of this system, and nor should you. Give up fast food for the rest of your life — if you value that life.

THE FOOD BABE WAY

SHUN FAST FOOD

The quickest, easiest way to break free from your chemical relationship to food is to give up fast food. Not only do I urge you to give up fast food, but I urge you to start making your own fast food at the same time. This is not difficult. If you want to be healthy, thin, and ageless, you've got to do this.

The best way to start this new habit is to be prepared. Spend a little time Sunday night preparing foods for the week. Use fresh, organic ingredients, cook in bulk, then divide your meals into glass containers and store in the freezer or fridge. This might take a little time, but it will be worth it when you need a fast meal after a very long day. I do this every week.

MAKE YOUR OWN FAST FOOD

I have a few recipes up my sleeve that taste better than any fast-food entrees you can buy: my Fast-Food Burritos, Chickpea Curry Wraps, Quick and Easy Home-Baked Pizza, and Sweet Potato Fries. You'll find them in the recipe chapter (Chapter 8).

STAY PREPARED

Wherever I go, I have food with me in case I feel hungry. This food might include packets of organic nuts, almond butter I can squeeze into my mouth, or pieces of fresh fruit. Packing simple, organic foods prevents me from making bad food decisions on the fly. You don't have to eat fast food if you prepare.

USE TIME-SAVERS

Another strategy is to go to the nearest grocery store that has a fresh salad bar with prewashed greens, lots of vegetables, and maybe some sushi. Buy one of the best "fast foods" ever—avocados—to slice over your salad. Voilà—you've got a superhealthy fast-food meal in no time.

YOU CAN DO THIS!

Everyone can employ these strategies, and it doesn't matter where you live. A few years ago, I visited the small town of Pickens, Mississippi, in Holmes County, considered the most obese county in the United States. Pickens is considered a food desert, a town or community with limited access to supermarkets and low-cost, nutritious foods. There is a strong link between food deserts and poor health. Adults in food deserts tend to be more obese, suffer from high blood pressure and diabetes, and have heart-related problems such as high cholesterol, elevated triglycerides, and a greater risk of heart and vascular disease. Kids who live in food deserts are also at very high risk of becoming overweight.

I discovered that although the local grocery store sold a lot of processed foods, it did carry fruits, veggies, organic tofu, and grains. I expected to see a lot of fast-food places in Pickens, but there were not that many. Then why was Holmes County the fattest county in America?

Although social and economic factors do play a part, the main culprit is the lack of credible nutrition education. Victims of obesity are being systematically brainwashed by corporate food company marketers. Dieters rely on calorie information on the labels of diet sodas, low-calorie processed foods, and low-fat products, and not on anything else. They don't pay attention to the chemicals that are making them fat, because they aren't aware of the harm that comes from these chemicals. And Big Food—a nickname for the food industry—doesn't want them to have this information.

I concluded from this trip that even in a so-called food desert, there are healthy alternatives to fast and processed foods. We have to learn how to make healthier choices, become aware of what's in our food by reading labels, and realize that Big Food is sending us messages that certain foods are healthy when, indeed, they may not be. Think about what you're eating, and know what's in it.

CHECKLIST

Today:

- ✓ I did my morning lemon water ritual.
- ✓ I enjoyed a green drink.
- ✓ I stopped drinking fluids with my meals.
- ✓ I drank, and bathed in, pure, clean, filtered water.
- ✓ I ate less dairy and made healthier dairy choices.
- ✓ I stopped drinking all sodas.
- ✓ I loved my liver by paying attention to alcohol consumption.
- ✓ I passed on fast food.

Day 9 — Detox from
Added Sugar

ONE OF THE MOST insidious ways the food industry poisons us is by dousing all sorts of foods with "added sugar." I'm talking about any sweetener that doesn't occur naturally in a food. Added sugar is one of the biggest perpetrators of our current health crisis, responsible for obesity, diabetes, disease, stroke, even cancer.

In fact, Americans eat close to 150 pounds of the stuff per person annually, probably because it's so addictive—eight times more addictive than cocaine, says a 2013 article by Dr. Serge H. Ahmed, published in *Neuroscience in the 21st Century*. And it doesn't matter if it is artificial or real sugar.

What added sugar does to the body is scandalous. It makes you fat by adding empty calories to your diet and jacking up your blood sugar— two processes that form excess body fat. It also screws with your appetite. According to Dr. Mark Hyman, writing in *The Blood Sugar Solution 10-Day Detox Diet*, sugar is different from other calories. "It scrambles all your normal appetite controls... driving your metabolism to convert it into lethal belly fat.... There is no doubt that sugar is a toxin."

Want to stay young-looking? Ditch added sugar. Excessive sugar makes your skin wrinkle. In a process called glycation, sugar molecules attach to collagen and elastin, two proteins that keep skin looking young, and create advanced glycation end products (AGEs). AGEs weaken your skin's support structure and lead to lines and wrinkles.

Added sugar sends your blood sugar sky-high—a reaction followed immediately by plummeting blood sugar. That low blood sugar triggers irritability and depression.

And it dumbs you down by interfering with communication among brain cells. A 2012 Mayo Clinic report found that people who eat a lot of sugar have a much higher chance of cognitive decline as they age. Too much added sugar can feed cancer, destroy the immune system, and promote cardiovascular disease.

Now is a good time to tell you that much of the added sugar on the market has been filtered through bone char. Often called natural carbon, bone char comes from the bones of cattle (and sometimes dogs). The bones are heated to very high temperatures, powdered, dehydrated, and turned into a charcoal filter to whiten cane sugar and remove impurities. I find this all pretty disturbing, especially if you are a vegan or a vegetarian who does not want to eat food contaminated in any way by animal parts.

Other types of sugar are subjected to bone char as well. Brown sugar is created by adding molasses to white sugar, which of course has been filtered through char. Confectioners' sugar—refined white sugar blended with cornstarch—also involves the use of bone char.

The largest sugar manufacturers in the United States all use bone char to refine and whiten cane sugar. I contacted C&H and Domino Sugar, both of whom responded to me via e-mail and confirmed they use it. These companies refine most of the sugar you'll find on store shelves in the United States.

Certain sugars are not processed with bone char. These include beet sugar, evaporated cane juice, turbinado, Demerera, muscovado, Sucanat, and all USDA certified organic sugars. I'm not saying any of these are good for you; I just want you to be aware of the bone char issue. After you detox from all added sugar, however, you won't have to worry about exposure to bone char.

If a food has any added sugar in it, you shouldn't be eating it. No one should be adding sugar to your food. Get away from the unnatural presence of added sugar and start this habit today!

DEVELOP A DISTASTE FOR ADDED SUGAR

Asking you to eliminate every type of "sugar" from your diet would be crazy, and any person trying to do this will fail in the long run. The key is to still include "good sugars" in your diet. These are forms of sugar that your body can easily assimilate and that provide vitamins, minerals, and other nutrients your body will use. They include naturally occurring sugar from fruits and vegetables, coconut palm sugar, honey, and maple syrup.

At the same time, you need to avoid the "bad sugars." Bad sugars are those processed from cane, corn, or beets. Table sugar and high-fructose corn syrup are the baddest of the bad. These sugars have been chemically stripped of their minerals. If you indulge in these sugars, you get no nutrition. You also make your body more acidic, because sugars devoid of minerals are acid-forming—and we know that it's better to eat mostly alkaline foods if we want to avoid disease.

THE FOOD BABE WAY

Here's how you detox from added sugar:

WATCH OUT FOR HIDDEN SUGARS

Don't buy, consume, or keep products in your house with the following ingredients in them: agave nectar, barley malt, beet sugar, brown sugar, buttered syrup, caramel, carob syrup, corn syrup, corn syrup solids, dextran, dextrose, diastase, diastatic malt, ethyl maltol, fructose, glucose, glucose solids, high-fructose corn syrup, invert sugar, lactose, malt syrup, maltodextrin, maltose, malitol, mannitol, raw sugar, refiner's syrup, sorbitol, sorghum syrup, sucrose, turbinado sugar, or yellow sugar.

AVOID ARTIFICIAL SWEETENERS

Don't replace these sugars with artificial sweeteners like aspartame, saccharin, and sucralose. These are off-limits, too! They are just as bad for the body—even worse, because some of them (e.g., saccharin) have been proven to be carcinogenic. Plus, artificial sweeteners have been linked to weight gain. They interfere with our satisfaction signals, causing us to crave even more sweet foods, and they're believed to promote surges in insulin, which can cause you to hold on to fat.

CONTINUOUSLY TRAIN YOUR PALATE FOR NATURAL SWEETNESS

Before you decide on a dessert or something else sweet to eat, consider natural options that will satisfy your sweet tooth. Over time, your distaste for refined sugar will naturally develop. Here's what I do:

When I crave chocolate: I go for a piece of a Righteously Raw bar, which is composed of 90 percent raw cacao and sweetened with coconut palm sugar and mint.

When I crave something fruity: I eat a couple of sulfur dioxide–free dried organic fruits—like apricots, prunes, cherries, golden berries, dates, goji berries, and figs—sometimes mixed with coconut. Dried coconut has a natural sweetness, but it has less than one gram of sugar per serving. Sometimes I drink cranberry or fruity herbal teas. Making a quick apple cobbler with just apples, cinnamon, oats, and a little sprinkle of maple syrup in a ramekin also does the trick.

When I crave something chewy, warm, and comforting: I make cookies from my Food Babe Sugar Blend, a mixture of prunes, banana, and dates blended with coconut oil (see my recipe for Forever Cookies on page 333). This blend serves as the perfect base for cookies, cakes, pies, and muffins. Also, I like to make warm almond milk blended with a date and vanilla, and sip on that while watching my favorite flick.

When I want ice cream or something cold: I make Homemade Coconut Milk Ice Cream (see the recipe on page 334) or have a bowl of frozen grapes.

When I crave something salty and sweet: I pop kettle corn with stevia (see below) or eat pieces of sprouted wheat pretzels dipped in raw-cacao chocolate.

When I want something fast: I reach for one of my favorite store-bought sweets:

Righteously Raw chocolate
Gnosis Chocolate
Alter Eco chocolate
Coco-Roons

Nutiva O'Coconut
Made in Nature dried fruit
Matt's Munchies dried fruit snacks (certain flavors)
Three Twins ice cream
Hail Merry snacks

CHOOSE GOOD SUGARS AND SWEETENERS

I'm talking about minimally processed sweeteners, in limited amounts, of course. These sugars contain various nutrients that are easily absorbed by the body and have numerous health benefits. Here are the four types of sweeteners that I use and recommend:

Coconut Palm Sugar

What it is: Derived from the nectar of the coconut palm tree flowers, this sweetener is one of the most natural unprocessed forms of sugar available.

Note: Some nasty Internet rumors claim that producing this type of sugar is environmentally irresponsible, but this claim is completely false. Highly abundant and thriving all over the world, coconut trees are not destroyed when tapped to obtain their sap. Nor does the tapping process impact the tree's ability to produce coconuts. By contrast, the farming of sugar beets—the main source of sugar in the United States—damages the environment because sugar beets are genetically modified and treated with the highly toxic weed killer glyphosate. GMO sugar beets are one of the least environmentally sustainable crops in the world.

Taste: Faintly like maple syrup or brown sugar.

Health benefits: Palm sugar has 10,000 times more potassium, 20 times more magnesium, and 20 times more iron than white sugar. Also, palm sugar has a lower glycemic index than traditional sugar. This means it can help keep your blood sugar more stable than white sugar.

Calories: 45 per tablespoon.

How to cook and bake with it: I love to use palm sugar for baking. Substitute it for granulated sugar at a 1:1 ratio in recipes.

Honey

What it is: A natural syrup made by bees using the nectar from flowers.

Taste: Varies depending on the flowers in the region.

Health benefits: Honey is the least refined sweetener in the world. You can get it right off the honeycomb, and it requires no processing. It contains antioxidants that have been shown to zap colon cancer–causing enzymes. It may also improve blood sugar control. Local honey has been shown to help fight seasonal allergies. Further, honey activates serotonin, the brain chemical that lifts the mood and encourages healthy sleep.

Calories: 64 per tablespoon.

How to cook and bake with it: Look for local and raw honey. Substitute it for granulated sugar at a 1:1 ratio in recipes. For best results with baking, cut back on the amount of other wet ingredients by ¼ cup for each cup of honey you use.

Maple Syrup

What it is: Derived from the sap of maple trees, this sweetener is boiled down, leaving the syrup.

Taste: A distinctive caramel-like flavor.

Health benefits: Maple syrup is full of minerals, vitamins, antioxidants, and amino acids. It has been shown in research to lower LDL ("bad") cholesterol and reduce abnormally elevated liver enzymes.

Calories: 52 per tablespoon.

How to cook and bake with it: Look for "Grade B maple syrup." It has more beneficial minerals than Grade A, because it is produced later in the harvesting season. Plus, it has a more robust maple flavor. Use ¾ cup maple syrup to replace 1 cup sugar, but reduce any liquids in recipes by 3 tablespoons per liquid to compensate.

Stevia

What it is: A noncaloric sweetener derived from a sweet-leafed plant that is typically grown in South America. But not all stevia is created equal.

In 1991, the FDA refused to approve stevia for use. Then, in 2008, the FDA approved the use of rebaudioside, a compound in the stevia plant. The Cargill Company figured out how to extract it, using a patentable process, then got rebaudioside approved. Coca-Cola uses rebaudioside in its Truvia sweetener. I don't know about you, but this scenario makes me suspicious. Think about it: Not until Big Food got involved did stevia become approved for use in food.

Truvia undergoes forty chemical steps to process the extract from the leaf. This process relies on chemicals like acetone, methanol, ethanol, acetonitrile, and isopropanol. Some of these chemicals are known carcinogens.

Truvia also contains a sweetening agent called erythritol. However, Big Food doesn't use natural erythritol. Instead, they start with GMO corn and take it through a complex fermentation process to create chemically pure erythritol. This erythritol has nasty side effects, like digestive problems. It can act as a strong laxative and give you diarrhea, for example. And in 2008, the Public Health and Medical Fraud Research Cooperative performed an extensive study showing that erythritol could drain your body of calcium and potassium—a problem that could damage your kidneys over time.

Maybe you've heard of Stevia In The Raw. It certainly sounds pure and natural, but take a careful look at the label and you'll see "dextrose" as the first item—so it's certainly not *just* stevia. PepsiCo's Pure Via isn't exactly pure, either: It lists dextrose first on its label, too. Dextrose is a sweetener likely made from genetically engineered corn, and like erythritol, it undergoes a long, complicated manufacturing process.

In light of these problems with commercial stevia, here's what I advise:

1. Buy a stevia plant for your garden, or purchase the pure dried leaves online. The leaves are naturally sweet. Just grind them up using a spice grinder or a mortar and pestle to make your own powdered stevia. Or you can float a few leaves in iced tea, hot tea, or any beverage that needs a little sweetening.

2. When buying commercial stevia or products sweetened with this herb, look for the designation "whole leaf stevia" on the ingredient label, rather than "rebaudioside" or "stevia extract." Also, look for a stevia extract that is 100 percent pure, without added ingredients (SweetLeaf & Trader Joe's have versions).

Try my recipe to make your own liquid stevia extract (see instructions on page 335).

Taste: Very sweet.

Calories: Noncaloric.

Health benefits: Stevia extract is 200 times sweeter than sugar, but it does not raise blood insulin levels.

How to cook and bake with it: 1 cup of sugar is the same as 1 teaspoon of liquid stevia or ⅓ to ½ teaspoon stevia extract powder. However, you must add a bulking agent to the recipe, since stevia alone can't perform a lot of normal cooking feats, such as softening cake batter, caramelizing, browning baked goods, or helping ferment yeast when baking bread. Good bulking agents include fruit purees, particularly applesauce. In this instance, you would use 1 teaspoon liquid stevia plus ⅓ cup applesauce or fruit puree to equal 1 cup of sugar.

**FOOD BABE ALERT:
AGAVE NECTAR IS NO SWEET DEAL**

Don't be tricked into thinking that agave nectar is a health food, especially you raw foodies. The real truth about agave nectar has been trickling out, and now we know that it's one of the most unhealthy and unnatural sweeteners you can eat.

Contrary to what the food industry has told us, agave nectar is not made from the sap of the agave plant. Instead, it is made from the starch of the plant's root. This starch, called inulin, is very similar to the starch in rice and corn. Inulin is made up of chains of fructose. As a result, agave nectar can contain between 70 percent and 90 percent fructose, which is more than you find in high-fructose corn syrup!

Although agave nectar doesn't cause a big blood sugar surge the way regular table sugar does, its fructose makes a beeline to your liver. The organ turns the fructose into triglycerides, which increase your risk of heart disease. Excessive fructose also interferes with the ability of cells to properly use insulin. This becomes a risk factor not only for diabetes, but also for a very serious condition called nonalcoholic fatty liver disease. This occurs when fat accumulates around the liver—a side effect of ingesting too much fructose.

Agave nectar is also a highly processed sweetener, produced in a way that very much resembles how cornstarch is processed into HFCS. Most commercially available agave is converted into fructose-rich syrup, by using genetically modified enzymes and a chemically intensive process that may include activated charcoal, resins, sulfuric and/or hydrofluoric acid, dicalite, and clarimex.

Does this sound healthy to you?

Agave nectar is unnatural and highly refined. It can make you gain weight, and it can affect your liver and your overall health. Do not swallow the marketing hype; leave this sweetener on the shelf.

I Did It the Food Babe Way

I love watching your videos and reading your stories; because of you I have changed the way and what we eat. Today I received a great review from my child's teacher, and it's because we removed all food dyes and sugar—he is able to focus and is doing great. Thank you and please keep up the great work. Keep the companies on their toes—your work is so important!

—Anne

If you develop this habit of staying away from added sugar and practice it on a regular basis, you'll be less likely to go overboard when presented with tempting refined sugar desserts. Even more, you'll naturally eat less sugar in the long run because your body will be getting real nutrition from food that hasn't been chemically altered. Eventually, you'll develop a distaste for refined sugar and your desire for ultimate nutrition will become instinctive. What a wonderful habit to develop and keep for life!

CHECKLIST

Today:

- ✓ I did my morning lemon water ritual.
- ✓ I enjoyed a green drink.
- ✓ I stopped drinking fluids with my meals.
- ✓ I drank, and bathed in, pure, clean, filtered water.
- ✓ I ate less dairy and made healthier dairy choices.
- ✓ I stopped drinking all sodas.
- ✓ I loved my liver by paying attention to alcohol consumption.
- ✓ I passed on fast food.
- ✓ I gave up refined sugar.

Day 10 — Eat Meat Responsibly

GROWING UP, I ATE meat almost every day. I scoffed at my mother's vegetarian cooking. Then, after learning about the horrible, inhumane treatment of farm animals, I completely changed direction and became a vegan. I ate no animal products of any kind and relied fully on vegetables, fruits, and grains.

After that, I felt great and looked great. Intuitively, though, I knew that I was more vulnerable to deficiencies in certain nutrients, such as vitamin B12, omega-3 fatty acids, iron, zinc, calcium, and vitamin D — all critical for energy and mood, among other things. So I gradually reintroduced meat into my diet. I now eat various types of meat, but I drastically limit my consumption. I have eight ounces or so a week, sometimes every two weeks, making my average around 20 to 30 pounds a year. Compare this to the typical American who eats 270 pounds of meat a year — it's a dramatic difference.

I also know the source of the meat I eat, and I make sure it fulfills the following criteria: It's raised under humane conditions, it's not pumped full of growth hormones and antibiotics, it's grown locally, and it provides all the vital nutrients I need for great health.

Today, I'd describe myself as nearly vegetarian. I'm still a fan of the vegan/vegetarian lifestyle, but I'm not a sanctimonious diehard who goes around bashing meat (unless it's of poor quality and raised irresponsibly). I know that if I eat too much poor-quality meat, I'm putting myself in harm's way. Such eating habits are a factor in heart disease, cancer, and diabetes, and can mean exposure to cancer-causing dioxins, which are found in chemical pesticides used to grow animal feed. I do advocate eating more plant-based foods than anything else. You can get all the protein you need from eating a mostly plant-based diet. Consuming less meat and eating it responsibly have been good for my health, the planet, and my dress size.

You can develop this wonderful habit by following the steps outlined below.

Cutting back on meat and eating it responsibly are easier than you think. Here's how to start.

EAT MEAT AS A CONDIMENT

I want to live to be a hundred and still be able to climb a mountain, don't you? One big secret to living longer and feeling great is to eat more veggies and less meat. When you plan your meals, put veggies center stage and relegate meat to the role of a condiment, not the starring attraction on your plate.

A slew of research has found we should be eating a diet that veers toward a plant-based one if we want to live longer and protect ourselves from a whole variety of cancers. If the habit of eating less meat feels new and uncomfortable to you, you might want to start by going meatless only a couple of times a week. Then progress to several meatless meals during a week. Or try becoming a weekday vegetarian, avoiding meat during the week but enjoying it on the weekends.

BOYCOTT FACTORY FARM MEAT

I'm an animal lover, so when I found out about the stomach-curdling practices of raising animals at "factory farms," I was incensed. Animals grown on factory farms subsist in horrific conditions. They live a life of cramped conditions, ill health, and injury or death during transportation, and they face the risk of not being properly stunned before they are slaughtered for human consumption. The majority of broiler chickens are raised in sheds, with sometimes as many as 100,000 crammed into one building. Pigs are given no anesthesia when their tails are cut off. Cows are given hormones that cause their udders to get so big that the animals can barely stand up on their own. Many animals never see the sun or feel anything but concrete under their feet. Many become crippled and feeble; others are unable to reach the feed or water and die.

Such inhumane methods affect our food chain, with terrible consequences. This level of animal cruelty causes stress to animals. They get sick, and then we consume sick animals, which in turn can cause us to become ill.

I'd rather see you buy meat that does not come from factory farms. Yes, that meat may cost more. But rather than judge the value of food in terms of dollars, think of its value in terms of nutrition—and your health. Food from factory farms might be cheaper, but not when you consider how much more nutrition you get from organic meat.

EAT LESS MEAT AND DAIRY AND CHANGE THE WORLD

Cut back on your consumption of these foods, and you will:

Feed more people. Our planet is home to more than 7 billion people, many of whom don't have enough to eat. Experts project we'll have another 3 billion mouths to feed within fifty years. However, we can feed 2,000 people with the same amount of grain that it takes to feed only 100 cows.

Reduce pollution dramatically. The meat and dairy industry generates 18 percent more climate-changing pollutants than all modes of transportation combined.

Save water. It takes 60 pounds of water to produce one pound of potatoes, but it takes more than 4,000 pounds of water to produce one pound of beef.

Improve your health. Overconsumption of meat has been proven to cause heart disease, cancer, and diabetes, and it's more likely to do so than any other food we eat—a fact supported by the acclaimed China Study, which examined the relationship between diet and chronic disease. And by cutting back on animal products, you can dramatically reduce your exposure to the cancer-causing dioxins that are found in the chemical pesticides used to grow animal feed.

BUY LOCAL

When I eat meat, I know its source: It's usually local and organic. One of the best ways to obtain the meat and other food that is optimum for your health is to buy directly from local farms, where you can shake the farmer's hand and talk to him or her about how his or her livestock is raised. You can connect online with farmers' markets or use a subscription-based community-supported agriculture (CSA) program to purchase organic meat.

When you're dining out, ask your server where the restaurant purchases its meat. If the answer is something like Tyson or Smithfield, that indicates the meat is probably processed to the hilt. The same goes for fish: Make sure it's wild-caught and not farm-raised. When I travel, I have less fear of eating local meat. I know it isn't coming from a factory farm operation—and therefore it's fresher and more likely to be contaminant-free. However, I always ask if the meat was raised without antibiotics and growth hormone.

Buying animal products directly from the farmer is becoming increasingly common. I like to know that food animals had a "free-range" life and weren't kept in a crate and pumped with antibiotics in some Big Ag operation. Ideally, meat should come from a healthy, contented cow that grazed on an open, green pasture its whole life.

ENJOY GRASS-FED VERSUS GRAIN-FED

Since the forties, most US cattle have been raised on grain so that they bulk up faster for mass production and earlier slaughter. The process has been helped along by hormones and antibiotics—a system fraught with environmental and health problems.

Raising cattle on grass takes too long for the typical factory farm. However, a grass-fed cow is ultimately healthier for you and for the animal. Scientific studies tell us that grass-fed meat is lower in artery-clogging saturated fat and higher in omega-3 fatty acids. Grass-fed meat is also a superior source of vitamins A and E, as well as the beneficial fat conjugated linoleic acid (CLA).

READ LABELS IN GROCERY STORES

When it comes to meat, milk, and eggs, look for the "USDA organic" label. This will help avoid the worst factory-farmed animal products in grocery stores. But just because a product is certified organic doesn't guarantee that it's 100 percent free of nonorganic ingredients, nor does it guarantee that the animals were treated humanely. You have to read and remember what the various labels mean. The chart below will help guide you.

GREEN LIGHT LABELS

These label claims are defined by a formal set of animal care standards that are publicly available. Compliance with these standards is verified by a third-party audit. Look for these labels when you're purchasing meat and dairy.

Label	Find On:	Standards
American Grass-fed Certified	Dairy, beef, lamb, and goat	A program certifying that meat and dairy come only from animals that ate nothing but their mother's milk and grass their whole lives. No hormones or antibiotics are permitted.
American Humane Certified	Dairy, eggs, chicken, turkey, beef, veal, bison, lamb, goat, and pork	This label signifies that the animals were raised under humane standards.
Animal Welfare Approved	Dairy, eggs, chicken, goose, duck, turkey, beef, bison, lamb, goat, pork, and rabbit	A program that audits and certifies family farms that raise their animals humanely.
Certified Humane	Dairy, eggs, chicken, turkey, beef, veal, lamb, goat, and pork	A certification and labeling program that sets rigorous standards addressing food, shelter, and compassionate slaughter for animals.
Certified Organic	Dairy, eggs, chicken, goose, duck, turkey, beef, bison, lamb, goat, and pork	Animals must be allowed to roam outdoors, with cows, sheep, and goats given access to pasture. The use of hormones and antibiotics is prohibited, but surgical mutilations (such as castration) without any pain relief are permitted.
Global Animal Partnership	Chicken, turkey, beef, and pork	A five-step animal welfare rating program that outlines specifics on how animals are cared for and raised.

YELLOW LIGHT CLAIMS

These claims are only somewhat reliable. Compliance with USDA's definition is not verified on the farm by the government or any independent third party.

Label	Find On:	Standards
Cage Free	Eggs	The poultry does not live in cages.
Free Range/Free Roaming	All products (including eggs)	The animals have been allowed to roam outdoors.

(Continued)

Grass Fed	Dairy, beef, bison, lamb, and goat	Animals that throughout their lives received 80 percent or more of their primary energy source from grass, green or range pasture, or forage.
Humanely Raised/ Humanely Handled	All products	This implies that farm animals received care above and beyond what the animal industries currently provide in factory farms.
Naturally Raised	Chicken, turkey, goose, duck, beef, bison, lamb, goat, and pork	This standard guarantees that no growth hormones or antibiotics were used and that no animal by-products were fed to the animals.
No Added Hormones/ No Hormones Administered	Dairy, beef, bison, and lamb	This label indicates that the animals were not given any added hormones over the course of their lifetimes.
No Antibiotics Administered/Raised without Antibiotics	All products	Affixed on milk and meat products, this label implies that the cows or chickens were never given antibiotics.
Pasture Raised/ Pasture Grown/ Meadow Raised	All products	Animals were raised outdoors and given continuous access to pastures.
Sustainably Farmed	All products	Food production techniques don't harm the environment and preserve agricultural land. But there's no guarantee that sustainable products are also organic.

RED LIGHT CLAIMS

These claims mean very little with regard to animal welfare.		
Halal	Chicken, turkey, goose, duck, beef, lamb, and goat	Products are prepared according to Islamic law and under Islamic authority. Halal products may have been slaughtered without first being stunned—a practice considered inhumane by animal welfare advocates.
Kosher	Chicken, turkey, goose, duck, beef, lamb, and goat	Products are prepared under rabbinic supervision. Kosher products may have been slaughtered without first being stunned—a practice considered inhumane by animal welfare advocates.
Natural	Chicken, turkey, goose, duck, beef, bison, lamb, goat, and pork	A USDA policy states that "natural" can be used on products that contain no artificial ingredients or added color and are only minimally processed. This label has no relevance to how the animal was raised.

United Egg Producers (UEP) Certified	Eggs	Meets minimum voluntary industry standards, which, according to the Humane Society of the United States, "permit routine cruel and inhumane factory farm practices."
USDA Process Verified	All products	This label indicates that the USDA has verified that a company is following its own standards in raising animals.
Vegetarian Fed	All products	The animal's diet did not contain any animal by-products. This label has no relevance to how the animal was raised. This also means the animal was likely raised on GMO grains like corn, soy, and cottonseed.

Adapted and condensed from: The Animal Welfare Institute, www.awionline.org.

BE CHOOSY ABOUT SEAFOOD

We know that eating fish is a healthy habit. Fish has virtually no saturated fat, and it's high in protein, omega-3 fatty acids, selenium, and vitamins D and B2. Eating fish from time to time helps prevent heart disease, stroke, and cancer, reduces hypertension, and boosts brainpower.

It's ironic, though: We turn to fish for a healthier diet, only to find that farm-raised fish and seafood are the subject of serious health concerns. Salmon is a good example. Farmed salmon are usually not fed their typical diet of krill, shrimp, and other fish, so it's hard for them to get the same amount of omega-3 fatty acids that wild salmon have. These fatty acids are crucial protection against heart disease, arthritis, and depression.

Farmed salmon are often fed a mixture of highly contaminated fish meal and fish oil mixed with corn and soy products, because it is cheap and helps fatten them up. This practice leads to horrible side effects. It turns the salmon gray, because they are not eating the creatures that make their flesh naturally pink. To fix this, salmon farmers are allowed to feed the fish supplements to help dye the salmon pink like wild salmon.

Farmed salmon are also less nutritious and contain a high level of toxins. Many species of farmed salmon are intentionally fattened, and this allows PCBs, or polychlorinated biphenyls, which are toxins, to accumulate more rapidly in their tissues.

Think farm-raised tilapia might be a better bet? Not really. Recent studies have concluded that eating tilapia may worsen inflammation, which can lead to heart disease, arthritis, asthma, and a world of other serious health problems. In fact, scientists have found that the inflammatory potential of tilapia is far greater than that of a hamburger or bacon!

What about shellfish? Not so fast. Shrimp actually holds the distinction of being the dirtiest of all seafood, according to Food & Water Watch. Ninety percent of the shrimp we eat is imported. This farmed shrimp is tainted with antibiotics, residues from chemicals used to clean pens, and filth like mouse hair, rat hair, and pieces of insects. Even E. coli has been detected in imported shrimp.

Holy mackerel! Who knew fish could raise such a stir?

SCOOP UP HEALTHY PROTEIN POWDER

If you cut back on meat and dairy, you might want to supplement with protein powders. There's something you need to know about these supplements. The food industry is making an absolute killing by selling protein powders that are filled with highly processed denatured proteins, chemicals, preservatives, and other additives. It's easy to fall prey to a protein powder that makes claims that no one is checking on or regulating. That is why it is critical to investigate your protein powders before taking that scoop.

Years ago, I used to buy a delicious vanilla whey protein from GNC to add to my smoothies. I was religious about using this particular brand. When it was suddenly discontinued, I became outraged. I called every GNC in town, searching for more. Eventually, I got to the bottom of why it was discontinued: The health department found rat droppings in samples of the protein at the manufacturing plant. It turns out I'd been drinking rat droppings all those years!

Needless to say, I've never looked at protein powders the same way again. I now do intensive research on a powder before I ever consider putting it in my body.

The key to finding a high-quality protein powder is asking the right questions: Is it organic and free of pesticides? Is it GMO-free? How is it processed? Does the processing allow it to retain its nutritional quality, its vitamins and minerals? Does it contain artificial or refined sugars? Does it have heavy metals?

Yes, I said "heavy metals." An eye-opening investigation conducted by *Consumer Reports* in July 2010 revealed that several popular, highly processed protein powders like Myoplex, Muscle Milk, Designer Whey, and GNC brand all contained arsenic, cadmium, and lead. Yikes.

I still love protein powder, so I've made it a point to use Nutiva hemp protein powder and Tera'sWhey organic whey. Both are free of pesticides, GMOs, and all those nasty chemicals. For more analysis on protein powders, go to foodbabe.com.

SKIP THE FAKE MEAT

Are you among those eating fake meat or eggs made in a laboratory petri dish? A lot of people aren't aware that meat replacements, especially the newer ones on the market, are loaded with chemicals and possibly GMOs.

One of the main ingredients in fake beef and chicken is soy protein isolate. It's processed by soaking soybeans in a chemical called hexane, whose emissions are a main constituent of smog. Hexane is also a known carcinogen and neurotoxin that has been linked to brain tumors. Despite this, the FDA doesn't regulate it.

Some of the newer fake meat and egg producers claim they don't use hexane as part of their production process. However, Beyond Meat gets its soy protein isolate from DuPont-owned Solae, whose Illinois plant spewed out 281,000 pounds of airborne hexane in 2011, according to the EPA.

Also, fake meats may contain maltodextrin, natural flavorings, gluten, canola oil, evaporated cane juice, dipotassium phosphate, titanium dioxide (for color), and potassium chloride, among other chemicals.

You might be tempted to ask who in their right mind would dare eat these products. The truth is that a lot of people who eat fake meats think they're eating healthy but don't actually know what they're ingesting. I worry that the food industry will continue to create these substitutes in laboratories, and then ten years down the road, we're going to find out that they cause cancer and other diseases.

Many people become vegans or vegetarians for health reasons, but fake meat doesn't strike me as contributing to a healthy lifestyle. Keeping your body healthy means staying nutritionally as close to nature as you can and as far away from fake foods as possible. I'm just not interested in eating something made in a factory and engineered to taste like something else. Choose the real thing a few times a week instead, and your health will soar.

BE CAUTIOUS WITH VEGGIE BURGERS

Should you eat highly processed veggie burgers as part of a healthy diet? I don't recommend it. I'm downright frightened of the ingredients in most frozen veggie burgers, and here's why:

Neurotoxins and carcinogens. The majority of store-bought veggie burgers contain some form of soy. As I stated above, nonorganic soy is extracted using hexane. The food industry uses the hexane extraction method because it is cheap, but it damages the environment and our bodies.

Cheap oils. If you see the words "canola oil," "soy oil," "corn oil," "sunflower oil," and/or "safflower oil," those products are likely extracted with hexane, too. But what further complicates this matter (if having a neurotoxin by-product in your burger is not enough) is that the overconsumption of these cheap oils is causing an abundance of omega-6 fatty acids in our diets. The imbalance of omega-6 fatty acids increases the risk of inflammation, heart disease, obesity, and prostate and bone cancer.

Textured vegetable protein, aka TVP. Several frozen veggie burgers are developed using soy products and textured vegetable protein. TVP is one of those foods I avoid at all costs; no one will ever convince me to eat something this processed. TVP is extracted from soy at a superhigh heat and made into a powder before it is "reshaped" into strips, chunks, and granules and then put back into food. The processing can also add artificial and natural flavors, MSG, colorings, emulsifiers, and thickening agents—including nitrosamine, which is a carcinogen no one should be consuming.

MSG. There are several hidden sources of MSG in vegetarian meat substitutes. MSG increases your insulin response, tricking your body into thinking you can eat more than you actually should. And this is exactly how scientists make rats obese, by feeding them MSG-laced food. Knowing that there is a potential substance that can trick me into eating more food is reason enough to avoid it at all costs. But MSG is also linked to terrible reactions in humans, like migraines, toxicity, and autoimmune disorders in people that have a sensitivity.

Genetically modified organisms (GMOs). If your veggie burger contains anything derived from corn or soy, you can almost guarantee it comes from genetically modified seeds, unless it is certified 100 percent organic. Genetically modified foods have been linked to toxicity, allergic reactions, and fertility issues and have not been studied for their long-term effects on our health.

A *veggie burger you can enjoy.* There are two delicious products that I rubber-stamp for quality and taste: Hilary's Eat Well burgers and Sunshine Burgers. These burgers contain none of the crappy chemicals I listed above and are actually really delicious!

Meat has its place in your diet, as long as you understand your options and make the healthiest choices—those that are good for your body and the land.

FOOD BABE SHOPPING LIST FOR MEATS AND PROTEINS

Organic, grass-fed beef
Organic chicken
Organic turkey
Applegate organic bacon
Wild salmon
Wild, locally caught fish

Organic, pasture-raised eggs
Hilary's Eat Well burgers
Sunshine Burgers
Nutiva hemp protein powder

CHECKLIST

Today:

✓ I did my morning lemon water ritual.

✓ I enjoyed a green drink.

✓ I stopped drinking fluids with my meals.

✓ I drank, and bathed in, pure, clean, filtered water.

✓ I ate less dairy and made healthier dairy choices.

✓ I stopped drinking all sodas.

✓ I loved my liver by paying attention to alcohol consumption.

✓ I passed on fast food.

✓ I gave up refined sugar.

✓ I ate less meat and I ate it responsibly.

Day 11 — Eat Raw More Than
Half the Time

I LOVE RAW FOODS. I'm talking about raw organic foods: natural, non-meat foods such as fruits, vegetables, nuts, and seeds that are uncooked. The absolute best thing about eating raw is that the food industry hasn't adulterated your food with chemicals, additives, preservatives, or BPA and other harmful packaging materials. It's worth mentioning, too, that cooking certain foods tends to deplete vitamins and destroy enzymes that aid in digestion and help defend the body against harmful inflammation.

When these foods are raw, you're getting some of the best possible nutrition—and it's the closest you can get to Mother Nature without growing your own food. Several years ago, before I was aware of the benefits of eating this way, raw foods made up around 5 percent of my diet. Today, 60 percent of my diet is composed of raw foods.

Once I made the change, I was no longer a prisoner of sweet cravings—those vanished, along with ravenous afternoon hunger. I craved vegetables instead. I couldn't get enough broccoli, spinach, kale, carrots, and fresh salads. I wanted green juice all the time. I dreamt of apples. My whole body was smiling. And I know that raw foods have been another factor in stabilizing my weight, leaving me with no need to rigidly diet.

Eating raw foods brings you a number of health benefits beyond weight control. One of those benefits is better heart health. A study published in 2005 in the *Journal of Nutrition* affirmed that a diet high in raw fruits and veggies reduced bad cholesterol, technically known as LDL cholesterol (the artery-clogging type).

Adding raw almonds to your diet scores big for heart health, too. In 1992, the *Journal of the American College of Nutrition* reported that eating 100 grams of raw almonds daily (about eighty nuts) could lower your overall cholesterol in just four weeks. This is because the fat in almonds is largely monounsaturated—so if you put the monos in your diet and subtract the saturated fat, your cholesterol will drop.

These findings made me wonder if we really need all those cholesterol-lowering drugs, with their potentially nasty side effects like liver damage. Maybe we should be popping almonds instead of pills.

Raw foods have a strong anticancer benefit. Certain fruits and vegetables act like protective shields to help prevent specific types of cancer—and there is a tremendous amount of research on this. Here's a roundup:

Cancer	Cancer-Preventing Raw Foods
Thyroid cancer	Raw vegetables, persimmons, and tangerines
Bladder cancer	Raw cruciferous vegetables (broccoli, Brussels sprouts, cabbage, cauliflower, kale, mustard greens, and radishes)
Ovarian cancer	Raw endive
Breast cancer	Raw vegetables, especially carrots
Rectal cancer	Raw fruits

The link between raw foods and fantastic health is just too strong to ignore. Start eating more raw foods today. It isn't hard—you just have to accustom yourself to the different methods of food preparation, such as juicing or tossing raw greens into your protein shake (which I hope you're already doing). It doesn't have to be a radical change, and it will feel simple once you get into the flow of things.

THE FOOD BABE WAY

BEGIN GRADUALLY WITH RAW FOODS

Start by adding one or two raw foods to your diet—today. This can be as simple as adding a fresh piece of fruit to your daily green juice at breakfast, or including ingredients like tomatoes, dark leaf lettuce, sprouts, onions, and cucumbers in your sandwiches. Move from there to having one or two raw vegetable salads daily—at lunch and dinner, for example.

Experiment with different types of salad greens, such as dandelion. My brother jokes with me every time I order a salad that doesn't resemble iceberg lettuce—he calls whatever I'm having a weed salad. Those weed salads are nutritional gold mines and usually contain one or two sprigs of dandelion leaves. Dandelion has amazing powers to detox your liver, and I'm always looking for ways I can include this supergreen in my diet. It's rich in iron and high in calcium, has more protein than spinach, and is packed with antioxidants (all the things that keep you looking and feeling young). And for the record, my brother now eats "weed" salads, too, because he sees the benefits firsthand!

COMBINE RAW WITH COOKED

Eating raw more than half the time is easy. I love this habit because you get a megadose of nutrition from raw, organic food, and you still get to enjoy cooked foods throughout the day. For instance, if you're having pizza for dinner, start your meal with a raw salad. Here's an example of how you can mix raw foods with cooked foods over the course of a day:

Breakfast: ½ cup cooked oatmeal, topped with 1 cup raw berries and 1 tablespoon raw walnuts.

Lunch: A big raw salad for lunch, topped with cooked lentils.

Snack: Fruit, veggie sticks, or a green smoothie or green juice.

Dinner: A small side salad of raw greens with dressing, organic chicken, sweet potatoes, and steamed broccoli.

SPROUT GOOD HEALTH

I've always loved sprouts—they're one of my recommended superfoods, and I try to eat them often. Every time I enjoy sprouts, I notice a huge burst in energy. I have even started my own sprout garden at home so I can have access to them all the time. Sprouts have an enormous amount of live enzymes compared to cooked fruits and vegetables. Their vitamin content is incredibly high, and they increase the alkalinity of your body (remember, an alkaline body avoids diseases like cancer).

Although many people are familiar only with alfalfa sprouts or mung sprouts (as found in chop suey), it's common today to see a whole range of sprouts on the grocery shelf: broccoli, clover, radish, lentil, sunflower, and more. Be adventuresome and see how many you can try.

SNACK IN THE RAW

When I used to work in a cubicle all day, I'd take time every Sunday to prepare five containers of chopped veggies to take to work. Every day, I'd eat one container of raw veggies before lunch. My body was getting the regular nutrition that it needed, so I had none of the 3 p.m. cravings that drive most people to the vending machine for an injection of sugary snacks.

For between meals, do the same: Snack on raw, cut-up organic veggies. Keep cut vegetables such as carrots, celery, broccoli, cauliflower, and peppers in the refrigerator for quick snacks. For a sweet bite, grab a piece of fresh fruit or a cup of fresh berries. And don't forget to juice. A veggie-fruit juice is one of the best all-around snacks you can choose. It staves off hunger without spoiling your appetite for a meal.

Continue adding raw food to your routine, and before long you'll achieve your 60 percent (or more) raw quota—and you'll discover how radiant health really feels.

CHECKLIST

Today:
- ✓ I did my morning lemon water ritual.
- ✓ I enjoyed a green drink.
- ✓ I stopped drinking fluids with my meals.
- ✓ I drank, and bathed in, pure, clean, filtered water.
- ✓ I ate less dairy and made healthier dairy choices.
- ✓ I stopped drinking all sodas.
- ✓ I loved my liver by paying attention to alcohol consumption.
- ✓ I passed on fast food.
- ✓ I gave up refined sugar.
- ✓ I ate less meat and I ate it responsibly.
- ✓ I increased the raw plant foods in my diet.

Day 12 — Break Some Bread — and Other Carbs

Remember when low-carb diets were all the rage? When people who snuck a slice of bread were at risk of doing hard time in a pasta factory?

I declare those days over! You can eat certain breads, pastas, and other grains on the Food Babe Way Eating Plan—as long as they're the right carbs—starting today.

Today's habit calls for you to cut out starchy *white* carbs—white rice, white flour, white pastas, and white flour products. These are high glycemic index foods, meaning they can jack up your blood sugar quickly. In response, your body churns out insulin, the hormone that escorts glucose into cells to be burned as energy, or stores excess glucose as body fat, particularly in your tummy—not a good reaction if you're trying to lose weight or stay healthy. White carbs are the devil in food form!

BEWARE: THE WHITE CARB ADDITIVES

Breads, pastas, and other white flour products are processed from wheat and thus are not always easy for your body to digest. Wheat can overwork your pancreatic enzymes and cause chronic inflammation. It can disrupt the good intestinal bacteria in your digestive system. It's addictive, too, making you crave more and ultimately eat more.

Wheat crops in this country have been through some serious genetic manipulation to make them profitable for the food industry and less healthy for us. Wheat products also contain the dreaded gluten, which is a protein found in wheat and other grains. If you are sensitive to gluten, eating foods that contain it can cause inflammation and damage to the lining of the small intestine—a condition that blocks nutrients from being properly absorbed.

If you don't have a sensitivity to gluten, there's still a big problem with wheat: We as a culture eat too much of it. Just take a look at the typical American diet: a white bagel or muffin for breakfast, a white bread sandwich for lunch, and white rolls or pasta for dinner—not to mention extracurricular carbs like crackers and cookies. That's a lot of white carbs in just one day.

The second big problem with wheat-based white carbs, namely, those sold in grocery stores and served in restaurants, is that they're full of nonfood ingredients. Take a look:

Dough conditioners. I can't complain about these enough, so here I go again. Although unnecessary in traditional or home baking, these additives are dumped into commercial recipes to make the process faster and cheaper for the food industry. The worst offenders are azodicarbonamide (the same chemical in yoga mats and shoe rubber), potassium bromate, DATEM, monoglycerides, diglycerides, and sodium stearoyl lactylate. All have been linked to health issues. And they're created from fats such as soybean oil or corn oil, which are most likely genetically modified.

Preservatives. Baked goods are meant to be eaten within a few days of baking unless frozen. Food companies, however, lace their products with preservatives to retard spoilage. If you see preservatives listed like calcium propionate, which is linked to ADHD, put the food down and keep searching.

GMOs. Most commercially available baked goods contain one or many genetically modified ingredients, such as soy lecithin, soybean oil, corn oil, cornstarch, or soy flour. Although GMOs have not been tested long-term on humans, it is well known that the pesticides sprayed on genetically modified foods are toxic and considered poisonous. Some GMOs are created by inserting a Bt soil bacteria into the seed itself so it "naturally" produces a pesticide that makes an insect's stomach explode when it tries to eat the seed. How's that for a yuck factor?

Added sugar. There's nothing wrong with a little honey to bring out the sweetness in bread and other carbs, but most manufacturers are using high-fructose corn syrup, a GMO sugar made from sugar beets, or artificial sweeteners like sucralose. "Light" breads, in particular, can be full of sweeteners, so proceed with caution on that front.

Artificial flavors and coloring. These additives are made from petroleum and are linked to several health issues, such as hyperactivity in children, allergies, and asthma. They will all appear on the label because the FDA requires it. However, ingredients like "caramel coloring" can fool you into thinking this ingredient is a real food. Most industrial caramel coloring is formed by heating ammonia and is considered a carcinogen when created this way.

WHY I LIMIT MY FLOUR CONSUMPTION

Typical flour is milled, and this process discards all the essential nutrients contained by the original grain. The wheat germ and cellulose (fiber) are removed and the heat that is generated to crush the grain into flour destroys any vitamin or mineral normally found in the grain, leaving a white powder devoid of life. It's essentially dead food. So the food manufacturers have to "enrich" it with added synthetic vitamins and minerals.

The next part is even scarier. Freshly milled flour usually isn't acceptable for consumption because of the look, feel, and smell of it. The FDA has approved over sixty chemicals for manufacturers to use to improve the aesthetics and shelf life of flour. Chlorine is used to bleach conventional flours to remove the smell and change the color. The flour is put into a gas chamber and treated with chlorine dioxide, which leaches out all the vitamin E and leaves a chemical called dichlorostearic acid.

Additionally, treating flour with chlorine can create more chemical by-products that have been known to react to other proteins and cause nervous system damage in humans. Wouldn't it be nice if the ingredient labels on food included all of these random chemicals, so we would actually know what's in our food?

As for whole wheat flour, it's more nutritious than white flour because the entire wheat germ stays intact and is not discarded. Wheat germ, however, has natural oils in it. These oils can turn rancid within just a few months. To prevent this, manufacturers often add chemicals to extend shelf life, making the flour less nutritious.

Thus, you'll find that a lot of brown breads—even those that are sold as 100 percent whole wheat—are laced with additives like refined sugar, artificial colors, dough conditioners, preservatives, and other questionable chemicals. Here are some prime examples:

NATURE'S OWN 100% WHOLE WHEAT

Stone-ground whole wheat flour, water, yeast, **brown sugar,** wheat gluten, contains 2% or less of each of the following: salt, **dough conditioners** (contains one or more of the following: **sodium stearoyl lactylate, calcium stearoyl lactylate, monoglycerides, mono- and diglycerides, distilled monoglycerides, calcium peroxide, calcium iodate, datem, ethoxylated mono- and diglycerides, enzymes, ascorbic acid), soybean oil,** vinegar, cultured wheat flour, **monocalcium phosphate, ammonium sulfate, citric acid,** sodium citrate, **soy lecithin,** natamycin (to retard spoilage).

THOMAS' 100% WHOLE WHEAT HEARTY MUFFINS

Whole wheat flour, water, yeast, wheat gluten, honey, farina, **cornmeal,** salt, cracked wheat, **preservatives (calcium propionate, sorbic acid),** grain vinegar, calcium sulfate, **soybean oil,** wheat starch, **mono- and diglycerides, datem, natural flavor, sodium stearoyl lactylate, ethoxylated mono- and diglycerides,** wheat sour, **dextrose,** calcium carbonate, guar gum, lactic acid, molasses, fumaric acid, whey, **soy flour,* caramel color,** acetic acid, **sucralose, citric acid,** sodium citrate, natamycin (a natural mold inhibitor), **potassium sorbate (preservative),** nonfat milk. *Trivial amount of soy flour.

PEPPERIDGE FARMS FARMHOUSE 100% WHOLE WHEAT BREAD

Whole wheat flour, water, nonfat milk (adds a trivial amount of cholesterol), **high-fructose corn syrup, soybean oil,** wheat gluten, yeast;

contains 2 percent or less of: honey, unsulphured molasses, oat fiber, salt, butter (adds a trivial amount of cholesterol), **vegetable mono- and digylcerides, calcium propionate (to retard spoilage), soy lecithin,** and enzymes.

THE FOOD BABE WAY

Before I share my top recommendations for the best (and healthiest) carbs on the market, I will tell you I eat bread only a few times a week, with some exceptions. When I travel, I like to enjoy the local culture (think croissants in France and pizza in Italy). I'm not about giving up whole food groups. The Food Babe Way is about balance and nutritious choices.

Here are the breads I feel good about buying:

GO FOR SPROUTED GRAINS

I love sprouted grains because they are technically vegetables, created when a grain is soaked in water and then sprouts into a little plant. These sprouts are then ground up to make bread. The body responds better to sprouted grain breads. There's not a huge insulin or sugar spike like you get from a refined flour product, so your body won't gain weight, produce inflammation, or experience the sugar metabolism problems that are common in diabetes.

Sprouted grains are much more easily digested and absorbed than starchy flour and contain more vitamins, minerals, and antioxidants than whole grains. My favorite sprouted grain bread is the classic Ezekiel 4:9 Sprouted Grain Bread by Food For Life—it's made from six organic sprouted grains and absolutely no flour! This combo of sprouted grains contains all nine essential amino acids, which makes up a complete protein. I use the cinnamon raisin version to make my yummy Cinnamon Raisin French Toast Crunch (recipe on page 302). There are no preservatives in these breads, so I keep them in my freezer and take out portions as I need them. I also love the sesame seed bread, wholegrain tortillas, corn tortillas, and English muffins by Food For Life.

Hands down, these are the healthiest breads on the market. They are available in most health food stores and some conventional stores in the freezer section. Other good sprouted breads are Manna Organics bread and Dave's Killer Bread sprouted wheat, which are both a healthy combo of organic sprouted wheat and seeds.

GET TO KNOW ANCIENT GRAINS

Cultivated for thousands of years, ancient grains represent some of the oldest grains consumed by humans. They include spelt, quinoa, amaranth, millet, and sorghum. Most are gluten-free and all are packed with vitamins, minerals, fiber, and protein. They offer tremendous benefits, such as preventing cancer, heart disease, and high blood pressure. Now you can find them in breads, which are a great way to reap these benefits. One of my favorite ancient grains breads is made by Manna. Gluten-free, it is baked with brown rice, sorghum, millet, amaranth, quinoa, and chia seeds.

GO GLUTEN-FREE WITH CAUTION

Make sure the bread you are buying is labeled "gluten-free" if you're trying to avoid gluten. I've been disheartened by many of the gluten-free breads on the market, however, because many are baked with various preservatives and additives. Please note, too, that almost all gluten-free breads contain added sugar in the form of honey, molasses, agave nectar, or evaporated cane juice.

For those of you cutting out gluten, here's a list of the healthiest gluten-free breads (note that all of these products contain added sugar):

- Seedy Buckwheat Molasses Bread—Happy Campers
- Gluten-Free Rice Almond Bread—Food For Life
- Gluten-Free Exotic Black Rice Bread—Food For Life
- Gluten-Free Super Chia Bread—Nature's Path
- Good Morning Millet Toaster Cakes—Ancient Grains Bakery
- Gluten-Free Deli Rye Style Bread—Canyon Bakehouse

CHOOSE ORGANIC

Last but not least, remember to always choose bread that is made with real certified organic ingredients. The wheat that is used to make most bread is heavily sprayed with pesticides. By choosing certified organic products, you will avoid exposure to GMOs.

DO PASTA RIGHT

I get a lot of questions about the products I buy at the grocery store and use on a daily basis because readers know I've done the investigative work. One of those questions is always "What are the healthiest pastas available and which ones do you recommend?" There are a lot of options out there, and it can be a daunting task to navigate the maze of choices. You might also wonder what is left when you take away wheat flour pastas. Fortunately, I can help. Here are my top pasta recommendations:

Zucchini noodles. You can turn zucchini and summer squash into noodles using a tool called a spiralizer. I admit these noodles aren't technically pasta, but they sure taste like pasta. If you're going grain-free or want a less heavy alternative to traditional pasta, this is a fantastic way to get your pasta fix. You can eat the noodles raw or warmed slightly in a skillet with sauce. Also, if you don't want to use a spiralizer, you can slice the zucchini or squash into thin slices like lasagna noodles and bake them. Remember to choose non-GMO and organic zucchini and squash, since the majority of these veggies are grown from genetically modified seeds.

Spaghetti squash noodles. Here's another veggie-based noodle and one of the most versatile pasta substitutes around. You simply cut the squash in half and bake the halves for about 45 minutes. Use a fork to pull out the strands, which resemble noodles—and taste like them, too. Spaghetti squash has a quarter of the calories of traditional pasta per cup, so you can eat it to your heart's content. One of my favorite ways to eat this squash is with homemade spicy tomato sauce and raw goat's milk hard cheese. Check out my recipe for Turkey Meatballs with Spaghetti Squash (page 320). Heavenly!

Bean pastas. Tolerant is a brand that makes lentil-based and black bean pastas. Their red lentil pasta mixed with some white wine, grass-fed butter, garlic, and raw-milk Parmesan makes an insanely good dish. A company named Explore Asian makes the most delicious pasta using 100 percent mung beans. The noodles are chewier than traditional pasta, but they are loaded with protein and fiber for a satisfying meal. The recipe for fettuccini on the back of the package works like a charm and is my favorite way to prepare these deliciously healthy noodles.

Soba buckwheat noodles. I love buckwheat! It's not technically a grain but a fruit seed. Suitable for gluten-free diets, buckwheat is high in protein and fiber. Look for 100 percent buckwheat, because there are a lot of impostors out there who use a blend of wheat and buckwheat. Eden Foods makes 100 percent buckwheat noodles, and Orgran offers 90 percent buckwheat, 10 percent rice spiral-shaped pasta. Both are delicious.

Sprouted grain pastas. These dense, hearty pastas are made from sprouted wheat kernels — not wheat flour. Sprouted wheat is high in protein and fiber. The sprouting process also increases the beneficial enzymes and vitamin and mineral content. My favorite brand is Food For Life, which is available in most natural food stores and online. I like the product's combination of ingredients, which includes other beneficial whole grains and beans: organic sprouted whole grain wheat, organic sprouted whole grain barley, organic sprouted whole grain millet, organic sprouted whole lentils, organic sprouted whole soybeans, and organic sprouted whole grain spelt.

Ancient grain pastas. Pastas such as elbow, penne, and spaghetti are now made from ancient grains such as quinoa, amaranth, brown rice, and combinations of these grains. A company called TruRoots makes delicious pastas. They're available in natural food stores and online. The elbow macaroni has been a staple in my house for a long time. Other ancient grain pastas I recommend include VitaSpelt pasta, Jovial einkorn pasta, quinoa pasta, and Eden Kamut & Quinoa blend.

SELECT INTACT GRAINS

If you haven't met already, let me introduce you to intact grains, which I distinguish from whole grains. Intact grains include barley, brown rice, buckwheat, farro, millet, oats, and quinoa. These grains contain 100 percent of the original kernel, which includes the bran, germ, and endosperm. All three kernel layers must be intact and present in their original form. Because of this, intact grains have a richer nutritional profile of antioxidants, B vitamins, protein, minerals, fiber, and healthful fats than grains that have been stripped of the bran and germ layers through processing.

An intact grain is not processed, whereas a "whole grain" may be processed. The FDA's definition of a whole grain is as follows: "cereal grains that consist of the intact and unrefined, ground, cracked, or flaked fruit of the grains whose principal components—the starchy endosperm, germ, and bran—are present in the same relative proportions as they exist in the intact grain." This definition covers breads, pastas, and other processed grains. It is so broad that even processed foods like Cheerios can still qualify as "whole grain"—which leads me to call "bull" on government definitions.

Intact grains have a lower glycemic index than whole grains, and they digest slowly, which helps you feel full longer so you won't overeat. Even people following a lower-carb diet can enjoy intact grains without worrying about blood sugar spikes and weight gain.

Dutch researchers analyzed the diets of more than 4,000 people and found that those who ate just one serving a day of intact grains weighed about seven pounds less than those who skimped on these healthy grains.

Before the 1950s, intact grains such as barley, brown rice, and millet were more commonly used in the Indian cuisine of my ancestors. As more Indians immigrated to the United States, they began to eat more refined carbohydrates, such as white rice and white flour. Consequently, type 2 diabetes, cardiovascular disease, and obesity among Indian Americans began to rise. These alarming changes were pointed out in an article published in *Nutrition Reviews* in 2011, and I have seen such changes firsthand in many of my own relatives. The article went on to cite research showing that if we can replace white rice with brown rice, whole wheat couscous, quinoa, barley, millet, or any ancient grains, the risk of diabetes, heart disease, and obesity goes down considerably. Great advice!

My bottom-line advice is to go with the grains — intact grains, that is.

Let's start this good grain/good carb habit today. We all deserve wholesome bread, pasta, and grains that will build great health.

CHECKLIST

Today:

- ✓ I did my morning lemon water ritual.
- ✓ I enjoyed a green drink.
- ✓ I stopped drinking fluids with my meals.
- ✓ I drank, and bathed in, pure, clean, filtered water.
- ✓ I ate less dairy and made healthier dairy choices.
- ✓ I stopped drinking all sodas.
- ✓ I loved my liver by paying attention to alcohol consumption.
- ✓ I passed on fast food.
- ✓ I gave up refined sugar.
- ✓ I ate less meat and I ate it responsibly.
- ✓ I increased the raw plant foods in my diet.
- ✓ I chose the best possible grains and carbs.

Day 13 — Balance Your Healthy Fats

I SWORE THAT MY marriage ceremony would not be a big fat Indian wedding.

Ours was to be a traditional Indian ceremony, and my husband-to-be, a Southern boy, was excited about the decision. Everything about an Indian wedding is huge: the marriage ceremony, the enormous spread of food, the flowers, the crowd, and the variety of entertainment. The only thing I didn't want to be huge was my belly, because I planned to wear a traditional Indian wedding gown called a *lengha*, a fitted, tummy-baring dress and long skirt of silk. Indian women tend to carry weight in their tummies, and I was no different back then.

Exposing my midsection to all my friends and family on one of the biggest days of my life terrified me. For weeks, I was motivated not to eat sweets. I shunned doughnuts and birthday cakes at the office. I exercised five times a week. And I ate two tablespoons of organic nut butter every day.

The day of my wedding arrived. I had flat, tight, six-pack abs, and I was in the best shape of my life. I breathed many sighs of relief. All of my cousins who flew into town for the wedding marveled at my abs. They said, "Wow, we thought Indian women couldn't get six-pack abs." They just kept staring at my tummy.

I credit this mainly to the almond butter. It kept me from over-indulging in other foods, and I knew from research that a good mono-unsaturated fat like almond butter could actually burn belly fat.

We have a love affair with fat, but it's a troubled relationship. We eat it, then we break up with it. Is fat good for us or bad for us? It turns out that it all depends on the type of fat you eat—and the balance of certain fats in your diet.

HOW THE FOOD INDUSTRY ADULTERATED OUR FATS

About 15,000 years ago, people ate wild game, wild plants, and fish. Their diets were well balanced in the ratio of omega-6 fats (from seeds) to omega-3 fats (from their wild food).

Another 5,000 years passed, and something happened.

Agricultural practices sprang up, and, along with them, agrarian communities. As grains and crops were domesticated and bread came into use, there was a gradual increase in the level of omega-6 fats and a gradual decline in omega-3 fats in people's diets. They just weren't eating as much natural food anymore.

Fast-forward to post–World War II. Starting in the 1950s, food-preserving technology that had been developed for the war drove the creation of processed mass-market foods, which were filled with oils and sugar.

The use of margarine swelled, too, because it was cheaper than butter. Margarine is produced through hydrogenation, which solidifies liquid at room temperature. To do this, vegetable oils are heated, subjected to semitoxic and toxic metals (such as nickel and aluminum), and exposed to hydrogen gas. This process also creates nasty trans fatty acids. Today, trans fats have been largely expelled from margarine, but they're still everywhere in processed food.

The vegetable oils used to manufacture margarine, like corn, soybean, cottonseed, and canola, contain large amounts of omega-6 fatty acids. These acids are found naturally in poultry, eggs, nuts, and avocados. Our bodies need this type of fatty acid, but today people are getting too much of it through processed foods—up to twenty times more than required, according to some estimates.

This imbalance between omega-3 and omega-6 puts the body in a state of chronic inflammation. It also tends to thicken the blood, potentially setting the stage for abnormal blood clotting. The longer you go with an imbalance of fats, the more likely you are to develop heart disease and its potentially deadly complications. Omega-3 fats, by contrast, maintain the safe and healthy consistency of circulating blood—and keep your cardiovascular system in good working order.

Researchers also claim that fats high in omega-6 promote tumor growth, while fats high in omega-3 block tumor growth. Omega-3 fats can actually slow down the spread of cancer cells to other organs. They also boost the immune system, making the body less vulnerable to diseases. Obesity, asthma, depression, premature aging, and other problems have been linked to an imbalance of these two fats. The more omega-6 fats we eat, the more omega-3 fats we require to counter the bad effects.

Today, omega-3 fatty acids have become the next "in" additive. Omega-3 is being put back in many foods, including cereals, eggs, peanut butter, milk, cheese, and orange juice. This is sad. We never had to worry about this back in the days before cheap oils and processed foods came on the scene.

I CAN'T BELIEVE IT'S SO UNHEALTHY...

Today's cooking oils are largely responsible for tilting the omega-3 and omega-6 ratio and inflaming our bodies. The offenders include the following:

CANOLA OIL

This oil is everywhere, from the hot food bar at my favorite grocery store to popular packaged foods like protein and granola bars. It's even mixed in with olive oil at major restaurants. We've been made to think canola oil is healthy, when it's anything but, thanks in part to some nutritionists and registered dietitians on the Canola Council.

Where does canola come from? Canola oil is extracted from rapeseed plants that have been genetically modified. The oil must go through extremely heavy processing with highly toxic hexane gas to even be edible, and it can go rancid very easily. It's also very high in omega-6 fats.

COTTONSEED OIL

You want to know about a really terrible oil? Let me tell you about cottonseed oil, a by-product of the cotton crop that is high in omega-6 fats and inundated with pesticides and chemicals. It is used to make potato chips and other processed foods. Kraft uses cottonseed oil in its Planters peanuts.

Cotton is a textile, so it is not regulated by the same standards as food crops. Pesticides and chemicals can be used on conventional cotton that can't be used on other conventionally grown crops. Ultimately, this puts our food supply in grave danger.

Cotton farming, which is particularly pesticide- and chemical-intensive, starts with the planting of GMO pesticide-impregnated seeds sold to farmers by Monsanto. The seedlings then require intense applications of fungicides, followed by pesticides and defoliants before harvesting.

To extract the oil and make it edible, the cotton plant must undergo intensive chemical refining, which includes using hexane as a solvent. Cottonseed oil is then used in livestock feed (along with the hulls) and put into many human foods, which is a possible route by which residual pesticides enter the food chain.

Cotton farming also may be killing India's farmers. Since 2002, thousands of Indian farmers have committed suicide—many after the costly genetically modified seeds they used failed. The seeds were produced with *Bacillus thuringiensis* (Bt toxin), a bacterium in soil that helps the crop ward off insects, particularly the bollworm. When the crops failed, the farmers lost all hope and ended their lives.

Being of Indian descent, I am saddened and infuriated by this unspeakable tragedy on a scale that is hard to express. There is nothing more insidious and despicable than an industry that preys upon the health, safety, and lives of innocent victims. Cottonseed oil does not belong in our food supply and should be strictly avoided.

OTHER HIGHLY REFINED OMEGA-6 OILS

For your own health and safety and that of your family, please be aware that there are other processed oils on the market that are highly refined and loaded with omega-6 fats. These include corn, soybean, grape-seed, safflower, sunflower, and peanut oils. Some of these are usually produced from GMO seeds and are unstable when exposed to heat. This instability causes oxidation, a process that generates free radicals. Free radicals are renegade molecules in the body that damage cells, triggering a host of diseases, from heart disease to Alzheimer's disease to cancer.

TRANS FATS

Trans fats, one of my Sickening 15, are created through the hydrogenation process. Trans fats are widely considered the worst kind for your heart and provide absolutely no benefit to human health. They can raise levels of "bad" cholesterol, increasing the risk of heart disease. In fact, in 2006 Harvard epidemiologists published research in the *New England Journal of Medicine* estimating that trans fats are responsible for between 72,000 and 228,000 cardiac disease events a year.

Fortunately, the FDA announced at the end of 2013 that it would require the food industry to phase out these heart-harmful fats. The agency ruled that trans fats no longer fall in the agency's GRAS category, which covers thousands of additives that can be used without FDA review. Once trans fats are banned, any company that wants to use them will have to petition the agency for a regulation allowing that use.

Until the phase-out is complete, trans fats still linger in our food, and they are killing people. Foods containing these deadly fats include:

- Pancake mix
- Packaged cookies
- Ready-made frosting
- Microwave pizzas
- Microwave popcorn

- Ready-to-bake garlic bread
- Pot pies
- Commercially baked pastries
- Fast foods (especially those that are fried)

The only way to know whether a food contains trans fats is to check the ingredient list for "partially hydrogenated" oils. If you see this, put it back on the shelf.

At the same time, be aware that some products claim to have "0 trans fat." Sounds good, right? Not so fast. These foods may still contain partially hydrogenated oils, a small amount of trans fat, and even a substantial amount of saturated fat. That's because the FDA defines "zero" as less than 0.5 grams of trans fat per serving. Thus, a serving could have as much as 0.49 grams of trans fat, which is a significant amount.

Restaurants are notorious for frying food in trans fats. Check with the kitchen before ordering and ask if they use any hydrogenated oils. Go so far as to ask them to read the actual ingredient list on the oil container. Nothing healthy comes from consuming trans fats in any amount.

WHAT ABOUT BUTTER?

While I was growing up, butter was a staple in my household. We thankfully never got into the margarine craze because my mother believed butter was good for the brain. It turns out she was right, and scientists have now concluded that butter is actually good for you in other areas, too. It's high in conjugated linoleic acid (CLA), a type of fat that protects you from tumor growth and cancer. Butter is not inflammatory like oils made from corn, canola, or soy, and it provides a nice dose of omega-3 fatty acids if you get it from the right source. But finding the right source can be tricky, given all the buzzwords and fancy marketing we face. Choosing the wrong type of butter can secretly ruin your health without your even knowing it.

Here's the problem: A lot of butter in the grocery store comes from cows fed almost entirely genetically engineered or GMO plant foods such as corn, soy, and alfalfa. Some farmers fatten up their feed with additional sugar from GMO sugar beets and cottonseed. As we've learned, cotton is the most toxic crop because it isn't treated as a food but rather as a textile and thus is less strictly regulated. Also, GMO crops are typically sprayed with astronomical amounts of pesticides.

There's more to worry about: Conventional dairy cow feed is sometimes fortified with additional protein, omega-3 fatty acids, and CLA from GMO rapeseed (used to make canola oil), because the cows are not getting these nutrients naturally from the grass. So in the end, conventionally raised cows are getting their food almost entirely from GMOs—food that was created in a laboratory, that hasn't been tested long-term, and that has produced horrific results in many animal studies. In a review of these studies published in 2009 in *Critical Reviews in Food Science and Nutrition*, researchers noted that GMO foods cause liver, pancreatic, kidney, blood, reproductive, and immune problems in animals that eat them. In short, GMOs make animals sick.

A certain type of butter, Land O'Lakes, was a favorite in my household when I was growing up. We'd use the whipped butter like nobody's business. My mom would use it on her infamous parathas (Indian stuffed flatbread), in countless desserts, and to make homemade ghee. But once I found out that Land O'Lakes was created from GMO-fed cows, my mom and I had a little chat. I explained to her that Land O'Lakes co-developed genetically engineered alfalfa, directly contributing to the GMO animal feed supply. I also explained that Land O'Lakes contributed nearly $100,000 to the "No on I-522 lobby"—lobbying against the bill to label GMOs in Washington State. This is in addition to the facts that Land O'Lakes is not organic and that they raise their cows with growth hormones that are linked to cancer, antibiotics, and harmful pesticide-ridden GMO feed. I told my mom she had to stop buying Land O'Lakes if we were going to change this world!

Beware, too, of butter blends with phrases on the labels like "with olive oil." These butters contain one or more GMO ingredients, such as soybean, corn, or canola oil. They may have questionable additives in them, too; check the ingredient list to protect yourself.

THE FOOD BABE WAY

Choosing better fats and correcting your omega-3 and omega-6 balance will improve every aspect of your health. After a few weeks, your hair will be glossier and stronger, your nails will grow more quickly, and your skin will be less prone to irritation. You may also find that small cuts will heal quickly and leave less scarring. After a few months, you'll have fewer aches and pains, your joints will be more mobile, and you'll probably be in a better mood. You'll greatly lower your risk of scary diseases, too.

Here are my guidelines for purchasing healthier butter and other fats and oils so that you can experience all these benefits and more:

LOOK FOR ORGANIC BUTTER

This will ensure that no growth hormones, antibiotics, harmful pesticides, or GMOs have been fed to the cows. Growth hormone, or rBGH, used to raise cows conventionally, is linked to cancer and often accumulates in the highest concentration in animal fat.

GO WITH GRASS-FED

Grass-fed or pasture-raised cows are going to produce more nutritious foods than cows raised with grains. The highest amounts of the most beneficial CLA and omega-3 fatty acids naturally come from grass-fed cows. In addition, grass-fed cows produce butter with 50 percent more vitamin A and E and 400 percent more beta-carotene (which gives the grass-fed butter a deeper yellow color).

TRY GHEE

Ghee is clarified butter from which all the proteins, milk solids, and lactose have been removed. This makes the butter more digestible, concentrated with nutrients, and great for immunity building. Ghee does not need to be refrigerated; it can stay on the counter for a few months without going bad. People with dairy allergies or sensitivities often do fine with this type of butter. Pure Indian Foods, Purity Farms, and Ancient Organics are my favorite choices because they are high-quality and organic and come from grass-fed cows.

PURCHASE THE HEALTHIEST OILS

Choose 100 percent coconut oil, olive oil, red palm oil (if it is sustainably harvested from Ecuador and does not hurt the rain forest), sesame oil, or hemp oil. Red palm oil has more vitamin A and E than any other oil. Another great choice is coconut manna. When warmed, it spreads just like butter.

ENJOY NUT BUTTERS

These are good dietary fats, too, but you have to be choosy. Take peanut butter, for example. Conventional peanuts are some of the most heavily sprayed crops. The amount of toxic pesticides sprayed on peanuts is suspected to have caused the increase in peanut allergies. As you know, peanuts have a very thin and porous outer shell, and this allows toxins in easily. And these toxins are not something you can wash off.

In addition, a substance called aflatoxin, which is produced by mold, is frequently present in peanuts. This toxin has been shown to cause liver cancer in people who live in developing countries where they eat a lot of corn, peanuts, and grains grown in poor-quality soil. Here in the United States, the FDA allows aflatoxin into our food system at varying levels. Aflatoxin is not something I want to consume on a regular basis, even in small "approved" doses.

I prefer almond butter to peanut butter any day. Almond butter is simply better for your health. According to an analysis conducted by *Prevention* magazine, almond butter has 69 percent more calcium, twice as much fiber, 86 percent more iron, and 169 percent more vitamin E than peanut butter. And remember, it may just trim your waistline.

Food Babe Shopping List for Healthy Oils

Nutiva organic coconut oil

Papa Vince's olive oil

Nutiva hemp oil

Organic Valley Pasture Butter (green foil wrapper)

Kerrygold butter

Eden Foods sesame oil

Once Again organic raw almond butter

Artisana nut butters

Nutiva Red Palm Oil

Pure Indian Foods ghee

CHECKLIST

Today:

   ✓ I did my morning lemon water ritual.

   ✓ I enjoyed a green drink.

   ✓ I stopped drinking fluids with my meals.

   ✓ I drank, and bathed in, pure, clean, filtered water.

   ✓ I ate less dairy and made healthier dairy choices.

   ✓ I stopped drinking all sodas.

   ✓ I loved my liver by paying attention to alcohol consumption.

   ✓ I passed on fast food.

   ✓ I gave up refined sugar.

   ✓ I ate less meat and I ate it responsibly.

   ✓ I increased the raw plant foods in my diet.

   ✓ I chose the best possible grains and carbs.

   ✓ I balanced my fats.

Day 14 — Supplement with These 10 Superhero Foods

A superhero is a fictional character who has extraordinary or super-human powers. What if nonfictional superheroes existed in real life in the form of food? Maybe they would have the extraordinary ability to provide your body with a high ratio of nutrition to calories, making them the most nutritionally dense foods available.

Or they might be able to combat evil villains like autoimmune dis-orders, depression, and cancer. How about a food that could protect your body from free radical and carcinogen invaders?

These foods do exist. They're called superfoods. They're the total opposite of weak foods, the ones with low nutrition, toxins, and tons of calories that make us sick and fat.

There are many superfoods around, but I've identified ten of the best ones to make today's habit even easier. Starting today, eat one or more of these foods daily to supercharge your health.

THE FOOD BABE WAY

INCLUDE FERMENTED FOODS

My stomach always gave me trouble when I was little. I'd wake up and not want to go to school because of it. My parents thought my complaints were completely made up — once when I was in second grade, my mom dragged me to the principal's office to teach me a lesson about not inventing ailments so I could miss school. But I wasn't making stuff up. I never felt well.

The digestive system remains a mystery to scientists even today, but the Chinese have said it is where disease starts — and they are right.

Inside your intestines, or gut, live trillions of bacteria. Most of these bacteria are beneficial and responsible for many of the processes that keep us healthy. They help fight infection, reduce cholesterol, manufacture B vitamins, detoxify the intestines, and more.

These "good bugs" also play a large role in preventing obesity. One reason is that they help prevent fat absorption in the small intestine—which means the body takes in fewer calories that could be deposited as fat. Scientists have found that overweight people harbor different types and amounts of gut bacteria than lean people do. Some bad bacteria seem to promote obesity, while good bacteria seem to fight it.

Fortunately, you can populate your gut with more of the good bacteria through diet. First, avoid sugar, refined carbs, and junk foods. They cause bad bacteria to thrive. Those bad bacteria then release endotoxins, which drive inflammation and cause metabolic changes that result in the overproduction of insulin, increased appetite, and greater fat storage. Second, eat fermented foods. They increase good bacteria and stop any bad bacteria from doing damage. As an added bonus, the fermentation process increases the vitamin and mineral content of food—making fermented foods the ultimate superfoods.

Here's how you can incorporate these foods into your diet:

- *Check out kimchi.* Kimchi is my favorite fermented food. It's a traditional fermented Korean side dish made of vegetables with a variety of seasonings. I like to eat it on top of quinoa, on wild rice, or on a sandwich.
- *Serve up some sauerkraut.* You probably know this finely cut, fermented cabbage best as a topping on ballpark hot dogs. But please don't put this amazing superfood on a casing full of pink slime! I like it on top of salads and sandwiches. It is supremely healthy for your gut.
- *Get to know miso.* Miso paste is created from a mixture of soybeans, sea salt, and rice koji (a yeast prepared in Japan from rice) that is then fermented. The fermentation process creates enzyme-rich compounds that are effective in eliminating bodily toxins from industrial pollution, radioactivity, and artificial chemicals in the foods you eat. Miso paste has been used for

centuries in Asian cultures as a form of probiotic, to strengthen the immune system, and to provide beneficial B12. My Miso Soup with Black Rice Noodles is a great way to work this superfood into your diet (recipe on page 315).

- *Try tempeh.* It's made through a culturing and fermenting process that binds soybeans into a cake form, similar to a very firm veggie burger. I like to marinate it and use it as a meat substitute.
- *Refresh with kombucha.* This is a lovely fermented drink that has natural carbonation. It is produced from SCOBY, which stands for symbiotic culture of bacteria and yeast. SCOBY is a culture that is used to brew the tea, which has detoxifying and immune-boosting benefits.
- *Yay for yogurt.* This cultured milk product is the ultimate fermented food, full of beneficial bacteria that maintain the health of your digestive system. I've been spoiled by being able to enjoy the purest yogurt on the planet, made by my mom. If you can't get homemade yogurt, make sure you choose a 100 percent grass-fed organic product. My favorite brands are Traderspoint Creamery, which comes in little glass bottles, and Maple Hill Creamery.

**FOOD BABE ALERT:
DON'T GET DUPED AGAIN: CONVENTIONAL
YOGURT IS JUNK FOOD**

In 2014, the Cornucopia Institute did a major exposé of yogurt, a food staple on which Americans spend $6 billion annually. The watchdog organization pointed out that giant food corporations, led by General Mills (Yoplait), Groupe Danone (Dannon), Walmart, and PepsiCo, are marketing conventional yogurt as healthy when in fact it is produced with chemicals and toxins under inhumane conditions.

Conventional yogurt comes from milk produced by cows that are confined and unable to graze in open pasture. They're fed GMO grains, not grass. As the yogurt ferments, chemical defoamers are added. Then

(Continued)

high doses of artificial sweeteners, sugar, or high-fructose corn syrup are added. That's not all: Artificial colors, synthetic preservatives, and the gut-harmful carrageenan are dumped in, turning most yogurts into junk food. These practices alarm me, since yogurt has been such a healthy, longevity-promoting food for ages.

The Cornucopia Institute recommends that we yogurt lovers buy minimally processed organic brands. These include Traderspoint, Maple Hill Creamery, Nancy's, Organic Valley, Kalona SuperNatural, Wallaby Organic, and Clover Stornetta, and regional brands such as Butterworks Farm, Seven Stars Farm, Straus Family Creamery, Hawthorne Valley Farm, and Cedar Summit Farm. By doing so, we support organic farmers, protect our environment, encourage humane treatment of animals, and ensure good health for ourselves and our families.

SWEETEN WITH RAW CACAO

Cacao is the raw ingredient from which chocolate is made, and it is a wonderfully complex substance. It contains more antioxidants than any plant food on earth. Plus, it's a cornucopia of natural compounds, including serotonin, endorphins, phenylethylamine, tryptophan, and anandamide, all of which have been shown to ease depression and create feelings of well-being and happiness. Extremely rich in antioxidants and minerals, especially magnesium, cacao is known to increase the overall pumping action of the heart muscle and help alkalize the body.

Raw cacao nibs are fantastic in desserts and can be used to add a nice little crunch to other foods. Here's how to incorporate raw cacao into your diet:

- Blend it into smoothies.
- Sprinkle it over cereal, yogurt, ice cream, or fruit.
- Bake it into cookies.
- Add it to trail mixes.
- Or just nibble on it!

GO FOR GOJI BERRIES

Used traditionally in Chinese medicine, goji berries can make your body glow because they allow your skin to absorb more oxygen. These little berries help improve circulation and move bacteria and viruses out of the body, thus strengthening your immune system. They can also help slow the growth of gray hair! Goji berries are a treasure trove of nutrition, containing more iron than spinach, more beta-carotene than carrots, and more protein than whole wheat.

Here's how to incorporate goji berries into your diet:

- Use them in place of raisins in any recipe.
- Eat them in cereals, such as my Perfect Porridge Parfait (recipe on page 297).
- Add them to trail mix.
- Or just snack on the berries for a chewy, nutrient-packed treat.

CHECK OUT CHIA SEEDS

Remember that funky Chia Pet—the one that sprouted a green coat after being watered? That pet was coated with chia seeds, which also happen to be a top superfood. The Aztecs ate chia seeds (whose name meant "strengthening") in times of famine to stay strong and would often survive just on these little seeds. Chia seeds are brimming with minerals and antioxidants. According to the USDA, just 2 tablespoons of chia seeds provide approximately 100 milligrams of bone-building calcium, 7.5 grams of dietary fiber, and 3 grams of protein (that's more protein than you find in most other grains and seeds). With the highest content of omega-3 fatty acids of any plant food, chia seeds fight inflammation in the body, thereby reducing the chances of heart disease, Alzheimer's, and depression.

Chia seeds are also thought to help keep your waistline trim. Once in your stomach, they expand to ten to twelve times their size and form a gel that makes you feel full. They also slow the digestive process in which carbs are broken down and converted to sugar, which means that fewer carbs end up feeding the fat cells around your belly.

Here's how to incorporate chia seeds into your diet:

- Add them to oatmeal, cereals, and yogurt.
- Sprinkle them over salads.
- Blend them into smoothies.
- Make them into a pudding by soaking them in milk.

SUPPLEMENT WITH SPIRULINA

This nutrient-packed water alga gets its superpowers through photosynthesis and has all the protein, vitamins, minerals, digestive enzymes, and chlorophyll your body needs for near-perfect nutrition. This means it's terrific for building muscle, losing weight, and fighting disease.

Spirulina is also a rich source of a phytochemical called zeaxanthin. This nutrient may reduce the risk of cataracts and age-related macular degeneration, which causes loss of vision due to damage to the retina.

Here's how to incorporate spirulina into your diet:

- Thoroughly mix 1 to 2 tablespoons of spirulina powder into 8 ounces of juice or water until it dissolves. Use an organic vegetable juice if you want to mask the sharp taste of the spirulina.
- Incorporate 1 to 2 tablespoons of spirulina powder in your smoothie and blend well.
- Sprinkle 1 to 2 tablespoons of spirulina powder into yogurt, mix it into soups, or sprinkle it over your cold or hot cereal for breakfast.
- Add spirulina powder to organic whole grain pasta, with a little olive oil.
- Sprinkle it over a salad to kick up the nutritional power of your raw greens.

SPRINKLE ON SOME HEMPSEEDS

I recommend hempseeds to everyone. (Yes—hemp is legal!) The quality of hemp protein is exceptional, and it provides the perfect proportion of omega-6 to omega-3 fatty acids (see Day 13) to reduce inflammation. The seeds are also full of vitamin E, which acts as an antioxidant in the body, and magnesium, which is needed for muscle growth.

These seeds also reduce cholesterol, strengthen your immune system, and could even help you lose weight, since they're packed with about 2 grams of fiber per tablespoon.

Additionally, hempseeds are high in the amino acid arginine. Research in the journal *Nutrition* suggests that eating foods abundant in arginine could lower your risk for cardiovascular disease.

If you eat hemp, can you still pass a drug test? That's a question I'm asked frequently. Both hemp and marijuana are varieties of *Cannabis sativa* and contain the psychoactive ingredient THC (delta-9-tetrahydrocannabinol). Hemp grown for food and fiber, however, contains only trace amounts of THC. You can safely consume hemp without any chance of getting high or testing positive for THC.

You can safely store hempseeds for up to a year at room temperature, but refrigeration extends their shelf life.

How to eat hempseeds:

- Toss them into salads.
- Coat salmon and chicken with the seeds; they work well as a light "breading."
- Blend them into shakes and smoothies.
- Stir them into yogurt or your morning oatmeal to kick up the protein content.
- Toss a handful into the batter for baked goods, such as quick breads, cookies, and muffins.
- Sprinkle them on just about any food and you'll elevate the dish to superfood status.

- Make your own hemp milk by blending ¼ cup seeds with 4 cups filtered water (no straining required). Hemp milk is a great option if you're a vegan or a vegetarian; if you have allergies to nuts, soy, whey protein, or casein; or if you're lactose-intolerant or want to reduce your dairy consumption.

ENJOY MACA

Grown atop the Andes Mountains in Peru, maca is a member of the cruciferous family, which includes broccoli, cabbage, cauliflower, kale, turnips, and radishes. The most popular way to eat maca is to use it in dried powder form. Dried maca contains 59 percent carbohydrates, 8.5 percent fiber, and slightly more than 10.2 percent protein, making it a well-rounded, near-perfect food. Maca is also rich in calcium, magnesium, phosphorus, potassium, sodium, and iron. Add to that the vitamins B1, B2, and C, and you can easily understand what makes maca a superfood.

Maca has been cultivated for more than 3,000 years, racking up an impressive list of benefits over that time, including:

- Increased energy
- Improved sexual function (maca has been touted as the natural Viagra)
- Improved mental clarity
- Healthier hair growth
- Enhanced thyroid health and improved metabolism
- Better-balanced hormones
- Protection against ultraviolet radiation
- Fewer PMS symptoms
- Improved skin tone
- Higher sperm count
- Prevention of osteoporosis
- Antidepressant properties

Maca is also a powerful stress reliever and may help rid your life of stress-induced problems. Not long ago, I was chatting with a close friend who was upset that she had gained fifteen pounds in two months. She had put on this weight even though she was doing nothing different in terms of her diet or exercise program. Alarmed by the sudden weight gain, she went to see her doctor, who checked her levels of cortisol (a stress hormone). Her cortisol was through the roof—a result of being stressed out from working on an important, time-consuming project.

Stress will jack up your cortisol levels and cause sudden weight gain, especially around your tummy. Fat tends to accumulate there because the cells in the abdominal region are highly sensitive to cortisol and are effective at storing excess calories.

Listening to my friend's story was a wake-up call for me. I'm a workaholic, and if I'm not careful, I can lose the balance in my life. That's when I decided to add maca to my diet on a regular basis.

In an exhaustive study of the maca plant, Dr. Gustavo F. Gonzales found that it can help improve homeostasis in the body. By definition, homeostasis describes your body's ability to regulate and control its inner environment physiologically, so that the body's functions remain stable even when exposed to certain fluctuating conditions in the external environment, such as stress.

It's easy to find maca at any natural food store or health food store, or online—which is a lot easier than hiking up the Andes Mountains to pick it yourself.

How to use maca powder:

- Toss a tablespoon into your smoothie for extra energy.
- Bake it into desserts such as brownies (it pairs well with chocolate).
- Try my Maca Hot Chocolate (recipe on page 296).

GET TO KNOW GOLDEN BERRIES

A wonderful benefit of traveling is that I get to sample the foods in every culture I visit. Several years ago, I was vacationing in Argentina, where I tasted a delightfully sweet but mouth-puckering fruit called the golden berry. It was love at first bite, and I've been eating these berries ever since. They are nature's Sour Patch Kids!

Grown in the mountains of South America, golden berries, also known as Cape gooseberries or Incan berries, have been prized for centuries for their nutritional benefits and sweet-and-sour citrusy flavor. A handful of golden berries packs a powerful punch of disease-fighting antioxidants. As a traditional folk remedy, these little berries have been used to help with weight control, stronger immunity, and good organ health.

Golden berries contain anti-inflammatory bioflavonoids (beneficial plant chemicals in fruits and vegetables) and are also an excellent source of vitamins A and C, both great for immunity. Unlike typical dried fruits, packaged versions of this superfood usually contain no added sugars or preservatives, which means you aren't loading up on unnecessary junk and additives.

To enjoy golden berries:

- Eat them straight out of the package (as you would with raisins).
- Mix the dried berries in trail mixes, oatmeal, or salads.
- Blend them into smoothies.
- Get adventuresome and turn them into a golden berry jam.

BE KEEN ON QUINOA

You've probably heard about this food or seen it in a grocery store. What is it? How do you cook it? And how the heck do you pronounce it?

It's quinoa (pronounced keen-wa), and it's been around since the time of the Incas. Quinoa is a major superfood; a nutritional breakdown shows it to be high in a variety of vitamins and minerals as well as protein. While visiting an organic quinoa farm in Peru, I met a farmer who insisted his mother, who is ninety-five years old, looks younger than him because she eats this wonderful superfood every day!

The starring nutrients in quinoa include vitamin B6, thiamin, niacin, potassium, and riboflavin, plus minerals like copper, zinc, magnesium, and folate, as well as the phytonutrients quercetin and kaempferol, which fight inflammation and disease. The reigning protein amino acid in quinoa is lysine, a nutrient not found in many other grains. This attribute puts quinoa on the level of milk when it comes to protein. Quinoa is low in fat, but it does contain omega-3 fats.

Technically not a grain (it is referred to as a grain because it resembles grains in appearance), quinoa is actually a seed. The kernels can be red, black, white, or golden. Quinoa does not contain gluten, making it a terrific carb if you're sensitive to gluten in any way, and it does not belong to the same plant family as wheat.

Quinoa's health benefits have been well validated by research. Eating quinoa reduces your chances of developing type 2 diabetes, but it can also help you keep those glucose levels balanced if you already have diabetes. This is because the complex carbohydrates in quinoa digest slowly and keep you satiated longer while keeping your blood sugar and appetite balanced.

Because quinoa is high in magnesium, the heart mineral, you'll protect yourself against heart disease and blood vessel problems. And do you ever suffer from migraine headaches? Quinoa to the rescue: It's high in riboflavin, or vitamin B2, which promotes blood vessel dilation in the brain and reduces instances of migraine headaches.

Quinoa is a near-cure for digestive ailments like constipation, too. This fiber-rich food scrubs the walls of the arteries, reducing plaque from the arterial walls that can otherwise eventually build up and cause a heart attack or stroke.

Quinoa is easy to prepare and cooks quickly. Always rinse it before cooking it. This washes away saponins that tend to give it a bitter taste.

There are many ways to enjoy this versatile superfood. For example:

- Enjoy it as a side dish, like a pilaf.
- Serve it as a breakfast cereal with some golden or goji berries.
- Bake it into meat loaf.
- Stir-fry it with veggies.
- Serve it as a salad ingredient.
- Mix it into soups, stews, or chilis.

CRUNCH DOWN ON SOME SPROUTS

Sprouts might look like baby or immature plants, but the concentration of nutrition in these tiny fresh beans and seed tendrils can range between 300 and 1,200 percent more than their full-grown counterparts. Sunflower, mung, and broccoli sprouts remain the best known and most popular. But today, you can get lentil sprouts, clover sprouts, snow pea sprouts, and radish sprouts—there's plenty of variety.

Sprouts are essentially the germinating part of a seed, bean, or whole grain. Within a few days of germination, they develop a high nutritional value, becoming rich in protein and high in vitamins C and E and many of the B vitamins. They're also very low in fat and calories. One cup of mung sprouts, for example, provides a mere thirty calories.

Sprouts are among the freshest vegetables you can eat. There are no preservatives or additives. They can be bought at the store or grown in your kitchen for pennies. Most store-bought sprouts are tested for bacterial contamination, but you should wash them just to be sure.

The easiest way to grow sprouts is as follows:

1. Place 2 to 3 tablespoons of seeds in a glass jar and cover them with water. Stretch some nylon mesh (like clean pantyhose) or cheesecloth across the neck of the jar and secure it with a rubber band. Let the seeds soak several hours or overnight.

2. Drain the water. Then rinse the seeds by adding warm water to the jar and swishing them around. Drain the water again. Repeat this process two or three times a day.

3. Keep the jar stored on its side in a dark place. Depending on the type of seed you use, sprouts will shoot up in three to five days. You can grow them to their desired size by repeating the drain-and-rinse method in step 2.

4. Store your sprouts in a food storage bag and refrigerate. Use them within a week.

Almost any seed and whole bean (and most whole grains) can be sprouted. Select only seeds that are graded for eating and have not been chemically treated. Never use tomato seeds or potato sprouts, since they are poisonous.

Sprouts are extremely versatile. Try them in salads, soups, stews, sandwiches, and stir-fries.

Power up with superfoods, and you'll give your body exactly what it needs, without fattening junk and additives. They are a simple, inexpensive way to supplement your diet, build your health, and feel energetic all day long.

Food Babe Shopping Guide for Superfoods

Superfoods can be found in natural food stores like Whole Foods, Earth Fare, Healthy Home Market, Sprouts Farmers Market, and Vitamin Shoppe and online via Amazon.com, the Green PolkaDot Box, and VItacost. Here's a list of my favorite superfood products for health:

Rejuvenative Foods kimchi	Earth Circle Organics
Zuké kimchi	Divine Foods
Farmhouse Culture sauerkraut	Navitas Naturals
Miso Master organic miso	Sunfood
Lightlife organic tempeh	The Maca Team
GT's kombucha	Alter Eco Foods
Synergy Kombucha	TruRoots
Nutiva	

CHECKLIST

Today:
- ✓ I did my morning lemon water ritual.
- ✓ I enjoyed a green drink.
- ✓ I stopped drinking fluids with my meals.

✓ I drank, and bathed in, pure, clean, filtered water.
✓ I ate less dairy and made healthier dairy choices.
✓ I stopped drinking all sodas.
✓ I loved my liver by paying attention to alcohol consumption.
✓ I passed on fast food.
✓ I gave up refined sugar.
✓ I ate less meat and I ate it responsibly.
✓ I increased the raw plant foods in my diet.
✓ I chose the best possible grains and carbs.
✓ I balanced my fats.
✓ I supplemented with at least one superfood.

CHAPTER 6

WEEK 3 — FEATS OF A REAL FOOD BABE

FIRST OF ALL, CONGRATULATIONS on completing Week 2. I'm proud of you—and you should certainly be proud of yourself. I'm sure you're feeling lighter and more energetic, and I bet the scales show a nice drop in pounds. You're probably thinking more clearly and feeling more creative, too. Booting chemicals from your body protects your brain and mental functioning. Eating more organic foods, having less meat and dairy, and forming all the Week 2 habits are changing your health for the better.

In Week 3, I'm going to make a real Food Babe (or Food Guy) out of you. You've formed some amazing habits already; now you're ready to graduate to what I call Food Babe Feats. These are lifestyle habits that will complete your transformation.

Let's go!

Day 15 — Know Thy GMOs!

WHEN I FOUND OUT that more than 70 percent of processed foods contained either corn or soy, I couldn't believe it. You don't have to be a rocket scientist to understand that eating too much of one type of food, to the exclusion of others, is not exactly healthy.

This trend in processed foods led me into a disturbing series of investigations. I began to read about a biotech company named Monsanto, notorious for developing Agent Orange and other controversial chemicals.

In 1996, Monsanto obtained a patent for a type of corn seed that is injected with genes drawn from bacteria to create a pesticide called Bt toxin within the corn. When insects eat this corn, their stomachs explode and they die.

When I found out about this, I was horrified. What was this type of genetically modified corn doing to us? Was it truly safe? Had anyone tested this new technology on humans yet?

The government has allowed the introduction of GMOs into the food supply without any required safety assessments. According to *Consumer Reports*, the "FDA, which regulates food safety, does not require any safety assessment of the GE crops, but invites companies to provide data for a voluntary safety review. This is in contrast to other major economies such as the European Union, Australia, Japan, and China, which all require that a premarket mandatory safety assessment of GE crops is conducted." Monsanto and the Environmental Protection Agency (EPA) both say GMOs are safe. They swear that Bt toxin hurts insects only and that it is neutralized in the human digestive system.

Research has proved otherwise. In one study, published in the journal *Reproductive Toxicology* in 2011, researchers at Sherbrooke University Hospital in Quebec found Bt toxin in the blood of pregnant women, and their fetuses, as well as in nonpregnant women. Another study, by the University of Caen, France, published in 2013 in the *Journal of Applied Toxicology*, found that Bt toxin showed toxic effects on human kidney cells.

Bottom line: It looks like Bt toxin can indeed be absorbed by humans, and that it may cause serious side effects.

Today, let's get serious about this whole GMO issue. Learn to identify GMO foods and get them out of your diet for good.

OMG: WHAT ARE GMOs?

A genetically modified organism (GMO) is a plant or an animal that has had DNA genes from another organism artificially forced into its own DNA. These foreign genes are extracted from bacteria, viruses, insects, and animals.

This kind of genetic modification does not use traditional crossbreeding techniques like hybridization. Hybrids are developed in the field using natural, low-tech methods. Genetically engineered crops are created in a laboratory using highly complex technology, such as gene splicing. These high-tech genetically engineered crops can include genes from several species—a phenomenon that almost never occurs in nature. The goal of mixing genes of different species is to create greater crop yields and increase pest resistance. With little understanding of how these alterations might adversely affect our health or the environment, the Big Ag industry has plowed ahead quickly in introducing these foods to the public. Today, 70 percent of all processed foods contain at least one GMO ingredient.

GMOs AND YOUR HEALTH

To date, there have been no long-term independent studies on the safety of GMO exposure to humans. "Long-term" and "independent" are the operative words here. Most GMO safety research has been funded by the very biotech companies that create GMOs. Independently funded studies are nearly impossible to conduct because researchers can't get their hands on proprietary GMO seeds, which companies claim are patent-protected. Scientific reviews have compared funding sources to study results, and they've found that when an industry funds its own research, it is sure to be positive.

We've learned quite a bit from this research, however. Studies in which animals were fed genetically modified corn have shown that GMOs cause a slew of liver disorders (for example, atrophied livers and altered liver cells) and several reproductive problems (infant mortality, altered sperm cells, infertility).

Clearly, we need more thorough research. Due to the careless injection of GMOs into the US food supply, the real test is being conducted on the millions of Americans who are consuming GMOs on a daily basis. As put by Gary Hirshberg, chairman of Just Label It: "An unprecedented agricultural experiment is being conducted at America's dinner tables."

A GMO BY ANY OTHER NAME...

You may hear GMOs referred to as genetically modified organisms or genetically engineered (GE) foods, and these terms mean essentially the same thing. The technology used to create GMOs may be called biotechnology, gene technology, or recombinant DNA technology.

Although we may not know enough about the long-term health effects of GMOs, we do know something about the toxicity of pesticides sprayed on GMO crops. For years, Monsanto has sold its flagship product, a weed killer known as Roundup, to farmers and consumers around the world. Roundup is used to selectively kill weeds while allowing genetically modified versions of sugarcane, corn, soy, and wheat crops to thrive.

The dominant ingredient in Roundup is glyphosate, which I mentioned in Chapter 2. Glyphosate is one scary chemical if it finds its way into the body. According to an article published in the May 2014 issue of *Alternative Therapies in Health and Medicine,* scientists have linked exposure to glyphosate to gastrointestinal disorders, obesity, diabetes, heart disease, depression, autism, infertility, and cancer.

Glyphosate is an endocrine disruptor. Endocrine disruptors mimic or block the action of natural hormones and wreak havoc with the body's endocrine system, a network of glands that includes the pituitary gland, adrenal glands, thyroid, thymus, pancreas, ovaries, and testes. These glands release hormones into our bloodstream to regulate many of our body's most important functions, including growth and development, reproduction, maintenance of healthy weight, maintenance of mood, and organ performance. When you ingest chemical endocrine disruptors, you are in essence altering your body's chemistry.

One of the most damaging effects of glyphosate is that it stimulates overproduction of estrogen. This in turn can fuel the growth of estrogen-dependent breast cancer—a fact uncovered by a groundbreaking study published in the journal *Food and Chemical Toxicology* in 2013. These researchers found that the risk of breast cancer was even greater in those exposed to glyphosate who supplemented their diet with soybeans (also known to stimulate estrogen).

Careless use of Roundup has caused a major health crisis in Argentina, where GMOs are big business. People in nearby farming communities have cancer rates up to four times higher than the national average. Monsanto, the manufacturer, blames the way the pesticides are being used: "If pesticides are being misused in Argentina, then it is in everyone's best interests—the public, the government, farmers, industry, and Monsanto—that the misuse be stopped."

A 2014 study led by scientists from the Arctic University of Norway detected "extreme levels" of Roundup in GMO soy. The study, published in *Food Chemistry*, analyzed thirty-one different soybean plants grown on Iowa farms and compared the accumulation of pesticides and herbicides on plants in three categories: (1) genetically engineered "Roundup Ready" soy, (2) conventionally produced (not GE) soy, and (3) soy cultivated using organic practices. The scientists found high levels of Roundup on 70 percent of genetically engineered soy plants.

One of the problems contributing to these extreme levels is that superweeds that are resistant to Roundup have evolved. In response, farmers spray even more Roundup on crops to try to kill these defiant weeds, and so more chemicals are infiltrating our food supply. So every time you eat GMO soy, you're probably taking a dose of Roundup with it.

Farmers are using other poisons, too, such as 2,4-D, which the US military used in Agent Orange to defoliate jungles during the Vietnam War. Dow Chemical Company has just received USDA approval for new 2,4-D-resistant GMO corn and soybean seeds, which compounds the problem.

Farming communities are coming to grips with these devastating problems. Many farmers are returning to planting non-GMO crops, yet they are continuing to spray with higher-risk herbicides to combat the superweeds. This means more chemical herbicide residues are ending up in the food you eat and poisoning our environment.

Big Ag wants us to believe that there is no difference between GMO and conventional crops, but that's BS. John Roulac, cochair of GMO Inside and founder and CEO of Nutiva, said, "One way [some] pesticide makers deceive regulators is by doing toxicity tests with just one ingredient found in their toxic concoctions. Yet in real life Americans and people across the world are subjected to hundreds of pesticides and synthetic chemicals which together increase the toxic load by a factor of ten times or more in one's immune system. How much Roundup do you want in your drinking water or in your blood? Or in expectant mothers' breast milk? Every time you buy food you choose to answer both vital questions."

THE HIDDEN TRUTH

What we sorely need are laws requiring clear labeling of foods with GMO ingredients. Currently, sixty-four countries regulate their GMO food, but the United States does not. Why?

Recent polling shows that Americans overwhelmingly support a labeling law, with upward of 90 percent demanding labels. Although two states have enacted GMO labeling laws, they have a trigger clause that prevents them from going into effect until four neighboring states enact similar laws.

GMO industry lobbyists have been caught red-handed using deceptive scare tactics to pressure states into not enacting labeling laws, calling such laws unconstitutional. The Organic Consumers Association obtained a leaked document written by the Grocery Manufacturers

Association (GMA) that explicitly threatens to sue the first state that enacts a labeling law. And this is exactly what happened in Vermont, after the citizens passed a GMO labeling law. Big Food backed by the GMA is currently suing the state.

Meanwhile, the Washington, DC, law firm Emord & Associates has concluded that such a law is constitutional and is well within our rights. Labeling initiatives in California and Washington were narrowly defeated, after the food industry and biotech companies (which develop GMOs and pesticides) spent almost $70 million on antilabeling propaganda. To add insult to injury, the GMA is currently attempting to push through a bill that will prevent other states from enacting GMO labeling laws. This is clearly not what Americans want.

 FOOD BABE ALERT: CORPORATIONS INVEST MILLIONS TO STOP GMO LABELING

Corporations have thrown their monetary weight around to defeat key pieces of legislation that would mandate labeling of GMO foods. California Proposition 37, which would have required packaged goods to be "clearly and conspicuously" labeled if they were genetically engineered or might have contained genetically engineered ingredients, was rejected in November 2012. A similar initiative in Washington, I-522, was defeated in November 2013, as was Colorado's Proposition 105 in November 2014.

Many companies you'd recognize contributed megabucks to lobbyists to defeat these statutes. Here are a few examples:

Nestlé and affiliated companies: $2,989,806
PepsiCo: $8,838,366
Coca-Cola: $5,765,851
General Mills: $3,614,571
Kellogg: $1,862,750
Kraft: $3,900,500
Monsanto: $24,201,606

Talk about million-dollar influence peddling! For a full list of companies that have contributed against your right to know, see Appendix C.

THE FOOD BABE WAY

Until some serious long-term research is conducted, I recommend going as GMO-free as possible, and I'm here to show you how.

LOOK OUT FOR HIGH-RISK INGREDIENTS AND FOODS

A quick scan of the ingredient label will tell you if a product contains any high-risk ingredients.

GMO crops currently being developed are soy, corn, cotton, canola, sugar beets, zucchini, yellow squash, Hawaiian papaya, and alfalfa. So, for instance, look for corn syrup, soybean oil, and canola oil on the label.

Become familiar with some of the names of ingredients and additives that are not so obvious, such as glucose derived from corn. Here is a list of common ingredients to use as a reference.

▶ Food Babe Alert: List of Possible GMO Ingredients			
Aspartame	Glucose	Malt extract	Soy milk
Baking powder	Glutamate	Maltodextrin	Soy oil
Canola oil	Glutamic acid	Maltose	Soy protein
Caramel color	Glycerides	Malt syrup	Soy protein isolate
Cellulose	Glycerin	Mannitol	Soy sauce
Citric acid	Glycerol	Methylcellulose	Starch
Cobalamin (vitamin B12)	Glycerol monooleate	Milk powder	Stearic acid
Colorose	Glycine	Milo starch	Sugar (unless specified as cane sugar)
Condensed milk	Hemicellulose	Modified food starch	Tamari
Confectioners' sugar	High-fructose corn syrup	Modified starch	Tempeh
Corn flour	Hydrogenated starch	Mono- and diglycerides	Teriyaki marinade
Corn masa	Hydrolyzed vegetable protein	MSG	Textured vegetable protein
Cornmeal	Inositol	NutraSweet	Threonine

Corn oil	Inverse syrup	Oleic acid	Tocopherols (vitamin E)
Cornstarch	Inversol	Phenylalanine	Tofu
Corn sugar	Invert sugar	Phytic acid	Trehalose
Cottonseed oil	Isoflavones	Protein isolate	Triglyceride
Cyclodextrin	Lactic acid	Shoyu	Vegetable fat
Dextrin	Lecithin	Sorbitol	Vegetable oil
Dextrose	Leucine	Soy flour	Vitamin B12
Diacetyl	Lysine	Soy isolates	Vitamin E
Diglyceride	Malitol	Soy lecithin	Whey
Equal	Malt		Whey powder
Erythritol			Xanthan gum
Food starch			
Fructose			

BUY USDA-CERTIFIED ORGANIC FOOD

Any food presented as certified organic, with the USDA organic label on it, is not allowed to have GMOs in any of its ingredients. So avoid all nonorganic foods or anything you might suspect has been sprayed with Roundup. Always read the ingredient lists just to be sure.

This means avoiding anything with added sugar, since a lot of sugar comes from Monsanto's genetically modified sugar beets. Also, steer clear of nonorganic flax, rice, and wheat. These have a moderate risk of being contaminated with GMOs and heavily sprayed with pesticides.

Be careful when choosing animal foods, too, since a majority of livestock in the United States are fed Monsanto grain and/or are treated with the GMO bovine growth hormone rBGH—another Monsanto invention. Do you really want to drink Monsanto Milk or eat Monsanto Butter?

PURCHASE FOOD WITH THE NON-GMO PROJECT VERIFICATION LABEL

The Non-GMO Project (www.nongmoproject.org) is the only organization offering independent verification of testing and GMO controls for products in the United States and Canada. Its verification label indicates that the product undergoes ongoing testing of all at-risk ingredients and the manufacturer complies with rigorous traceability and segregation practices. The Non-GMO Project verification is audited every year to ensure compliance. You can download the Non-GMO Shopping Guide onto your smartphone to help you out while shopping.

CHECK OUT FRUIT AND VEGETABLE LABEL NUMBERS

In the fresh produce section, you'll notice that every fruit and vegetable has a sticker on it with a PLU (price lookup) number, designated by the Produce Marketing Association. Any five-digit number beginning with an 8 is a GMO, but such labeling is optional and not in wide use. No surprise as most Americans say that they would avoid GMOs. If you see a five-digit number beginning with a 9, the fruit is organic and not GMO. Four-digit numbers indicate that the produce was conventionally grown, nonorganic, and possibly GMO.

EAT LESS PROCESSED FOOD AND COOK YOUR MEALS FROM SCRATCH

If all you did was to stop eating processed food, you'd shield yourself automatically from most GMOs. An overwhelming amount of processed food—70 percent—contains GMOs, so one of the biggest changes you can make is to eliminate these foods. If you don't enjoy cooking, try it out just one or two nights a week. Before you know it, it will become more of a habit and you'll begin to enjoy homemade meals more than anything that comes out of a box.

Also, commit to #GMOFreeFridays, on which you encourage your coworkers to bring non-GMO foods to work. This action will help raise awareness of the problem in your workplace. Or, for family, friends, and others who don't work, ask them to buy non-GMO foods and prepare a non-GMO meal on Fridays. Use the hashtag #GMOFreeFriday on social media to share your food and spread the word.

When you go out to eat, ask your server if the food is non-GMO. He or she might not know, but at least you'll start educating your favorite restaurants and their workers.

SHOP LOCALLY AT FARMERS' MARKETS AND CO-OPS

Most GMOs are produced on large industrial farms and shipped out to big food manufacturers. When you buy from your local small farmers, you're less likely to come across GMOs. Seek out opportunities to ask farmers about GMOs and whether or not they use them. Use the Local Harvest website at www.localharvest.org to find local farmers' markets, co-ops, and family farms, which are great sources of organic produce, grass-fed beef, fresh herbs, and other non-GMO goodies.

STICK IT TO MONSANTO WHERE IT HURTS

Contact your mutual fund manager and make sure you aren't blindly investing in Monsanto's destructive acts. Many Fidelity, Vanguard, and State Street mutual funds own and control enormous volumes of Monsanto stock. You may even wish to contact these companies yourself and tell them why you're dumping their funds. Stock evaluations are a powerful leverage point for activism against corporations.

Once you put these actions into play, you'll find that it is entirely possible to live a GMO-free life. And that's a huge feat for a Food Babe.

ASK YOUR FAVORITE BRANDS TO GO NON-GMO

Call, e-mail, tweet, or post a message on your favorite company's Facebook page and ask them to go non-GMO. Some of the biggest news in the food industry last year was the General Mills conversion of Cheerios to a non-GMO cereal. This cultural milestone signals not only the swelling consumer exodus from industrial GMO foods, but also the rise in the use of social media by concerned citizens to educate the public and demand non-GMO foods.

CHECKLIST

Today:

    ✓ I did my morning lemon water ritual.

    ✓ I enjoyed a green drink.

✓ I stopped drinking fluids with my meals.

✓ I drank, and bathed in, pure, clean, filtered water.

✓ I ate less dairy and made healthier dairy choices.

✓ I stopped drinking all sodas.

✓ I loved my liver by paying attention to alcohol consumption.

✓ I passed on fast food.

✓ I gave up refined sugar.

✓ I ate less meat and I ate it responsibly.

✓ I increased the raw plant foods in my diet.

✓ I chose the best possible grains and carbs.

✓ I balanced my fats.

✓ I supplemented with at least one superfood.

✓ I avoided GMO foods as much as possible.

Day 16 — Dine Out the Food Babe Way

I MET MY HUSBAND at work on a Wednesday and by Friday, he was already asking me out. It was love at first sight. Our first date was at the Cheesecake Factory.

At the time, the Cheesecake Factory had just opened at the mall. It was the new hot spot in Charlotte, and people were flocking to it. After waiting more than an hour to get a seat, we headed to our table. The server plopped down a loaf of delectable hot pumpernickel bread. I dove in, thinking I was eating nutritious whole grain. It would not be until much later during my work as the Food Babe that I learned that these delicious-looking dark restaurant breads were made with one of the same ingredients as yoga mats, used as a dough conditioner, as well as other nasty, suspect chemicals.

When you dine out at huge franchises such as the Cheesecake Factory, you need to know that the food is not really fresh; it is trucked in from big food suppliers, where even vegetables are preshredded, losing vital nutrition in the process. They may also have undergone a process called crisping, in which they're washed with sodium hypochlorite phosphate to release dirt and residues; this substance is commonly used as a disinfectant or bleach and is considered a pesticide. As for something like Parmesan cheese, it's shredded with wood pulp, aka cellulose, thrown in. Most of the food is treated with preservatives such as sodium benzoate to help it hold up during the trip from its source to the restaurant. Once at these types of chain restaurants, the food is cooked, microwaved, or rewarmed in ways that cause chemicals to leach into it. And it may not be cooked right away; restaurants typically slap stickers on plastic bags of food that show their "cook by" date. All of this is done so that the franchise saves money and makes big profits.

Even seasonings come premade. I was at a Thai restaurant recently and about to order red curry vegetables. I asked the server if the dish contained MSG. He explained that although the restaurant does not add MSG, the curry seasoning it uses contains the ingredient. It's so difficult to avoid these things, yet it is very important that we do.

BIG CHAINS, BIG FOOD POLLUTION

Some of the most popular chain restaurants in the country are serving up unbelievable concoctions of chemicals (see my alert below), and for this reason, I avoid dining at these establishments. You've got to be informed about what you're being served at these places.

If you want a real insider's look at how the big restaurant chains operate in this regard, read *The American Way of Eating: Undercover at Walmart, Applebee's, Farm Fields, and the Dinner Table* by journalist Tracie McMillan. McMillan goes undercover as a California farm worker, as a Walmart produce handler, and later as a kitchen assistant in an Applebee's in Brooklyn, New York. At Applebee's, she chronicles how the food is frozen or prepackaged, and reports that everything on your plate is portioned from plastic bags that the "cooks" in the back do nothing more to than microwaving or boiling them, then assembling the food to make it look appetizing.

 FOOD BABE ALERT: A PLATE OF CHEMICALS COMING RIGHT UP

Eat at any of the major restaurant chains at your own nutritional risk. Here's a look at what you might be eating if you order the following popular dishes.

Applebee's — Sampling of menu items exposes you to at least 10 of the Sickening 15 ingredients

Spinach Artichoke Dip: Skim milk, spinach, **soybean oil**, artichoke hearts, water, salt, **citric acid,** dehydrated onion, **modified corn starch, bleached wheat flour,** Romano cheese (cow's milk), pasteurized milk, cheese culture, salt, **enzymes,** dehydrated garlic, seasoning, **xanthan gum, maltodextrin, flavor, enzyme modified butter fat.**

Lemon Parmesan Shrimp (Weight Watchers endorsed menu item): Blackened shrimp sautéed with tomatoes, onions and basil. Served over creamy rice with a decadent lemon and Parmesan cream sauce.

Lemon Parmesan Cream Sauce (aka "Homestyle Sauce"): Water, cream, chicken broth, seasoning, **corn starch, xanthan gum, natural flavors,** spices, parmesan cheese, pasteurized part skim milk, cheese culture, salt, **enzymes,** butter roux, onions, roasted chicken base (chicken meat, chicken juices, salt, **autolyzed yeast extract, flavors,** sugar, potato flour), chicken base (chicken meat including chicken juices, salt, **hydrolyzed soy and corn protein).**

Weight Watchers nonstick spray: Canola oil, **soy lecithin.**

Blackened seasoning (used on 41/50 shrimp): Blackened Seasoning: spices, salt, chili peppers, dehydrated onion, dehydrated garlic, **dextrose, soybean oil.**

Creamy rice: White rice.

Cheesecake Factory—Sampling of menu items exposes you to at least 12 of the Sickening 15 ingredients

Wheat bread (complimentary bread): Enriched wheat flour (niacin, reduced iron, thiamine mononitrate, riboflavin, folic acid), **malted barley flour,** water, **whole wheat flour,** rolled oats, **rye meal, yeast, brown sugar, sugar, high-fructose corn syrup,** molasses, wheat bran, wheat gluten, **vegetable oil shortening (partially hydrogenated soybean oil, cottonseed oil and/or canola oil),** salt, **caramel color, diglycerides, diacetyl tartaric acid esters of mono- and diglycerides,** sorbic acid, **enzymes, azodicarbonamide, L-cysteine,** guar gum, **corn syrup,** wheat.

Herb Crusted Salmon Salad: *Salmon:* Salmon, yellow mustard, sage, parsley, rosemary, thyme, green onion (cooked in **canola**/olive oil blend). *Salad:* Baby lettuce mix, cucumber, red onion, asparagus, Roma tomato, endive, lemon slices.

Balsamic vinaigrette: Balsamic vinegar, red wine vinegar, Dijon mustard, **soy sauce,** garlic, shallots, sugar, salt, pepper, **canola oil, canola oil blend** (extra virgin olive oil/**canola oil).**

Ultimate Red Velvet Cheesecake: Cream cheese (pasteurized cultured milk, salt, stabilizers [**xanthan,** carob bean, and guar gums]), butter (pasteurized cultured milk, salt, stabilizers [**xanthan,** carob bean, and guar gums]), **sugar, powdered sugar, corn oil (fully refined and dewaxed corn oil),** whole egg, sour cream, **modified corn starch, sodium tripolyphosphate,** guar gum, calcium sulfate, locust bean gum, buttermilk, white chocolate (**sugar,** cocoa butter, whole milk powder, skim milk, whey powder, lactose, **soy lecithin,** natural vanilla), water, **invert sugar, red color (maltodextrin, xanthan gum,** guar gum, **FD&C red 40),** dark chocolate powder (100% cocoa beans processed with alkali), baking soda, mascarpone cheese (pasteurized milk, cream, **citric acid),** salt, vinegar, baking powder, vanilla extract, **artificial vanilla flavor.**

Crust: Flour (**enriched bleached wheat flour, malted barley flour,** niacin, iron, thiamine mononitrate, riboflavin, folic acid).

Chili's—Sampling of menu items exposes you to at least 12 of the Sickening 15 ingredients

Memphis Ribs: (100% pork ribs, and rib spice made of salt, dehydrated garlic, **brown sugar,** spices, **yeast extract,** dehydrated onion, **sugar, citric acid, corn starch, natural flavor, disodium inosinate, disodium guanylate,** with not more than 2% silicon dioxide added as an anticaking agent), Memphis Dry Rub (**brown sugar,** spices, paprika, garlic powder, salt, onion powder, and **silicon dioxide** [anticaking agent], salad oil (**soybean oil with citric acid** added as a preservative), classic BBQ sauce (**high-fructose corn syrup,** tomato paste, distilled vinegar, water, **corn syrup,** molasses, salt, red wine vinegar, contains less than 2%

(Continued)

of spices, **modified food starch, sugar, potassium sorbate** and **sodium benzoate** as preservatives, onion, paprika, garlic, turmeric, **caramel color**).

Original Ribs: (100% pork ribs, and rub spice (salt, dehydrated garlic, **brown sugar,** spices, **yeast extract,** dehydrated onion, **sugar, citric acid, corn starch, natural flavor, disodium inosinate, disodium guanylate,** with not more than 2% **silicon dioxide** added as an anticaking agent), classic BBQ sauce (**high-fructose corn syrup,** tomato paste, distilled vinegar, water, **corn syrup,** molasses, salt, red wine vinegar, contains less than 2% of: spices, **modified food starch, sugar, potassium sorbate** and **sodium benzoate** as preservatives, onion, paprika, garlic, turmeric, **caramel color**).

Boneless wings: *Chili's boneless buffalo wings:* **Enriched wheat flour,** spices, dried garlic, dried onions, dried egg whites, bread crumbs, **enriched wheat flour,** wheat gluten, **soy flour, soybean oil,** spice extract, yeast, **corn syrup,** salt, **yellow corn flour.** (Wings are fried in **vegetable oil shortening**). *Buffalo wing sauce:* Cayenne pepper, vinegar, salt, water, **vegetable oil,** garlic, **dextrose,** molasses, **corn syrup, xanthan gum, caramel color,** spices, **modified food starch, sugar,** tamarind, **natural and artificial favor.** *Blue Cheese dressing:* **Soybean oil,** water, blue cheese (pasteurized milk cheese culture, salt, **enzymes**), red wine vinegar, egg yolk, **sugar,** salt, spice, garlic, **potassium sorbate,** buttermilk solids, **natural flavors.** *BBQ Sauce:* **High-fructose corn syrup, corn syrup,** tomato paste, distilled vinegar, water, molasses, salt, red wine vinegar, onion, paprika, garlic, turmeric, **sugar, potassium sorbate, sodium benzoate.**

Olive Garden — Sampling of menu items exposes you to at least
12 of the Sickening 15 ingredients

Olive Garden salad dressing: Water, **soybean oil,** distilled vinegar, **high-fructose corn syrup,** salt, egg, Romano cheese, dehydrated garlic, **sugar,** spices, **xanthan gum, dextrose, calcium disodium EDTA, annatto color, natural flavors.**

Olive Garden breadsticks: Enriched flour, wheat flour, **malted barley flour,** reduced iron, riboflavin, folic acid, water, **high-fructose corn syrup,** salt, yeast, **soybean oil, sodium stearoyl lactylate, calcium stearoyl lactylate, monoglycerides, diglycerides, distilled monoglycerides,** calcium peroxide, **enzymes,** ascorbic acid, calcium sulfate, **calcium propionate.**

> **Olive Garden breadsticks topping (varies):**
>
> *Butter:* Margarine (**liquid unhydrogenated soybean oil,** water, salt, **vegetable monodiglycerides,** sodium, **sodium benzoate, canola oil, citric acid**).
>
> *Butter:* **Hydrogenated soybean oil,** water, salt, vinegar, **sodium benzoate, citric acid, natural and artificial flavor, calcium EDTA,** beta carotene, vitamin A palmitate.
>
> *Garlic salt:* Garlic powder, granulated salt.

Olive Garden marinara: Ground peeled tomatoes, tomato puree, salt, **food starch, modified citric acid,** mushroom base (mushrooms, water, salt, **corn maltodextrin,** unsalted butter, **sugar, hydrolyzed soy and corn protein, yeast extract, hydrolyzed wheat gluten,** onion powder, corn oil, **hydrogenated soy oil,** lactic acid, calcium lactate), onions, marinara base concentrate (onions, **yeast extract,** salt, **soy oil, hydrolyzed soy and corn protein,** water, butter, garlic, dehydrated onion, **disodium inosinate, disodium guanylate,** mushroom juice, onion powder, **xanthan gum**).

Alfredo sauce: Heavy cream, butter, parmesan, salt, pepper, garlic, milk, base (wheat, nonfat milk solids, parsley, **hydrogenated soybean and cottonseed oils,** salt, **sugar, corn starch,** onion powder, parmesan cheese, Swiss cheese, buttermilk solids, blue cheese, creamed butterfat, spice).

Meatballs: Beef, water, egg whites, **textured soy protein concentrate,** Romano cheese, sheep's milk, bread crumbs (**enriched flour, wheat flour,** niacin, reduced iron, thiamine mononitrate, riboflavin, folic acid, **corn syrup, sugar, vegetable shortening [hydrogenated soybean oil, hydrogenated cottonseed oil],** salt, **yeast, whey, soy flour, dough conditioner [sodium stearoyl lactylate], calcium propionate**), dehydrated onions, **soy protein concentrate,** salt, spices, **sodium phosphate,** garlic powder, parsley.

Olive Garden Pasta Fagioli: Beef, yellow onions, carrots, celery, oregano, pepper, cayenne pepper, hot water, beef base (beef, water, beef stock, salt, **corn, soy,** wheat protein, **canola oil, hydrolyzed corn gluten,** onion powder, **caramel color, dextrose,** lactic acid), kidney beans. Pasta for the soup is made in the restaurant with flour, eggs, and sugar.

Nonetheless, I love to eat out and will continue to do so. I'm simply careful about the selections I make.

So, eating out and eating healthy: an impossible order? Not if you remember who's in charge: you. Take control today, using these strategies.

THE FOOD BABE WAY

In a perfect world, we would all know exactly what we were eating while dining out. While at present this is nearly impossible, there are things you can do to make sure you get the healthiest choices. Here are my general tips:

MAKE DINING OUT A SPECIAL OCCASION

Your meal will be memorable and you'll save money by avoiding food that isn't good for you.

EAT HALF OF A GRAPEFRUIT

Unless you're taking certain medications that can be compromised by grapefruit, eating this fruit before a meal can bring some surprising benefits. In 2006, the *Journal of Medicinal Food* reported that half of a fresh grapefruit eaten before meals triggered significant weight loss in overweight people. The grapefruit blunted a rise in insulin two hours after the meal, and this may have accounted for the weight loss, since spikes in insulin can be fat-forming.

SUPPRESS YOUR APPETITE WITH WATER

Drink a large glass of water about twenty minutes before going out to eat. This will curb your appetite and keep you from overindulging.

ORDER A SALAD AS YOUR FIRST COURSE WITH DRESSING AND/OR CHEESE ON THE SIDE

This will help alkalinize the body and get your digestive enzymes working. If the menu doesn't indicate what kind of lettuce is used, ask, and then request that your salad be made of mixed greens, arugula, or romaine, not iceberg. Simply dip your fork in the dressing and spear pieces of salad before each bite; you'll minimize the fat and calories this way but still get the flavor of the dressing.

QUIZ YOUR SERVER

Servers have probably seen or sampled all the dishes and can tell you if your fish or other entrée is swimming in oil or covered in cream sauce.

COMMUNICATE YOUR ALLERGIES OR FOOD SENSITIVITIES

Don't be shy about telling your server that you don't want to eat butter, dairy, soy, corn, or other foods. Butter really isn't bad for you if it's organic, but restaurants can go overboard and drown dishes in butter. Soy and corn oils are the cheapest oils available, so many restaurants use them, but as I've discussed, they will dump an overdose of omega-6 fatty acids into your body. They're also probably not organic and have been genetically modified. Ask the chef if he or she can use olive oil instead in your dish.

CHECK THE SOUP

Before you order soup at a restaurant, ask if it's homemade or if it contains additives. One cold, rainy day last year, I was hungry for soup. I live right across the street from a gourmet food shop called Dean & Deluca that serves delicious-looking soups. The restaurant was calling my name. In I went. I asked for a list of the soups' ingredients, and I was shocked! The shop orders their soups premade from Sysco, a huge manufacturer of processed foods. These soups contain a lot of soy oil, and the hidden version of the obesogen MSG.

ORDER ORGANIC PROTEINS

Don't order the meat unless you know it's organic and grass-fed. No such choices? Fish is your next-best bet, as long as it's not farmed salmon. This type of salmon is often fed a mixture of highly contaminated fish meal and fish oil mixed with corn and soy products because these substances are cheap and help fatten up the fish. As I mentioned, salmon is fed supplements to make the flesh more pink. Farmed salmon is loaded with antibiotics, pesticides, and other toxic chemicals.

If there are no good meat or fish choices on the menu, try a bean and/or veggie dish instead. If available, goat cheese or nuts can be added to your salad as protein. Avocado is a nice addition as well; it's filling and full of good fats.

MIX AND MATCH

Don't see anything you like on the menu? Check out the specifics for each dish and ask the waiter to create a custom plate. Once I was stuck in an airport with one food option—Ruby Tuesday. The restaurant had fresh guacamole, served with chips, and a platter on the menu included fish. I asked them kindly to make me a plate of fish and a large scoop of that guac. It was delicious and satisfying, and I made it home without biting off the arm of the passenger seated next to me.

ORDER OFF (NOT FROM) THE MENU

Ask the chef to create something for you. This request can be made easily at a fancier or more established restaurant where chefs are highly skilled and can experiment for you. I remember once I attended a work dinner at a fancy steakhouse inside a casino. Because I rarely eat steak and nothing else really appealed to me, I asked the chef to create a vegetable plate. He got really creative with veggies and whole grains, tossed with a little olive oil. The dish was so fabulous that one of my bosses looked over and said, "Wow — I wish I had ordered that."

BUILD A RELATIONSHIP WITH A FAVORITE RESTAURANT

When I'm too busy to cook but still want to eat healthy, I head to my favorite standby. I've gotten to know the staff, and they make everything perfect for me every time. For example, the sushi chef prepares a special roll with all veggies and no white rice or fatty sauces. He calls it the Food Babe Roll. He also knows that I like my ponzu sauce on the side of my sashimi, not poured on top. I always start with a big bowl of romaine with extra cucumbers and the ginger dressing on the side, and they serve great hot green tea. My meals there are fail-proof, and I never have to stress about what I'm eating.

EAT ETHNIC

Ethnic dining is wildly popular, but be vigilant about:

MSG. This ingredient, commonly found in Chinese, Thai, Malaysian, and processed foods, is a flavor enhancer that is recognized as a safe additive by the FDA. But the pesky ingredient is known to cause numerous adverse symptoms, including obesity, headaches, facial pressure, chest pain, nausea, and more. Even if you aren't sensitive to this additive, it is used to make food more tasty and addictive, which isn't a good thing since portion sizes in a lot of these restaurants are enormous.

Sauces: Ethnic dishes usually come with seriously tasty sauces. Although they're not additives per se, it's difficult to know what's in them. Sauce is something you may want to skip unless you're familiar with the ingredients.

Here are my tips for wise, healthy dining at various types of ethnic restaurants.

Tips for Eating Chinese Food

Avoid tofu unless it's organic.
Opt for steamed vegetables and rice instead of stir-fry dishes, which could use oils containing GMOs.

If you must have stir-fry, ask if they can make it with coconut oil. If not, rice-bran, sunflower, or sesame oil can be used (100 percent with no other vegetable oils added).

Make sure meat is organic, and if not, choose vegetarian dishes, as long as they aren't drowning in sauce.

Avoid dishes with GMO crops such as corn, soy, canola, sugar beets, cotton, zucchini, squash, and papaya.

Make sure food is MSG-free.

Tips for Eating Thai Food

Instead of opting for pad thai, which is cooked with vegetable oil, choose a vegetable dish without sauce or with a sauce you can have on the side, so you can control the amount you consume. The fewer toxins, the better! You can also ask for your dish to be steamed rather than stir-fried, which is always a healthier option.

Make sure meat and tofu are organic.

Tips for Eating Mexican Food

Stay away from GMO-laden corn chips; consider asking for veggies to dip in salsa or guacamole.

Opt for vegetarian and bean dishes unless organic meat and cheese options are available.

A taco salad with vegetables, avocado, and salsa is your best bet.

Tips for Eating Indian Food

Opt for vegetable dishes without sauce unless the meat and dairy are organic.

A few great choices at an Indian restaurant:

Daal. A protein-rich dish made of lentils, peas, or beans that is typically eaten with rice and vegetables.

Channa masala: Chickpeas cooked in an exotic blend of north Indian spices.

Navratan korma: Mixed vegetables cooked in a gravy made from cashew nuts.

Mushroom mutter: Fresh sliced mushrooms cooked with green peas, tomatoes, and spices.

Whole wheat paratha or chapati: Handmade flatbread. Some restaurants will gladly make the switch to whole grain if you ask.

Tips for Eating Japanese Food

Order only organic edamame. Nonorganic varieties are full of pesticides and have been genetically modified. Forget fish roe (*tobiko*). These tiny little fish eggs are cultivated and then dyed beautiful colors to seem more appealing. Look, but don't touch!

Eliminate imitation crab. This is the typical "fish" found in the California roll and many other rolls. A stick of processed crap, it is really composed of minced fish left over in some factory somewhere, combined with egg whites, gluten, artificial colors, sorbitol, and a bunch of other ingredients like hydrolyzed soy protein and disodium inosinate — forms of MSG.

Freak out about farmed salmon. I would say the majority of sushi restaurants serve farmed salmon. This stuff is dreadful, filled with chemical pesticides. Farmed salmon also has about fifty more calories per three-ounce serving than wild salmon does and half as much omega-3 fatty acid. Choose other types of fish — and make sure they're wild-caught.

Limit your dip. One tablespoon of soy sauce has roughly 500 milligrams of sodium. Given that you might eat up to three tablespoons of soy sauce, this is a ridiculous amount of sodium to be consuming at one meal. Wonder why your skin is puffy or your stomach bloated after a meal of sushi? I personally don't even use soy sauce anymore; I ask the chef for ponzu sauce instead. It's a little sweeter than soy sauce because it contains some mirin (Japanese cooking wine) but has less sodium overall.

Certain foods don't belong in Japanese cuisine, such as cream cheese or mayo (often found in spicy tuna). These foods probably contain nonorganic dairy and other ingredients not found in the typical Japanese diet.

What's up with the fake wasabi? Real Japanese horseradish is amazing for you. It can help detoxify your body and prevent many forms of cancer. It is also antimicrobial and helps protect you from bacteria that might be present in raw fish. But most sushi restaurants are using a cheap alternative they can get in the form of powder. This powder contains harmful additives like artificial food coloring (yellow and blue make green!). High-quality restaurants will have the real deal, but you have to ask for it.

Recognize your rice. Sushi rice is typically short-grain rice that is polished white, cooked, and then mixed with rice wine vinegar. When you add vinegar to rice, you decrease its glycemic index, or GI. GI is a measurement of how quickly a food is converted to sugar in your body. By lowering the GI of rice, vinegar prevents the rapid surge in blood sugar you would normally get if you ate rice alone. Aha! This is how the Japanese get away with eating white rice without worrying about blood sugar spikes, but does that mean you go crazy with the rice? No. Because I prefer to consume my lower-quality carbs as dessert, I order my vegetable roll sans rice and add asparagus. Brown or black rice are better options too.

Don't be tempted by tempura. Think twice about ordering any roll or other menu item that is fried or has the word "tempura" in its description. What kind of oil are they using to fry? Do they fry it in trans fat? Opt for sashimi, which is simply raw fish served on a platter with sliced pickled ginger.

Do not order the seaweed salad, unless you know it doesn't contain food coloring. Artificial food coloring is what gives the salad that bright green color. Yellow #5 can cause severe allergic reactions, and Blue #1 has caused brain cancer in lab animals.

Tips for Eating French Food

Before ordering a cheese plate, ask if the cheese is imported from France. A cheese from France means you are safe from rBGH—genetically engineered growth hormone—and genetically modified ingredients, as France has banned GMOs altogether.

A goat cheese salad is a good option. So are tuna Niçoise salads or vegetable crepes.

Use your judgment when it comes to choosing meat. Ask how the restaurant sources their meat. If it is organic, you should feel at ease when ordering meat dishes.

Tips for Eating Vietnamese Food

Order vegetarian pho, and make sure to ask for a vegetarian broth. Pho usually comes with beef or chicken broth. Make sure the restaurant doesn't use MSG.

Order a vegetable curry with steamed rice.

Order a wooden steamer basket with veggies such as broccoli, cauliflower, carrots, Napa cabbage, snow peas, asparagus, and bean sprouts, among others, with steamed rice.

Tips for Eating Ethiopian Food

You should be fine ordering almost anything at an Ethiopian restaurant. This cuisine is one of the healthiest ethnic options because dishes contain a lot of lentils and vegetables. Be sure to ask about the oils used in the preparation of each dish.

Tips for Eating Italian Food

Ask for plain pasta drizzled with olive oil, salt, and pepper and topped with steamed vegetables. Other good choices include buffalo mozzarella salad, fish, and steamed vegetables. If the Parmesan is imported from Italy, it won't contain growth hormone, because it is illegal to treat cows with hormones in Italy.

Tips for Eating Pizza

If your pizza restaurant does not offer organic cheese, ask for a cheese-free pizza loaded with vegetables.

Most pizza places have a salad option; choose a garden salad without meat or cheese.

EATING AWAY FROM HOME: DINNER PARTIES AND HOLIDAY GATHERINGS

I have to be honest: During the holidays, it's hard for me not to give in to nostalgic cravings and indulge in foods I typically avoid the rest of the year. It's the holidays, for goodness' sake, and I want to celebrate like everyone else.

But every January, I'd find my skinny jeans tighter and my waistline generally uncomfortable when I sat down. And let's not even talk about how I felt mentally—tired all the time and not self-confident at all. I hate those feelings!

After I started learning about what was really in my food, I made a conscious decision to avoid eating processed food regardless the time of year because I knew the toxic chemicals were responsible for making me gain weight. If there was something I really wanted to eat that I knew was filled with additives, artificial ingredients, or other questionable substances, I would make it at home with my own organic ingredients so I could indulge.

Because we live in an overly processed world, it's important to learn how to navigate holiday parties, whether during a conventional family meal or at the annual cocktail party your neighbor generously hosts. Whatever the occasion, here's what to do:

1. Eat before you arrive. Before you get to the party, have a good organic meal at home. Fill up on one of my green smoothies or dig into a salad loaded with lots of veggies so that you don't arrive at the party feeling ravenous.

2. Don't sample everything. Just because it's there doesn't mean you have to eat it. When choosing what to put on your plate, stick to familiar foods and avoid foods you normally wouldn't eat outside of a holiday party. Load up your plate with plant foods, and keep it simple. Sampling the entire buffet is dangerous. According to Susan Roberts, professor of nutrition and psychiatry at Tufts University, studies have shown that "the higher the variety of items you are confronted with, the more people consume without even realizing it."

3. Watch out for nuts. I used to think grabbing a handful of nuts was a good idea at parties, until I learned that most party nut mixes are doused with GMO oils, MSG, and other nasty additives. No thanks!

4. Bring your own dish. There's a rule in etiquette that says "never show up at a party empty-handed." Use this rule to your advantage and bring along your favorite healthy dish. That way, you have the option of eating at least one healthy item while you're at the party. You'll also have the opportunity to share a healthy dish with friends and family and teach them that good food can be good for you.

5. Socialize more and snack less. To keep your mind off all the dangerous goodies and temptations, move away from the buffet table and socialize elsewhere. Keeping your mind focused on something other than food will help prevent you from overindulging. I love spending parties socializing rather than eating. If I'm still hungry afterward, I know I can always get a clean meal at my go-to restaurant or at home later. Besides, sometimes it's fun to grab a group of people for a late-night meal or after-party.

6. Keep track of your drinks. Remember, your liver is your main fat-burning organ. If you're trying to lose weight or even maintain your ideal weight, alcohol is one of your worst enemies—so slow down and keep your alcohol intake on the low end, especially if you have multiple gatherings per week. A sparkling water with lime looks like a vodka tonic. No one will know you choose not to drink alcohol. Personally, I love to bring wine to a party so I know I have organic red wine available to drink and share. As I mentioned earlier, I don't mind the occasional tequila on the rocks with lime; it's one of the cleanest liquors.

7. *When all else fails, eat when you get home.* I promise you won't starve to death waiting a couple of hours to eat. And if you have special needs (say, you are diabetic or hypoglycemic), you already know what you need to do to make sure you stay steady. Simply not eating has been my saving grace in many situations—not just at parties, but in airports, too. Later on, I always thank myself for putting my health first.

8. *Lead by example.* Most important, while attending a party, go in with the understanding that not all of the guests will share your sentiments regarding your real-food lifestyle. Friends and family members who follow a conventional diet may not understand why you make the choices you do. If you're questioned about your diet, try to give your friends and family an honest and informative answer about your decisions without berating them about their own decisions.

As Mahatma Gandhi said: "Be the change you wish to see in the world."

CHECKLIST

Today:
- ✓ I did my morning lemon water ritual.
- ✓ I enjoyed a green drink.
- ✓ I stopped drinking fluids with my meals.
- ✓ I drank, and bathed in, pure, clean, filtered water.
- ✓ I ate less dairy and made healthier dairy choices.
- ✓ I stopped drinking all sodas.
- ✓ I loved my liver by paying attention to alcohol consumption.
- ✓ I passed on fast food.
- ✓ I gave up refined sugar.
- ✓ I ate less meat and I ate it responsibly.
- ✓ I increased the raw plant foods in my diet.
- ✓ I chose the best possible grains and carbs.
- ✓ I balanced my fats.
- ✓ I supplemented with at least one superfood.
- ✓ I avoided GMO foods as much as possible.
- ✓ If dining out, I made healthy, organic choices.

Day 17 — Do a Kitchen Cleanout

HERE'S A HABIT THAT will turn you into a Food Babe (or Guy) in no time at all: regular kitchen cleanouts. I don't mean a simple cleaning where you throw out a few items. I mean the kind where it's more like surgery. You're going to surgically remove some of the junk that has fossilized deep in the back of your pantry, refrigerator, and freezer. And as with surgery, you don't just rush into this. You have to be methodical.

Honestly, before I developed this habit, I wasn't really sure what I would find in my kitchen. There have been enough layers in my pantry and refrigerator that geologists would have a field day. I've found an ominous collection of chemical-filled junk, stuff that lasts so long that even bugs don't eat it; a box of baking powder with added aluminum dating back to the Bush years; and an art project made out of jelly beans, relics of my candy-eating days.

Even after I started eating organic foods, there was still a lone container of Crisco perched on a shelf near my stove. My friends were aghast: "What are you doing with that evil fat?" they asked. Fortunately, it had not been opened. Any unopened foodstuff like my errant Crisco container can be returned to the supermarket, depending on the purchase date and whether you have the receipt. I was able to return the Crisco, but not before explaining to the store manager why. If more people admonished their grocery stores for carrying poisons, there'd be less of this stuff on their shelves. Some grocery stores carry organic products you might never have seen where you live. Costco in Northern California convinced Frito-Lay to go organic and offer their customers organic "Ruffles," and even offer a "Doritos" without MSG. Grocery stores are our friends — if we communicate our needs to them, they will start to listen to us and ask manufacturers to develop safer and healthier products. This is exactly why Walmart is going to start offering a wide array of organic products under the Wild Oats brand.

If you're looking to change your diet for good, this is a great habit to develop. Here's how I did it.

THE FOOD BABE WAY

CLEAR OUT

Take everything out of your pantry and refrigerator, shelf by shelf. Clearing the shelves is the only way you can inventory what you have on hand—and what you want to toss. Then sort through the toxic debris by checking the ingredient list and cross-referencing it with the Sickening 15 on page 38. Toss out items that are full of chemical additives. Again, if they have a "satisfaction guarantee" on them, you might be able to get a full refund or store credit. It's worth asking your local grocery store about this—especially if you are finding a lot of toxic foods in your cabinets.

RESTOCK

Restock the shelves with what you've kept, if anything, and place the things you use most within the easiest reach. Keep all of the items in the same place all the time. Follow my pantry essentials below and organize items according to drinks; breakfast cereals and grains; bread, pasta, and whole grains; beans; dried fruits, nuts, and seeds; snacks; desserts and sweets; freezer items; and condiments and other staples.

Here's a look at what I consider "pantry essentials" (*All items should be certified organic unless otherwise noted*):

Drinks:

Suja juices (the green varieties like Twelve Essentials)

Harmless Harvest coconut water

Kombucha

Sparkling water

Almond milk (homemade or without carrageenan)

Coconut milk (homemade or without carrageenan)

Larry's Beans coffee

Numi tea

Traditional Medicinals tea

Yogi tea

Breakfast cereals and grains:

Food For Life Ezekiel English muffins — cinnamon raisin

Oat groats

Buckwheat

Steel-cut oats
Gluten-free rolled oats
Nature's Path Qi'a cereal
Food For Life Ezekiel cereal

Kaia Foods raw buckwheat granola dark
Purely Elizabeth granola
2 Moms in the Raw cereal

Bread, pasta, and whole grains:

Food For Life Ezekiel bread — sesame
100% buckwheat noodles
Tolerant Foods lentil pasta
Food For Life Ezekiel penne pasta
Food For Life Ezekiel linguine
TruRoots sprouted quinoa
Quinoa flakes
Farro
Brown rice

Red Himalayan rice
Black Forbidden rice
Almond flour
Coconut flour
Oat flour
Whole wheat stone-ground flour
Mary's Gone bread crumbs
Spelt flour

Beans:

Dry or canned chickpeas, also known as garbanzo beans (in BPA-free cans)
Dry or canned red kidney beans (in BPA-free cans)
Dry or canned black beans (in BPA-free cans)
Dry or canned cannellini beans (in BPA-free cans)
TruRoots sprouted lentils
Green lentils
Yellow lentils

Dried fruits, nuts, and seeds:

Goji berries
Golden berries
Currants
Dried figs
Dried plums
Dates
Dried mango
Walnuts
Almonds
Pistachios
Brazil nuts

Pecans
Cashews
Chia seeds
Flaxseeds
Hempseeds
Sesame seeds
Sunflower seeds
Pumpkin seeds
Tahini
Almond butter
Sunflower butter

Snacks:

Brad's Raw Foods chips and crackers
Unique Splits sprouted wheat pretzels
Mary's Gone Crackers
Mary's Gone Crackers sticks and twig pretzels
Late July tortilla chips
Suzie's Thin Cakes—flax and spelt
479° popcorn

Desserts and sweets:

Gnosis Chocolate
NibMor chocolate
JJ's Sweets Cocomels—coconut milk–based chocolates
Alter Eco quinoa chocolate
Dark chocolate chips
Righteously Raw bars
Three Twins vanilla ice cream
Luna & Larry's Organic Coconut Bliss Ice Cream
Go Raw coconut cookies
Kur organic bite-size bars
Erewhon brown rice cereal

Freezer items:

Food For Life Ezekiel whole wheat sprouted tortillas
Food For Life Ezekiel corn tortillas
Hilary's Eat Well burgers
Wild-caught salmon
Frozen mango
Frozen strawberries
Frozen blueberries
Frozen mixed berries
Frozen acai
Frozen pineapple
Frozen artichokes

Condiments and other staples:

Organic ketchup
Yellow mustard
Stone-ground mustard
Apple cider vinegar
Cold-pressed olive oil
Nutiva hemp oil
Nutiva hemp protein
Nutiva extra virgin coconut oil
Tamari
Ponzu sauce
Mirin
Balsamic vinegar
Organic rice wine vinegar
Maple syrup
Raw local honey
Pickles
Olives
Himalayan sea salt
Dry nonirradiated spices (Simply Organic or Frontier Co-op)
Low-sodium vegetable broth
Low-sodium chicken broth
Yellow Barn Organics spaghetti sauce
Nutiva coconut manna

Coconut palm sugar

Date sugar

Stevia extract

Raw cacao powder

Unsweetened coconut flakes

Aluminum-free baking powder

POST A CHECKLIST

Last but not least, post a checklist on the inside of your pantry door, using my list as a reference. Cross off items as you deplete them. Not only will the checklist remind you of your inventory, it will alert you to what you don't have and help you plan your weekly shopping trip. You can find a printable version of this checklist here: foodbabe.com/pantry-list/.

A clean pantry, fridge, and freezer are easily attainable. You can do it!

CHECKLIST

Today:

✓ I did my morning lemon water ritual.

✓ I enjoyed a green drink.

✓ I stopped drinking fluids with my meals.

✓ I drank, and bathed in, pure, clean, filtered water.

✓ I ate less dairy and made healthier dairy choices.

✓ I stopped drinking all sodas.

✓ I loved my liver by paying attention to alcohol consumption.

✓ I passed on fast food.

✓ I gave up refined sugar.

✓ I ate less meat and I ate it responsibly.

✓ I increased the raw plant foods in my diet.

✓ I chose the best possible grains and carbs.

✓ I balanced my fats.

✓ I supplemented with at least one superfood.

✓ I avoided GMO foods as much as possible.

✓ If dining out, I made healthy, organic choices.

✓ I cleaned out my kitchen—and will keep it that way.

Day 18 — Change Your Little
Grocery Shop of Horrors

THE SURROUNDINGS WERE UNFAMILIAR. It was like someone had dropped me from a helicopter into a strange land, and I was lost. Only this wasn't a strange land; this was a grocery store called Earth Fare. It was my first-ever visit to a natural food store.

I was accustomed to shopping at regular, mainstream supermarkets, and I was surprised by what I saw at Earth Fare. There was a natural meat counter. The chicken, beef, and lamb had been allowed to roam and graze naturally. Most of the meat had been given organic feed. The animals had not been given antibiotics or hormones. The eggs were fresher than those I bought elsewhere. The fruits and vegetables, unsprayed, were fresh and colorful. I carted my way through the bulk food section, seeing bin after bin of staples and grains, many of which I'd never heard of.

But where was the regular stuff? Coca-Cola? Rice Krispies? Doritos? I was totally confused. All I found were products I didn't recognize, so I roamed the aisles forever, reading labels and inspecting ingredient lists. I discovered real granola bars for the first time; I tossed a box of them into my shopping cart.

This maiden trip turned into many trips. From that day on, I began to shop exclusively at stores where I could find organic, additive-free foods. I realized that where you shopped could affect how you looked and felt.

When you're trying to eat nutritiously, grocery shopping can be a little bit like searching for buried treasure. With nearly 50,000 product choices in the average grocery store and around 17,000 new items introduced each year, you wonder if it's even possible to find anything healthy and organic. I'm here to tell you that it is.

Today's new habit will make grocery shopping a cinch: Change your supermarket to a grocery store that specializes in natural, organic, chemical-free foods.

WHAT WHOLE FOODS DOES THAT WALMART DOESN'T!

Consumer reporter Ben Blatt, writing for the online magazine *Slate*, did an exposé, comparing foods at Walmart with foods at Whole Foods. Whole Foods bans foods that contain certain ingredients—around seventy-eight blacklisted ingredients to date, all of which frequently show up in processed foods and many of the Sickening 15. Here are some examples:

- Artificial colors
- Artificial flavors
- Aspartame
- Azodicarbonamide
- Benzoyl peroxide
- Dimethylpolysiloxane
- High-fructose corn syrup
- Hydrogenated fats
- Monosodium glutamate (MSG)
- Nitrates/nitrites
- Sodium benzoate
- TBHQ (tertiary butylhydroquinone)

Because Walmart doesn't ban any of the ingredients on the Whole Foods list, Blatt calculated some scary statistics for consumers who shop at the giant retailer:

- Approximately 14 percent of food products sold at Walmart would be banned from the shelves at Whole Foods, on the sole basis that they contain high-fructose corn syrup.
- About 54 percent of food items sold at Walmart would be vetoed by Whole Foods, if all seventy-eight ingredients were taken into account. Let me give you a visual here: If someone did a sweep of Walmart's grocery section to remove all foods containing those banned ingredients, more than half the shelves would be empty. The soft drink aisle in Walmart would be virtually bare, since

97 percent of Walmart's soft drinks are laced with ingredients Whole Foods deems unacceptable.

- Not a soda drinker (good!)? More than 36 percent of the waters at Walmart contain ingredients that would prohibit them from being sold at Whole Foods.

In all fairness, I understand that some big-name conventional grocery stores are making an effort to include more organic produce and convenience foods. That's a good thing. In these cases, take some time to read labels and decipher the names of ingredients. What looks like a wholesome food might turn out to be a disaster. Take breads labeled "100% whole wheat," for example. Often they contain artificial sweetener, dough conditioners, colorings, preservatives, and other chemicals. Even cereal isn't safe. Many packaged cereals, advertised as being good sources of whole grains and fiber, contain a highly processed sugar called maltodextrin and other preservatives. Thankfully, many conventional grocery stores, like Walmart, are starting to carry organic brands under their own private label. Choosing these brands over conventional brands will save you from a lot of toxic chemicals. Check for Wild Oats at Walmart, Simply Balanced at Target, GreenWise Market at Publix, and HT Naturals at Harris Teeter, for example.

It's easier and safer to shop at a store or market that has high-quality, organic foods. Change your grocery store, and you'll change your health for the better. For more tips on specific grocery stores, visit foodbabe.com.

THE FOOD BABE WAY

SHOP WELL

Shop where you can get the best-quality groceries and produce available. Stores like these have been around forever, but in the recent past they've become more mainstream, allowing anyone who wants a healthier lifestyle to make the transition.

I recommend the following grocery stores because they're committed to banning certain ingredients from their shelves:

- Whole Foods Market
- Earth Fare
- Sprouts Farmers Market
- Trader Joe's (with caveats; see below)
- Wild Oats Marketplace
- Mother's Market & Kitchen
- Healthy Home Market
- Erewhon

FOOD BABE ALERT: WHAT IS TRADER JOE'S HIDING?

For the record, I love shopping at Trader Joe's. It's fun and the employees are super nice and helpful. However, Trader Joe's won't share any information with me, and they are cloaked in secrecy regarding their business practices. Take the company's position on GMOs, for example: "Our approach to Genetically Modified Organisms is simple: we do not allow GMO ingredients in our private label products (anything with Trader Joe's, Trader José's, Trader Ming's, etc. on the label)."

Given this policy, we should trust them, right? Not necessarily. During my research, I found that no independent third-party certifier regularly verifies that Trader Joe's products are non-GMO. It is completely up to Trader Joe's product supply team to regulate GMOs from suppliers—not the Non-GMO Project or the USDA (for organics), both of which require high standards and third-party testing before a company can state that a product is GMO-free. If there are complaints about a product, Trader Joe's will conduct verification with an undisclosed, secret third party, but it's up to the consumer to complain.

Trader Joe's says they review affidavits (the documents that prove an ingredient is not made or contaminated with GMOs) from their suppliers who make their store-branded products, but there is no way to verify this. I asked Trader Joe's if they would send me an affidavit showing proof of non-GMO corn or soy in at least one of their products that wasn't labeled certified organic. They refused, saying, "Unfortunately we don't share those documents: they are confidential." They wouldn't even tell me what country some of the packaged products were produced in, as they do not provide "country of origin" labeling.

(Continued)

The denial of my request was maddening! We have the right to know where our food comes from and what's in it, and Trader Joe's is refusing to give us this information.

I understand that many people might shop at Trader Joe's due to low costs, but considering Trader Joe's lack of transparency, there's only a limited list of products I would personally buy:

- Certified organic fruits, vegetables, nuts, and seeds
- Certified organic branded Trader Joe's products (USDA certified), for example, their organic popcorn made with olive oil
- Certified organic milk products
- Certified organic meat—a lot of conventional meat is still sold at Trader Joe's; reports suggest that up to 90 percent of the meat products sold there can be raised with antibiotics
- Certified organic coffee and teas (like Yogi tea)
- Certified organic frozen produce, like berries
- Some conventional items (like kimchi) that do not have high-risk GMO crop ingredients
- Paper products; Trader Joe's uses environmentally friendly practices and recycled paper

The most important thing to remember when shopping at Trader Joe's, or anywhere else for that matter, is to read the ingredient lists.

BE A STRATEGIC SHOPPER

Once you get to your store of choice, shop strategically. Buy mainly whole foods, like fruits, vegetables, beans, sustainable meats, and grains. Most grocery stores stock these foods in the outside aisles. Your purchases should come from these aisles.

Check out the Clean 15 and Dirty Dozen lists available on the Environmental Working Group's website at ewg.org to help you learn which fruits and vegetables have the least pesticides. The Dirty Dozen lists the twelve most chemical-laden produce, whereas the Clean 15 identifies those with the lowest chemical residue. I use cucumbers in one of my favorite smoothies, and because they are on the Dirty Dozen list, I buy organic. It's important to buy organic versions of anything on the Dirty Dozen list. These lists change from time to time, so always consult the EWG website.

Here's my version of the foods you must absolutely buy organic if you can:

1. **Dairy** (milk, cheese, yogurt, ice cream, etc.)
2. **Meat** (look for 100 percent grass-fed, antibiotic-free, and growth hormone–free, fed an organic and non-GMO diet)
3. **Corn, soybeans, zucchini, yellow squash, canola, sugar beets, papaya, and cottonseed oil.** All of these are high-risk GMO crops. Remember to check the ingredient list on all packaged goods for these foods.
4. **The following fruits and vegetables:**
   - All leafy greens (kale, arugula, collards, spinach, cilantro, parsley, dandelion, chard, etc.)
   - All berries (strawberries, blueberries, raspberries, blackberries)
   - Sweet bell peppers
   - Apples
   - Celery
   - Cherry tomatoes
   - Cucumbers
   - Potatoes
   - Grapes
   - Hot peppers
   - Nectarines
   - Peaches
5. **Eggs** (stick to pasture eggs and chickens fed an organic diet)
6. **Tea and coffee**
7. **Dried herbs and spices** (nonorganic herbs and spices are irradiated, reducing medicinal quality)
8. **Chocolate**

Choose meats and dairy wisely: You want to purchase foods that are labeled "organic," "grass-fed," "free of hormones," "not produced with antibiotics" "wild," and so forth.

Fats or no fats: Fat is an essential part of your diet, and it will help keep you slim—especially around your tummy. But you've got to consume fats and oils that come from unrefined vegetable sources or oily fish such as salmon. Avoid trans fats at all costs. And stay away from oils like soy, corn, canola, and cottonseed in any product.

Don't buy genetically modified foods, ever, if you can help it. Look for "organic" or "non-genetically modified" on the label.

By all means, avoid ingredients you can't pronounce or that you've never heard of. Put that product back!

HAVE THE GOODS DELIVERED

Most of the time, I prefer comparing prices and selecting my groceries in the store, but you might feel differently and want to shop online. It's a great option if you're short on time, sick in bed with a cold, or running all over town with your kids. With a few mouse clicks, you can order organic food without fueling up your car or getting dressed. Here are some of my recommendations:

- Buy direct from your favorite brands. If there are staples you routinely buy, get them sent to your house.
- Instacart. Use this service for the ultimate convenience. Pick out the items you want online, and a personal shopper will go to your selected supermarket, do your shopping, and deliver it to your door. Right now the service is available in fifteen cities at supermarkets including Whole Foods, Costco, and Kroger.
- Abe's Market. This is an online retailer specializing in organic and natural goods. You can find everything here, from packaged foods to green household items.
- Vitacost. This is a great low-cost website that has a wide variety of organic and healthy foods, plus vitamins and other supplements.

- Herbspro. Here's another money-saving site, with low prices on all sorts of organic foods and products.
- Green PolkaDot Box and Thrive Market. These services deliver organic and non-GMO food directly to your doorstep. It's a membership club like Costco and Sam's Club, with some of the lowest prices available for organic staples, meat, dairy, and other goods, but you don't have to leave your house. Even for someone like me, who lives in close proximity to several natural food stores, the convenience of having an organic food delivery service is exciting. The time saving is one thing, but the money saving makes it a slam dunk.
- Organic produce delivery (Door to Door Organics, Absolute Organics, FreshDirect, or Simply Fresh). Every Tuesday I receive a delivery of organic produce right to my door. Not only does this keep my kitchen stocked with plant-based goodness, it also keeps things interesting: I get seasonal produce that I might not choose on my own, and this gives me reasons to come up with new recipes. If you aren't that daring, you can certainly request what you like from these services. But I suggest you let them surprise you every week; it makes opening that big box that much more rewarding and fun.

BUY LOCAL: FARMERS' MARKETS AND CSAS

Purchasing food from local sources in your own community is the best way to obtain seasonally fresh food. Local food can be significantly cheaper than food shipped from miles away. Find a farmers' market near you through localharvest.org or the USDA; get to know your local farmers, develop a personal relationship with them, and negotiate prices.

Ask your local farmers about their farming practices. Do they spray their crops with pesticides? Do they grow organic produce and raise organic livestock? What sustainable farming practices do they follow?

Be the last person to leave the farmers' market, too. Farmers will likely cut their prices at the end of the day so they don't have to take their produce back to the farm.

Or buy a share in a community-supported agriculture (CSA) program. The CSA farmer provides you with a basket of seasonal vegetables that you pick up or have delivered to your home each week. With CSA-provided food, you know it's not transported from many miles away.

GROW YOUR OWN

You might think this is a crazy suggestion, but hear me out: Growing your own food isn't as hard as you might think. My mother has always had a large vegetable garden. She takes great joy in cultivating her vegetables and preparing meals with them. She always encouraged me to have my own garden, too.

Here's how to get started:

- Plant an herb pot in your kitchen or somewhere convenient so you can always have fresh herbs on hand. Organic herbs are one of the most overpriced items at the grocery store.
- Refer to the Organic Consumers Association for tips on how to grow organic food inside your home year-round.
- Remember to buy non-GMO seeds; check out Sow True Seed for lots of options.
- If you have a garden, learn how to can or otherwise preserve the produce you grow so that you don't waste excess.

SAVE A WAD OF CASH

The biggest concern I hear about living an organic lifestyle is the cost. It's likely the only immediate downside, because everything else about living organically is pretty magical. You know by now that nonorganic food often contains cancer-causing hormones, immunity-destroying antibiotics, and dangerous pesticides. Buying high-quality organic food and eating the most nutritious foods on the planet will save you big bucks down the road in prescription drugs, doctor visits, and other medical costs.

Here are my top strategies to mitigate the money pains of buying organic. Let the savings begin!

LOOK FOR HEALTHY DEALS

If you find a good sale, stock up on key organic, nonperishable, and frozen items.

Take advantage of any special where you can "buy one, get one free" or buy one and get the other for a discounted price. (This trick only works if you really love the product and it is a staple in your home—otherwise it could lead to wasted food.)

Check out the store brands to save money. They're significantly cheaper than national brands.

Always use your rewards cards. Most convenience stores, grocery stores, and drugstores offer rewards or savings cards that help you save money on certain items at the checkout counter. Swiping your rewards card may save you an extra $.50 on most items.

Check the websites of your favorite companies for coupons and special promotions. Almost all of them have some. You can also find coupon deals on companies' social media pages.

Check out various coupon sites for organic products. Some of my favorites are Mambo Sprouts, Saving Naturally, Organic Deals, Organic Food Coupons, Healthsavers, Organic Deals and Steals, and Simply Organic.

Before you check out at an online store, visit www.retailmenot.com for online promotional codes and discounts for all your favorite online stores and sources.

START AT HOME AND IN YOUR KITCHEN

Stay organized. Plan your meals for the week according to what's on sale or what you have coupons for.

Write out a weekly and monthly budget to help keep track of your spending.

Make your own organic granola bars, kale chips, smoothies, juices, etc., to replace store-bought.

Invest in at least a two-stage water filter, which is installed directly under your sink, to avoid having to buy bottled water. Check the

Environmental Working Group's guide on choosing the right water filter for you.

Finally, check out the book *Wildly Affordable Organic* by Linda Watson for menu planning on $5 a day or less.

USE YOUR FREEZER

Organic frozen produce is usually cheaper than fresh, especially for out-of-season fruits and vegetables.

Freeze the following:

- Local in-season produce
- All leftovers (doubling recipes is a good idea), using inexpensive mason jars or silicone ice molds for smaller portions
- Homemade cookie dough and treats like my Almond Chocolate Freezer Fudge (recipe on page 334)
- Kitchen staples like butter, cheese, and bread scraps for bread crumbs or homemade croutons

MAKE MONEY-SAVING CHOICES

Reduce meat and dairy consumption if you cannot afford to go 100 percent organic. One way to do this is to be vegan before 6 p.m., as Mark Bittman suggests in his book VB6. For example, have a green smoothie for breakfast with Ezekiel toast, eat a large salad with lentils at lunch or a wrap made with hummus, and for dinner choose high-quality meat in small portions.

Cut back on the amount of organic meat used in a recipe by replacing half with organic beans.

Buy a whole organic chicken rather than breasts, legs, or wings for a lower cost per pound. You can use the carcass to make your own chicken broth.

Do not buy prewashed and ready-to-eat fruits and veggies, as they can cost twice as much.

Buy organic coffee and tea such as Larry's Beans organic coffee and

Numi tea, rather than going to expensive coffee shops. You'll save time in the morning, too.

Eat out only twice a week—eating organic at home is significantly less expensive than eating at organic restaurants.

BUY IN BULK

Because the manufacturer doesn't have to pay for the cost of designing the label and making packaging materials, bulk foods are often cheaper. I save a ton of cash by buying everything—from oat groats, to nuts, to dried fruit and lentils—in bulk.

Bring measuring cups with you to the grocery store if you are buying from bulk containers. That way you can get exactly the amount you need for a specific recipe and you won't pay for extra.

Buy the whole animal from a local farmer and freeze the portions you don't use. Consider splitting the cost with some friends.

To satisfy your sweet tooth, skip the full-size packages of organic candy and chocolate. Buy a few pieces in the bulk section; for example, go for a few pieces of organic dried fruit or ten organic chocolate-covered almonds.

Find out what fruits and vegetables are in season and buy those in bulk, since they are significantly cheaper. Freeze or can whatever is left over.

Join a buying club with your neighbors, friends, or family and buy large quantities at a discount. For example, United Buying Clubs (unitedbuyingclubs.com) serves more than 3,000 clubs in 34 states.

SELECT ORGANIC BRANDS THAT SAVE YOU BUCKS

Choose less expensive grocery store brands like Trader Joe's, Earth Fare, 365 Everyday Value, ShopRite, Wegmans, Kroger, Publix, and Harris Teeter. Regardless of the brand, these are all required to follow the same guidelines set forth by the USDA organic certification program if they bear the USDA organic seal, and chances are that you won't be able to tell the difference between a brand name and a store brand.

Remember that if you are not satisfied with your organic product, most grocery stores and organic food companies offer you a money-back guarantee.

CHECKLIST

Today:

    ✓ I did my morning lemon water ritual.

    ✓ I enjoyed a green drink.

    ✓ I stopped drinking fluids with my meals.

    ✓ I drank, and bathed in, pure, clean, filtered water.

    ✓ I ate less dairy and made healthier dairy choices.

    ✓ I stopped drinking all sodas.

    ✓ I loved my liver by paying attention to alcohol consumption.

    ✓ I passed on fast food.

    ✓ I gave up refined sugar.

    ✓ I ate less meat and I ate it responsibly.

    ✓ I increased the raw plant foods in my diet.

    ✓ I chose the best possible grains and carbs.

    ✓ I balanced my fats.

    ✓ I supplemented with at least one superfood.

    ✓ I avoided GMO foods as much as possible.

    ✓ If dining out, I made healthy, organic choices.

    ✓ I cleaned out my kitchen—and will keep it that way.

    ✓ I changed my shopping habits.

Day 19 — Cook Outside the Box

WHEN I WAS A little girl, the kitchen was off-limits. My dad wouldn't let me near a stove, for fear I would burn my little fingers off. I despised helping my mom set the table. Going to the farmers' market was torture. Indian food was scary. Burger King and McDonald's were so much more enticing.

After I went away to college, contemplating dinner involved not opening up the refrigerator or turning on the stove but picking up a phone and dialing for takeout. I knew this couldn't be good for me. I really needed to master some culinary basics, so in my midtwenties, after my wake-up call, I decided to tie on an apron and learn.

At first, I was intimidated. I didn't think I could boil an egg without burning it. But my overachieving nature took over. I saw learning to cook as a challenge. I relied on cookbooks, the Food Network, online information, and guidance from friends. I made a lot of mistakes, burned a lot of dishes, and totally botched what looked like easy recipes.

Practice makes perfect. Through trial and error, I learned how to cook and even to create my own recipes. I love collecting recipes from my travels and meeting people from around the world who share their cooking styles. These experiences have made me an adventuresome cook.

Most days I cook on the stove, and I don't *always* burn myself. My favorite chore is setting the table. I can spend countless hours at the farmers' market. I love Indian food. I think food from Burger King and McDonald's is evil. How things have changed.

Cooking at home is exceedingly healthy for you, because you have total control over the ingredients you use. Regardless of income, the best predictor of a healthy diet is how much food is cooked at home. You don't adulterate your food with preservatives, colorings, or MSG. You control the kind and the amount of fat, sugar, and salt used. You don't risk leaching plastic into meals. If you are buying organic ingredients, you don't cook with pesticides. You know exactly what you're eating.

Contrary to what you might have been led to believe, cooking at home also saves you time and money. You can make many dishes in less time than it takes to jump in the car and go to a fast-food restaurant. You can cook in bulk and reheat dishes when you're ready for a meal. By planning what you'll make and having the ingredients on hand, you'll save money. And you can be creative with leftovers, either recycling them into new dishes or packing them in containers and sending them off as lunch the next day—an option I fully explore in my household. If you have a well-stocked pantry, it's easier and cheaper to reach into the cupboard and cook than it is to shop for additional ingredients.

Buy It Cheap, Make It Keep

Quick fact: Americans waste an estimated 1,400 calories of food per person *every single day*. Don't be among them. Here are my suggestions:

Keep raw nuts and flours in your refrigerator to prevent them from going rancid.

Line your refrigerator's crisper drawer with paper towels to absorb excess moisture. This will help keep produce fresh.

To repel bugs, place a bay leaf in containers of rice, flour, and pastas.

Buy and keep bananas separated from one another; they won't spoil as fast.

Do not throw away nut meal from homemade nut milk. Use it for smoothies or baked goods like biscotti for extra nutrition and flavor. Or make nut flour by spreading the pulp out on a baking sheet and drying it in a 250°F oven or dehydrator.

Use vegetable pulp from juicing to add fiber to soups or smoothies, or to make crackers or bread.

Place limp celery, carrots, and radishes in water with a slice of potato to make them crunchy again.

Keep all organic citrus fruits in the fridge—they will last one to two weeks longer.

Do not wash organic dark leafy greens or berries until you are ready to eat them.

Store herbs, spring onions, and asparagus upright in a large glass filled with an inch of water.

Use "aging" food wisely. For example, use stale bread in panzanella and overripe bananas in banana bread. You can also freeze overripe bananas and later blend them into smoothies.

Choose to eat less; use a smaller plate to help you control the amount of food you eat.

Compost all food waste to put nutrients back into your garden (and save money on fertilizer).

When my husband and I go out for a nice dinner, our restaurant bill is around $50 or $60, easily. That's just for two meals! How many meals do you think I could make at home with $50? Plenty. I can buy raw organic cheese, organic beans, salsa, romaine, and sprouted tortillas for a taco dinner for $15 or less, and have plenty of leftovers for lunch or dinner the next day or more. Cooking at home—and saving money in the process—is a no-brainer.

Once you get used to preparing foods in a healthy way, you're hooked for life.

THE FOOD BABE WAY

START SLOWLY AND KEEP COOKING SIMPLE

My advice to anyone learning to cook is not to be overly ambitious. If you've just started climbing mountains, you don't attempt Mount Everest, so don't try to serve something like crepes suzette.

As a novice cook, I relied on websites such as cooks.com or allreci pes.com. Choose a few recipes from cooking sites that you think you can handle, and follow the steps to the letter. These sites stay on top of cooking trends and cater to time-crunched home cooks, so they're good places to turn to. (Please note: you might need to modify the ingredients based on what you've learned in this book so far!)

Cruise your local bookstores for interesting cookbooks and stock up. I have a library full of them to inspire me to cook with new ingredients or make dishes in an innovative way. My favorites are in Appendix B at the back of this book.

Watch television cooking shows, but don't make cooking a spectator sport. In his book *Cooked*, Michael Pollan revealed that Americans spend more time watching people cook on popular shows than actually cooking.

A trick for beginners is to keep it simple. Find recipes that use only a few ingredients—for example, a veggie omelet. You can knock this out in minutes and cook it in one pan to save dishwashing time.

Once you get four or five recipes under your belt, consider yourself a graduate of Cooking 101. The recipes in this book are perfect for beginner and intermediate cooks. They don't take long—because I don't have a lot of patience—so you can whip them up in no time.

You don't have to cook every single meal at home. I suggest that you cook at least fifteen meals a week and feel free to eat out the rest of the time. My 21-Day Food Babe Way Eating Plan is designed around this concept; it will help you plan your cooking and your restaurant eating.

COOK FRESH CUISINE

Whenever possible, cook outside the box. By that I mean cook fresh, using foods as close to nature as possible. Once a food goes into a box or bag, it loses some or much of its nutritional value.

PREP AHEAD OF TIME

Do as much prep work as you can the night before or first thing in the morning. Wash and cut carrot sticks and other veggies and make organic pudding or desserts. Make a whole casserole or pot of soup so all you have to do is pop it into the oven or heat it up on the stove.

GET INTO THE SPIRIT OF COOKING

Finally, enjoy the aromas as you cook or bake. Notice how the whole atmosphere of your home changes as people you love start to gather.

Your meal doesn't have to be perfect, but because you put your heart into it, the *experience* will be truly perfect in the end.

FOOD BABE ALERT: TWO REASONS TO TOSS OUT YOUR MICROWAVE

It pops corn perfectly. Zaps a cup of cold coffee. Nukes the kids' oatmeal. But guess what? That hunk of electronics hogging counter space in 80 to 90 percent of America's kitchens is not good for us. Here's why:

Microwaves create carcinogenic compounds in your food. Heating meat, dairy products, plastics, and paper has been shown to create carcinogens. The Center for Science in the Public Interest (CSPI) reported leakage of chemicals such as BPA, polyethylene terepthalate (PET), benzene, toluene, and xylene from the packaging of common microwavable foods, including pizzas, chips, and popcorn. The term "microwave safe" is not regulated by the government. The safest course of action is not to use any plastic containers or plastic film in microwave ovens.

Microwaves have been associated with the increase in obesity. The microwave has made it extremely easy and convenient to eat processed foods while destroying their nutritional content and exposing you to unnecessary toxins. The more toxic, dead food people eat, the more calories they consume trying to get the nutrition their bodies so desperately need. The result: weight gain.

Michael Pollan, in his book *Cooked,* sums up the microwave problem best: "The microwave oven, which stands at the precise opposite end of the culinary (and imaginative) spectrum from the cook fire, exerts a kind of antigravity, its flameless, smokeless, anti-sensory cold heat giving us a mild case of the willies. The microwave is as antisocial as the cook fire is communal."

Spice Up Your Health

Spices have incredible medicinal properties. They curb hunger (cayenne), boost metabolism (paprika), kill cancer cells (turmeric), and fight inflammation (cinnamon). But these benefits are more likely to be

(Continued)

realized if the spices are pure. Before I started investigating what was in my food, I had no idea there were several harmful ingredients lurking in my spice cabinet.

Conventional spices are treated with chemicals and contain GMOs. What's more, virtually all conventional spices sold in the United States are fumigated (sterilized) with hazardous chemicals that are banned in Europe.

Conventional spices are also irradiated. Radiation is used to kill bacteria and other contaminants, but the finished product has decreased levels of vitamins and natural enzymes. Irradiation also changes the chemical composition of a spice, potentially creating carcinogenic by-products and increasing our exposure to free radicals, which cause aging and disease.

With that said, it's extremely important to fill our pantries with spices that promote health. Below are strategies for buying spices:

- **Always buy organic spices.** Organic spices are not irradiated and are free from pesticides, GMOs, artificial colors, preservatives, and synthetic anticaking agents. (Try Simply Organic, Frontier Co-op, and other organic brands.)
- **Check the expiration date.** Spices, unlike wine, do not get better with age. They lose their powerful benefits. Make sure you clean out your pantry often to avoid using expired spices. Buy smaller organic spice packets or jars; spices lose their flavor and medicinal qualities quickly. Earth Fare, for example, has little preportioned plastic bags of herbs and spices available at a fraction of the cost of whole jars.
- **Replace conventional spices as soon as possible.** If your spice cabinet is full of conventional spices, start to buy organic spices for each new recipe you make. Eventually you'll have a whole new assortment of organic spices to choose from.

CHECKLIST

Today:

✓ I did my morning lemon water ritual.

✓ I enjoyed a green drink.

✓ I stopped drinking fluids with my meals.

✓ I drank, and bathed in, pure, clean, filtered water.

✓ I ate less dairy and made healthier dairy choices.

✓ I stopped drinking all sodas.

✓ I loved my liver by paying attention to alcohol consumption.

✓ I passed on fast food.

✓ I gave up refined sugar.

✓ I ate less meat and I ate it responsibly.

✓ I increased the raw plant foods in my diet.

✓ I chose the best possible grains and carbs.

✓ I balanced my fats.

✓ I supplemented with at least one superfood.

✓ I avoided GMO foods as much as possible.

✓ If dining out, I made healthy, organic choices.

✓ I cleaned out my kitchen — and will keep it that way.

✓ I changed my shopping habits.

✓ I committed to cooking more meals at home.

Day 20 — Fast Every Day

SO HERE WE ARE on Day 20. Now what?

How about this: Fast every day. What? Fast every day? I know what you're thinking: That's insanity! But it's not. Here's what I mean: Do not eat anything for at least twelve hours, from the time you eat dinner until the time you break the fast with breakfast. This may not seem like a big deal, or a real fast, but basically, I'm recommending that you eat no late-night snacks or indulgences after dinner—just twelve straight hours of no food.

Why?

From practicing this habit, I learned that my body needs a break from eating to restore itself and reenergize. This habit has allowed me to eat at regular intervals, too, and I sleep better at night. When I don't practice this habit, I feel lethargic, heavier, and bloated.

Fasting every day has magical benefits, trust me. For one thing, it heals your digestive system—one of the most important parts of your body. If anything goes wrong with your digestive system, the rest of your body will suffer—your mood, behavior, skin, energy, detoxification, and more.

It takes roughly eight hours for your body to completely digest your last meal of the day. During the next four hours or longer, your body goes into detoxification mode, giving your body more time to clear out dead and dying cells as well as regenerate new cells. This process is the true fountain of youth, since aging occurs when more cells die than are being produced. If you intermittently fast for twelve hours overnight, you'll grow younger as you sleep.

Another benefit of overnight fasting is fat burning. When you fast for twelve hours, your body has to use up stored glucose for fuel, burning excess fat from your body.

A third benefit is heart health. Intermittent fasts lower body temperature, blood pressure, and heart rate and increase levels of good cholesterol.

What's good for the heart is good for the brain. Intermittent fasts help you sleep better, so that your brain can process stress hormones such as cortisol. These fasts also help you focus and improve memory and sensory perception. Short fasts also promote the production of beta-hydroxybutyrate, a protective brain chemical that can make you less sensitive to excitotoxins like MSG.

One of the most amazing things I noticed right after I adopted this habit was that I woke up with more energy and was better rested. If you've ever gone to bed with a full stomach, you know what I mean.

Adopting this habit can be so rewarding. It helps restore your health, slow aging, and renew your energy.

THE FOOD BABE WAY

Intermittent or overnight fasting has been extremely easy for me and can be easy for you, too. Some guidelines:

HAVE A SCHEDULE

Keep a regular, established dinnertime. I try to have dinner between 7 p.m. and 8 p.m. every day. Do not eat anything after dinner is over.

Go to sleep around the same time each night. For me that's usually around 10 p.m. Regular sleep times improve sleep quality and help prevent insomnia.

DON'T FORGET DAY 1'S HABIT

Upon waking, drink your lemon water (see Day 1). Then it's time to break your fast. Have breakfast no earlier than twelve hours after the last morsel passed your lips. I usually have breakfast between 8 a.m. and 9 a.m.

BREAK YOUR FAST

Don't skip breakfast. Here's your chance to power your body with nutrition—and keep hunger and overeating at bay for the rest of your day.

Finding the right time frames might be different for you based on your schedule, but once you find your flow, this habit is easily sustainable for life. So here's to fasting every day and waking up feeling lighter, more rested, and reenergized.

 FOOD BABE ALERT: THE DANGERS OF EATING AFTER DARK

From a health perspective, there are a number of reasons to stop nighttime nibbling:

Heart problems: According to an American Heart Association study published in *Circulation* in 2013, men who reported that they ate late at night (after going to bed) had a 55 percent higher risk of coronary heart disease than those who were not late-night noshers.

Acid reflux: Technically called gastroesophageal reflux disease (GERD), acid reflux occurs when a valve between the esophagus and the stomach doesn't close properly. Acid from your stomach then flows upward into your esophagus but is not squeezed back into the stomach. Acid reflux is potentially dangerous, leading to esophageal problems and possibly cancer. One way to reduce your risk of acid reflux is to avoid eating late at night.

Digestive consequences: Digestion slows down after dinner and while you're sleeping. If your system is overfed late in the evening, digestion and absorption of nutrients may be delayed and impaired. The consequences could be indigestion and a decrease in nourishment.

Night eating syndrome (NES): This is a peculiar eating disorder, in which sufferers have irrepressible urges to eat several times during the night when they should be sleeping. NES begins innocently enough, with night eating as a response to stress and emotional problems. But it can progress to a full-fledged psychological disorder that needs to be treated with therapy.

CHECKLIST

Today:

   ✓ I did my morning lemon water ritual.

   ✓ I enjoyed a green drink.

✓ I stopped drinking fluids with my meals.

✓ I drank, and bathed in, pure, clean, filtered water.

✓ I ate less dairy and made healthier dairy choices.

✓ I stopped drinking all sodas.

✓ I loved my liver by paying attention to alcohol consumption.

✓ I passed on fast food.

✓ I gave up refined sugar.

✓ I ate less meat and I ate it responsibly.

✓ I increased the raw plant foods in my diet.

✓ I chose the best possible grains and carbs.

✓ I balanced my fats.

✓ I supplemented with at least one superfood.

✓ I avoided GMO foods as much as possible.

✓ If dining out, I made healthy, organic choices.

✓ I cleaned out my kitchen—and will keep it that way.

✓ I changed my shopping habits.

✓ I committed to cooking more meals at home.

✓ I "fasted."

Day 21 — Travel Organically

PICTURE THIS: You're on one of the most beautiful and remote islands in the world, with the best scuba diving, the richest biodiversity of marine life, the most crystal-clear water, and the nicest people — basically heaven on earth.

Then you find out that most of the food offered at the island resort is highly processed and tainted with MSG, artificial colors, flavors, preservatives, and other additives.

This happened to me when my husband and I celebrated our sixth wedding anniversary at a resort on Mabul Island, off the east coast of Borneo in Malaysia. The island was formed by a spectacular coral reef atop an extinct volcano and is home to more than 3,000 species of fish. It took two days of traveling, a one-and-a-half-hour car ride, and a one-hour boat ride to get there from Thailand — quite a trek.

Mabul Island is known, too, for its lovely stilt houses rising from the sea. We spent a week in one of these homes, from which we could see an astonishing array of multicolored reef fish swimming in the blue water below. It was idyllic, and we felt like we were honeymooning all over again.

So isolated was the resort that we did not have access to bakeries, farmers' markets, or restaurants. The only place to purchase food was at the resort store, which sold only highly processed snacks, candy, and soda. The best we could do was buy coconut water and fruit from a nearby village. Fortunately, I had managed to pick up seven lemons in Kuala Lumpur on the way into Borneo, so I would at least be able to have my lemon water with cayenne.

I had packed food for the journey, of course, but the resort was our last stop at the end of a three-and-a-half-week journey. Our organic stash had dwindled. To say I was a bit worried about what I would be eating is an understatement!

For dinner our first night, the hot food looked tasty but suspicious. I asked the manager if she knew whether MSG or other additives were used to prepare the food. She said she was almost positive they weren't. In my gut, I didn't believe her. She suggested that after dinner, I speak to the kitchen staff directly, meet the chef, and make sure my questions were answered definitively. After dinner? I thought that was odd, but I rolled with it. After all, I was on vacation and didn't want to start an argument.

Unless we know the source of meat, my husband and I try to eat vegetarian meals while traveling. At dinner that night, no vegetarian entrees were offered on the buffet, so we asked for a special order. Out came fried tofu, covered in a thick brown sauce, with vegetables and white rice. I tried some but filled up on raw vegetables and fruit instead. After dinner, I went back to the kitchen to meet the chef. He was more than accommodating and showed me the packages of spices and powdered sauce mixes they used on almost all the food. As I read through the ingredients, my head started to spin. The brown sauce used to make my tofu definitely included MSG, along with probably every other harmful ingredient I've blogged about.

I made a polite request to have our food prepared with salt and pepper and nothing else. The chef graciously complied, and our worries were over. Rosy, the lead cook, made us incredibly delicious additive-free food from scratch, from special soups to a popular Malaysian dish called *roti canai* with vegetables that blew us way.

To think that we could have been eating potentially toxic food for a week. But I learned that it's possible to eat toxin-free, even in a faraway land. You just have to ask for what you want.

Also, I like to be prepared while traveling, so that I don't have to eat nutritionally dead food on my trips. That's why I pack many of my own foods.

THE FOOD BABE WAY

Before you leave for the airport or jump into your car for a road trip, take the time to do the following:

CALL AHEAD

Whenever I travel and know my food options might be limited, I call or send an e-mail to the hotel ahead of time, requesting my food selections, letting them know ingredients I avoid, and giving them my preferences for preparation. Upon arrival, I confirm all of this with the kitchen staff.

DO YOUR HOMEWORK

Before you go anywhere, do some research to find restaurants and businesses that use local and/or organic products. Before traveling to Turks and Caicos one year, I discovered a café called Fresh Bakery and Bistro that specialized in organic breads and other goods. Its menu was delightful.

PACK YOUR OWN "AIRPLANE FOOD"

My favorite options are smoothies (on the way to the airport), oatmeal or yogurt for morning flights, and hummus sandwiches on sprouted wheat tortillas packed with organic greens for later flights. Yogurt is technically a liquid according to the TSA, but if you premix it with fruit, you won't be caught when you go through security. Other good packable meals are an assortment of raw veggies (think carrots, celery, peppers, broccoli), whole grain crackers like Mary's Gone Crackers, or a filling, high-fiber avocado. All of these will keep your hunger in check so that you can avoid the snack cart when it rolls around. Important: Don't pack your food in aluminum foil. It will set off alarms in the X-ray machine.

PACK SMALL BAGS OF ORGANIC QUICK-COOKING ROLLED OATS, CINNAMON, AND DATES

I place a mixture of ¼ cup instant plain oatmeal and a few sprinkles of organic cinnamon in a Ziploc bag. In another Ziploc bag, I carry one date and a few walnuts. When I'm ready to make my oatmeal, I get a cup of hot water from the hotel, a gas station, a coffee shop, or wherever I happen to be. Then I break or cut up the date into pieces and add it with the oatmeal to the hot water, do a quick stir, and let it sit until it's warmed through and the oats have soaked up all the water. Before eating my oatmeal, I add the walnuts as a crunchy topping. The cinnamon and the date, which dissolves quite a bit in the oatmeal, bestow amazing natural flavor and sweetness.

This recipe varies depending on what I have access to. Often, I'll add banana, raisins, goji berries, almond butter, and other nuts. Many toppings travel well.

BUY SMALL PACKS OF DRIED ORGANIC GREEN POWDER

When I can't get my usual green juice or smoothie, I like to carry powdered green mixes that are loaded with dark leafy greens, which contain chlorophyll and algae to keep you alkaline throughout your travels. Mix the powder into a small carton of coconut water for a quick hydrating treat. This makes a perfect snack when you don't have access to a lot of green vegetables.

PACK SOME DETOXIFIERS

These include a few organic apples, lemons, and cayenne pepper to detox after a long flight or drive. Mix lemon juice and cayenne in hot water for your morning ritual (see Day 1). The apples provide fiber and keep your hunger at bay until you have your first meal after arrival.

STAY HYDRATED

Pack a water bottle to be filled at the airport, or buy water after you've cleared airport security. I like to bring at least 32 ounces of water with me. I can't tell you how many times the airlines have been stingy about giving me water. Drink at least 16 ounces of water a few hours before your flight, and limit alcohol and caffeine. Drink 8 ounces of water for every hour of flying time.

TRY MY ENERGIZER FOR LONG PLANE RIDES

My secret is fresh ginger tea. It stimulates my circulation and makes me feel terrific after I deplane. Take a thermos, and toss in ¼ cup of freshly chopped gingerroot. After passing through security, head to an airport coffee shop and request a large cup of hot water. Be sure to give the barista a nice tip for serving you free hot water. (Do not wait until you get on the plane to get hot water; water on planes is notoriously dirty.) Pour the hot water into the ginger-filled thermos and let it brew. Once you're on the plane, sip your ginger tea. You'll feel so energized when you arrive at your destination.

POP SOME ALMOND BUTTER

For an energy treat, try Artisana organic almond butter, available in single-serve packages. Just open and squeeze into your mouth or spread on celery sticks or a whole wheat cracker.

PURCHASE A TRAVEL BLENDER AND PACK HEMP PROTEIN POWDER

Cuisinart and Vitamix make good travel blenders. Ask the hotel for fresh veggies and fruit, and prepare quick, healthy meals in your hotel room.

TACKLE THE TRAVEL MUNCHIES

Pack Ziploc bags of organic cereal, sprouted wheat pretzels, or home-made trail mix. Try a mixture of organic raw nuts like almonds, cashews, and walnuts; organic seeds like sunflower and pumpkin; and something sweet like organic raisins, golden berries, or dates. Trail mix doesn't need refrigeration and can last forever in your suitcase. I've made several individual servings to last me throughout long travels; you never know when you'll need them.

CHECK A COOLER

Here's a great way to enjoy endless possibilities: Pack organic veggies, homemade hummus, and other goodies in a cooler with frozen soups, which double as refrigeration. Hopefully, your destination has a stove or a toaster oven you can use to warm up food. Otherwise, you might have to resort to a microwave—just make sure not to microwave your food in plastic!

When I used to travel every week for work, I'd spend a little time on Sunday preparing my cooler. As soon as I'd get to the office, I'd unpack the cooler in the break room, put the food in the fridge, and have home-made snacks and meals for the next three days. While everyone else was eating Subway or Salsarita's Fresh Cantina, I was having hot tomato white bean soup and marinated kale salad.

AVOID FACTORY-FARMED MEAT

Don't eat meats unless the restaurant or grocery store assures you that they're free of growth hormone and antibiotics. I don't eat any meat while vacationing unless I know it's additive-free.

WATCH OUT FOR "FRESH BREAD" IN LOCAL GROCERY STORES

It's horrendous, with a laundry list of ingredients that your body can't process. Buy bread from the local bakery or look in the freezer section at the grocery store for higher-quality bread. While vacationing in the Caribbean, I once found Ezekiel cinnamon raisin bread in the freezer section and made great sandwiches for the dive boat. I grabbed a few bananas from the breakfast table every morning and used almond butter from single-serve packets to make the sandwiches. This saved us from eating the dive boat's free catered selection of white-bread ham sandwiches and the Funyuns, Doritos, and Cheetos they offered.

DO A POST-TRIP DETOX

After a trip, my body is screaming for a detox. (My mind, on the other hand, has a different plan, like planning my next trip…ahhh.) Even though I follow healthy habits on the road, I don't always watch what I eat, nor do I stick to my usual exercise program—which is why I take some simple steps to get back on track after traveling.

Eat at home. This should be your *numero uno* priority. While on your trip, you probably took in more fat, calories, sugar, and toxins than you'd normally eat. While that's not terrible, it's a good idea to cook your own food again to obtain more nutrition.

Sip dandelion tea. This stuff is dynamite for reducing swelling or bloating from traveling or eating too much salt. I've found that eating out almost always guarantees salt bloat, even though I ask servers to reduce the salt in my food. Dandelion flushes out excess salt. It also stimulates the liver, which helps the body clear out toxic invaders you might have been exposed to while traveling. My favorite brand of dandelion tea is Traditional Medicinals.

Have daily wheatgrass shots. A quick method of detoxing is to enjoy a daily shot of this wonderful juice. It's a surefire way to help speed up your energy and metabolism.

Eat raw vegetables at every meal. Pump up your intake of raw fruits and veggies at most meals, and be sure to drink your daily green juice or smoothie. Raw produce is known for its ability to remove toxins and heal your body fast.

Plan a juice fast. When you get back to your normal routine, say after a week or so, consider a juice fast for one to three days: Drink several types of freshly made juice five or six times a day, but no other food. A fast will also help you lose any weight gained on your trip. Check out more on juice fasting at foodbabe.com.

Hot yoga. For me, hot yoga is an effective physical detox. No other activity gives me more pleasure and peace of mind, because yoga helps improve digestion, circulation, and brain function. With hot yoga, you exercise in a hot room—for two main reasons. First, the heat helps make your muscles more supple so that you can flex more deeply into the poses. Second, the heat helps increase sweat, which then efficiently releases toxins. A lot of naysayers claim that you can't sweat out toxins, but I don't believe them. I know that when I haven't been eating right or have been exposed to some element that is not good for my body, my skin will literally sting after sweating. If I'm practicing clean living, I don't feel this. I've become so in tune with my body, I know exactly what's going on. Yoga helps me listen to, and tune in to, my body even more. If you haven't tried hot yoga, or any kind of yoga, I highly recommend it.

CHECKLIST

Today:

✓ I did my morning lemon water ritual.

✓ I enjoyed a green drink.

✓ I stopped drinking fluids with my meals.

✓ I drank, and bathed in, pure, clean, filtered water.

✓ I ate less dairy and made healthier dairy choices.

✓ I stopped drinking all sodas.

✓ I loved my liver by paying attention to alcohol consumption.

✓ I passed on fast food.

✓ I gave up refined sugar.

✓ I ate less meat and I ate it responsibly.

✓ I increased the raw plant foods in my diet.

✓ I chose the best possible grains and carbs.

✓ I balanced my fats.

✓ I supplemented with at least one superfood.

✓ I avoided GMO foods as much as possible.

✓ If dining out, I made healthy, organic choices.

✓ I cleaned out my kitchen—and will keep it that way.

✓ I changed my shopping habits.

✓ I committed to cooking more meals at home.

✓ I "fasted."

✓ I committed to traveling organically.

PART III

THE 21-DAY FOOD BABE WAY EATING PLAN AND RECIPES

CHAPTER 7

THE 21-DAY FOOD BABE WAY EATING PLAN

I CREATED THIS MEAL plan to illustrate how simple it is to break your relationship with questionable food additives and live an organic lifestyle. Along with my twenty-one-day habit change program, this twenty-one-day eating plan is a catalyst to losing weight, feeling great, and looking great.

The 21-Day Food Babe Way Eating Plan is designed for all types of people: those who are in need of a smooth transition from the conventional to the organic lifestyle, those who just want a dietary plan to follow, and those who have veered off track and seek a reset.

The plan is set up to give you fifteen home-cooked meals; the rest you can eat out, provided you follow my guidelines for dining out organically.

The recipes here are plant-based and organic. They are largely geared to be vegan, vegetarian, and gluten-free. Where I've called for chicken or salmon, please feel free to substitute beans or legumes—or any vegetarian or vegan protein of your choice. In the next chapter, I've included recipes specifically for this plan, along with recipes that I've mentioned throughout this book.

Keep in mind that my eating plan is flexible. If there's a breakfast you like, enjoy it several times a week. The same goes for lunches and dinners. Feel free to eat fruits and vegetables other than the ones I mention, but make it your goal to eat at least six servings of fruits and vegetables each day. Your daily green drink will give you a head start on this.

I've found my passion in sharing what it takes to live a healthy, organic lifestyle, and I'm excited to share this meal plan and its recipes with you. Enjoy!

Every day:
Begin your day with a hot lemon-cayenne drink before breakfast.
Drink a green drink daily, either before breakfast, as a snack, or before dinner. I have six options for you:
Green smoothies: Hari Shake (page 292), Ginger Berry Smoothie (page 293), or
    Pineapple Grapefruit Shake (page 293)
Green juices: Ravishing Red Juice (page 294), Kickin' Kale Juice (page 294), or
    Lemon Lime Cooler (page 295)

WEEK 1

Day 1
Breakfast: 1 whole wheat English muffin, spread with 2 tablespoons almond but-
    ter, plus 1 sliced peach or other seasonal fruit
Lunch: On the Go Pasta Salad (page 305)
Dinner: White Bean Chili (page 312) and a small green salad topped with sprouts
    (use any of the three dressings listed in the recipe section, page 310)

Day 2
Breakfast: ½ cup cooked steel-cut oatmeal with 1 cup fresh berries, topped with
    almond milk
Lunch (restaurant): Order a vegetable plate or a large salad and ask for olive oil
    and lemon juice on the side to dress it. Ask your server for some nuts, seeds,
    avocado, or quinoa to add to your salad.
Dinner: Mac 'n' Cheese (page 313), plus some raw cut-up veggies

Day 3
Breakfast: Quinoa Veggie Scramble (page 297)
Lunch: 1 cup organic lentil soup, plus 1 small side salad drizzled with apple cider
    vinegar and hemp oil

Dinner: One filet of baked wild-caught salmon with organically grown green vegetables such as spinach or green beans; ½ cup wild rice, plus a side of kimchi

Day 4

Breakfast: ¼ cup Nature's Path Qi'a cereal, ½ cup almond milk, and ½ cup berries

Lunch (restaurant): Order a vegetable plate or a large salad and ask for olive oil and lemon juice on the side to dress it. Ask your server for some nuts, seeds, avocado, or quinoa to add to your salad. Or, if you eat at home, have some leftover Mac 'n' Cheese, plus some raw cut-up veggies.

Dinner: Masala Burgers (page 314) over a bed of greens with ½ avocado sliced on top

Day 5

Breakfast: Perfect Porridge Parfait (page 297)

Lunch: 1 cup raw spinach salad (baby spinach, chopped carrots, chopped celery, and cucumbers drizzled with fresh lemon juice and sprinkled with sea salt), topped with ¼ cup shredded goat cheese

Dinner (restaurant): Order grilled wild-caught fish and a side salad. Ask for olive oil and lemon juice on the side to dress your salad.

Day 6

Breakfast (restaurant): Order grass-fed organic yogurt, 1 tablespoon chia seeds (if the restaurant has them), and fruit of your choice.

Lunch: Hilary's Eat Well veggie burger topped with ½ avocado, sliced, and a piece of seasonal fresh fruit on the side

Dinner: Chicken with Sautéed Kale (page 315), plus a side of kimchi

Day 7

Breakfast: ⅓ cup Purely Elizabeth granola with almond milk, plus ½ cup berries or other seasonal fruit of your choice

Lunch (restaurant): At a Chinese restaurant, order steamed vegetables and brown rice.

Dinner: 1 cup Ezekiel penne pasta, topped with Yellow Barn Biodynamic or Eden Foods spaghetti sauce, plus a side salad of greens and raw cut-up veggies (use any of the three dressings listed in the recipe section, page 310)

WEEK 2

Day 8

Breakfast: Chia Seed Pudding (page 298)

Lunch: Avocado toast: Top 1 piece of Ezekiel bread with Dijon mustard, ½ avocado, and sprouts. On the side, have a handful of Brad's Raw Foods kale chips, plus one piece of fruit.

Dinner: Miso Soup with Black Rice Noodles (page 315)

Day 9

Breakfast: Ezekiel cereal or Purely Elizabeth granola, with almond milk and seasonal fresh fruit

Lunch (restaurant): Order a vegetable plate or a large salad and ask for olive oil and lemon juice on the side to dress it. Ask your server for some nuts, seeds, avocado, or quinoa to add to your salad.

Dinner: Moroccan Veggie and Chickpea Soup (page 316)

Day 10

Breakfast: ½ cup cooked steel-cut oatmeal with 1 cup fresh berries, topped with almond milk

Lunch: Hilary's Eat Well veggie burger with ½ avocado, sliced, and a piece of seasonal fresh fruit on the side

Dinner (restaurant or grocery store): Sushi—1 roll with brown or black rice, plus a small side salad with ginger dressing

Day 11

Breakfast: 1 whole wheat English muffin, spread with 2 tablespoons almond butter, plus 1 sliced peach or other seasonal fruit

Lunch (restaurant): 1 cup organic lentil soup or vegetarian chili, plus a small side salad drizzled with apple cider vinegar and hemp oil

Dinner: Vegetable Lasagna (page 317), plus a small side salad with sprouts (use any of the three dressings listed in the recipe section, page 310)

Day 12

Breakfast: Walnut Breakfast Bars (page 299)

Lunch: 1 cup raw spinach salad (baby spinach, chopped carrots, chopped celery, and cucumbers drizzled with fresh lemon juice and sprinkled with sea salt), topped with ¼ cup shredded goat cheese

Dinner: Black Bean and Sweet Potato Soup (page 318) with Mary's Gone Crackers

Day 13

Breakfast: Nature's Path Qi'a Cereal topped with ½ cup cashew milk and ½ cup fresh berries

Lunch: Avocado Sauté Mushroom Wrap (page 305)

Dinner (restaurant): At Chipotle, order the black bean salad with guacamole and any type of salsa.

Day 14

Breakfast: Carrot Cake Pancakes (page 301)

Lunch (restaurant): A slice of cheese-free pizza loaded with vegetables, along with a side salad of greens (use any of the three dressings listed in the recipe section, page 310)

Dinner: Ginger Garlic Salmon (page 320), plus steamed vegetables of your choice or side salad (use any of the three dressings listed in the recipe section, page 310)

WEEK 3

Day 15

Breakfast: Breakfast Burritos (page 301)

Lunch (restaurant): Order a vegetable plate or a large salad and ask for olive oil and lemon juice on the side to dress it. Ask your server for some nuts, seeds, avocado, or quinoa to add to your salad.

Dinner: Turkey Meatballs with Spaghetti Squash (page 320)

Day 16

Breakfast (restaurant): Choose either oatmeal with fresh fruit or a vegetable omelet with fresh fruit.

Lunch: Chicken Salad Sandwich (page 307)

Dinner: Quick and Easy Home-Baked Pizza (page 322)

Day 17

Breakfast: Cinnamon Raisin French Toast Crunch (page 302)

Lunch (restaurant): Order a vegetable plate or a large salad and ask for olive oil and lemon juice on the side to dress it. Ask your server for some nuts, seeds, avocado, or quinoa to add to your salad.

Dinner: Mexican Casserole (page 322)

Day 18

Breakfast: Quinoa Veggie Scramble (page 297)

Lunch: Open-Faced Crunchy Veggie Sandwich (page 308)

Dinner: Eggplant Parmesan (page 324) plus a small side salad with sprouts (use any of the three dressings listed in the recipe section, page 310)

Day 19

Breakfast: Mini Frittatas over greens (page 299)

Lunch (restaurant): Order a vegetable plate or a large salad and ask for olive oil and lemon juice on the side to dress it. Ask your server for some nuts, seeds, avocado, or quinoa to add to your salad.

Dinner: Grilled Chicken with Rhubarb-Cucumber Slaw (page 325)

Day 20

Breakfast: 1 whole wheat English muffin, spread with 2 tablespoons almond butter, plus 1 sliced peach or other seasonal fruit

Lunch: Spicy Tomato Kale Soup (page 306), plus a small side salad (use any of the three dressings listed in the recipe section, page 310) or raw veggie sticks

Dinner (restaurant): Order organic grilled chicken with steamed vegetables and a side garden salad (ask for olive oil and lemon juice on the side to dress your salad).

Day 21

Breakfast: Blueberry Lemon Hempseed Muffins (page 303)

Lunch (restaurant): Order a vegetable plate or a large salad and ask for olive oil and lemon juice on the side to dress it.

Dinner: Veggie Sloppy Joes (page 326), plus Sweet Potato Fries (page 332)

SNACKING ON THE FOOD BABE WAY EATING PLAN

Feel free to enjoy one or two snacks a day on this plan. Good choices are seasonal fresh fruit or one of my juices or smoothies. If you're in the mood to cook, you can find delicious snack recipes—both savory and sweet—on page 327, or on my website, foodbabe.com. If not, here is a list of time-saving store-bought snacks you can enjoy between meals, if you desire:

- Fruit of your choice
- Raw veggies
- Raw nuts or nut butter
- Organic Homemade Frappuccino (page 327)
- Power Snacks by Navitas Naturals (serving size: 3 bites)
- Brad's Raw Foods chips and crackers

- Mary's Gone Crackers — plain, onion, herb, etc. — with goat cheese
- Late July chips with Field Day salsa
- Raw Crunch bar
- Kur Superfood Delights (serving size: 2)
- Eden Foods Wild Berry Mix (serving size: 3 tablespoons)
- Dry-roasted pistachios (1 ounce or 1 handful)
- Go Raw cookies (1 serving)
- Organic prunes (6)
- Organic carrots with organic hummus
- Sprouted wheat pretzels (1 serving)
- ½ cup instant oatmeal, made with water, topped with ½ cup blueberries
- Trader Joe's organic olive oil popcorn (1 serving)

CHAPTER 8

THE FOOD BABE WAY EATING PLAN RECIPES

Since I became the Food Babe, I've been creating organic and easy-to-make recipes that will help you maintain a healthy diet. My recipes are also geared toward the budget-conscious person in all of us, so you won't find pricey ingredients here. Healthy, organic eating doesn't have to be expensive.

Although I love to cook, I don't like to spend a lot of time cooking— I'd rather be eating—so you'll find that my recipes don't take very long to prepare.

This collection of recipes complements my 21-Day Eating Plan and features a number of recipes I mention in various parts of the book. You'll find delicious renditions of old favorites here, too, such as lasagna, macaroni and cheese, pizza, French fries, ice cream, and more. Feel free to change them up, add new ingredients, substitute other organic ingredients, or experiment in any way.

When you cook organically, you have so much more control over what you and your family eat. You take more responsibility for your well-being and that of those you love.

I hope you enjoy these recipes as much as I do, and that they become a permanent part of your repertoire and an integral part of a healthful, satisfying diet. They're truly delicious, nutritious, and quick to prepare, while energizing you inside and out.

Here's to your health!

A NOTE ON INGREDIENTS

Here are some basic guidelines to follow when shopping for the 21-Day Food Babe Way Eating Plan. As a general rule, please purchase all certified organic ingredients if they are available.

Baking powder: Choose the aluminum-free kind.

Bread: Choose bread, tortillas, or rolls that are made from sprouted wheat, whole grains, or sprouted corn. Avoid white flour and check for added preservatives, dough conditioners, and sugars.

Broth/stock: Choose chicken or vegetable broth without hidden MSG additives (see page 54). You can also make your own broth or stock at home using leftover vegetables or chicken bones.

Butter: Choose grass-fed.

Canned foods: Choose sauces, condiments, and other preserved foods in glass jars or cans that are BPA-free.

Cereal: Choose whole grain cereals with no added sugars or fortified vitamins.

Cheese: Select goat cheese.

Chocolate: Choose fair trade. Raw chocolate has the highest nutritional value.

Dairy: Choose grass-fed if possible. Try raw and goat cheeses. Nut milk and almond yogurt are great alternatives to traditional dairy products. Make sure these are unsweetened.

Flour: Choose whole wheat flour over white flour. You can also use spelt flour, almond flour, coconut flour, or a sprouted grain-based flour.

Honey: Choose raw and local if possible.

Meats: Purchase chicken that is hormone-free and beef that is grass-fed. If you can find these items at a local farmers' market, that is always a great option.

Oats: Choose steel-cut oats, oat groats, or gluten-free oats for optimal nutrition.

Oils: When buying olive oil or coconut oil, always choose extra virgin. Hemp oil and sesame oil are also great alternatives.

Pasta: Choose sprouted-grain, buckwheat, or whole wheat pasta. When choosing gluten-free pasta, look for varieties made from brown rice, quinoa, or corn.

Rice: Choose sprouted, brown, wild, black, or red Himalayan rice over white rice.

Salt and pepper: Choose sea salt over kosher or table salt and grind your own pepper in a mill.

Soy sauce: Choose low-sodium and non-GMO soy sauce.

Sugar: Choose coconut sugar, dates, or stevia extract to sweeten dishes instead of refined white sugar.

Tea: Choose non-GMO certified teas without added flavors, and make sure the tea comes in safe packaging. You can also buy loose-leaf tea.

Thickeners: Use arrowroot powder instead of cornstarch to thicken sauces.

Vinegars: Choose raw and unfiltered vinegars. Apple cider vinegar and balsamic are great choices.

Water: Choose filtered water in glass bottles if purchasing from a store, or water filtered at home.

Smoothies, Juices, and Beverages

My Basic Green Smoothie

SERVES 2

2 cups water, coconut water, almond milk, or coconut milk

3 cups vegetables: spinach, kale, romaine, collards, chard, celery, and/or cucumber, ends removed as they can be bitter

1 cup fruit (preferably frozen because frozen fruit will thicken your smoothie and make it cold and refreshing): strawberries, blueberries, raspberries, pineapple, cranberries, peaches, mango, and/or banana

Optional: If you're using this smoothie as a breakfast meal replacement, add 1 tablespoon ground flaxseeds, grass-fed yogurt, hempseeds, protein, chia seeds, or almond butter; for extra sweetness, add 1 pitted date

1. Put the liquid and 1 cup of the vegetables in a blender.

2. Blend for 30 seconds until well combined.

3. Add the rest of the vegetables and blend for another 30 seconds.

4. Add the fruit and blend for 30 seconds to 1 minute.

5. Serve immediately or store in an airtight container for up to 2 days. Shake or stir before serving.

My Perfect Green Juice

SERVES 2

8 cups dark leafy greens: spinach, kale, collards, chard, parsley, dandelion, arugula, and/or cilantro

2 apples, cored (or 2 carrots; 2 beets, washed thoroughly; 2 oranges, peeled; or 2 cups fresh pineapple, peeled and coarsely chopped)

1 cucumber, ends removed (or 8 stalks celery, 2 fennel bulbs, or 2 cups
   romaine)

Optional flavorings: juice of 2 lemons, 4 slices gingerroot, or 2 cloves garlic

1. Feed the dark leafy greens into your juicer, cup by cup.
2. Juice the apples, carrots, beets, oranges, or pineapple. Then add the rest
   of the ingredients.

Note: If you don't have a juicer, you can blend all the ingredients in a blender
and strain using a strainer lined with cheesecloth to squeeze the juice out of
the pulp.

Hari Shake

SERVES 2

8 ounces water

Juice of ½ lemon

4 cups kale, stems removed

3 sprigs parsley

3 sprigs cilantro

4 large stalks celery, chopped

1 apple, cored and chopped, or 1 cup strawberries or fruit of your choice

1 pear, cored and chopped

Optional: 1 tablespoon hemp protein, chia seeds, or hempseeds if you're using
   this shake as a breakfast meal replacement

1. Put the water and lemon juice in a blender with the first 2 cups kale.
2. Blend for 30 seconds until well combined.
3. Add the additional kale, parsley, cilantro, and celery and blend for
   another 30 seconds.
4. Add the apple and pear and blend for another 30 seconds to 1 minute,
   until well combined. (Do not overblend.)
5. Pour the mixture into 2 glass storage jars and chill for at least
   15 minutes before serving.

Ginger Berry Smoothie

SERVES 2

4-inch piece gingerroot (peeled if not organic)

4 cups leafy greens (kale, collards, romaine, spinach, chard, etc.), stems removed

4 large stalks celery, chopped

2 cups mixed frozen berries (strawberries, blueberries, cranberries, etc.)

1 cup water

Optional: 6 tablespoons hemp protein powder, if you're using this smoothie as a breakfast meal replacement

1. Put all the ingredients in a blender and blend for 1 minute, or until smooth.

2. Serve immediately or store in an airtight container in the refrigerator for up to 1 day. Shake or stir before serving.

Pineapple Grapefruit Shake

SERVES 2

12 ounces water

4 large stalks celery, chopped

I cucumber, ends removed

½ grapefruit, peeled and segmented

4 cups kale, stems removed

2 cups frozen pineapple

1. Put the water, celery, cucumber, and grapefruit in a blender.

2. Blend for 30 seconds until well combined.

3. Add the remaining ingredients and blend for another 30 seconds to 1 minute. Serve immediately or store in an airtight container in the refrigerator for up to 1 day. Shake or stir before serving.

Ravishing Red Juice

SERVES 2

½ bunch kale

½ bunch parsley

5 carrots

1 beet, with stems and leaves

4 stalks celery, chopped

1 green apple, cored

2-inch piece gingerroot (peeled if not organic)

1 cucumber, ends removed

1. In a juicer, juice each vegetable in the order listed.
2. Serve immediately or store in an airtight container in the refrigerator for up to 1 day. Shake or stir before serving.

Kickin' Kale Juice

SERVES 2

1 bunch kale

½ bunch cilantro or parsley

4 stalks celery, chopped

2-inch piece gingerroot (peeled if not organic)

1 cucumber, ends removed

1 lemon, peeled

Optional: 1 green apple, cored (for added sweetness)

1. Juice the ingredients in the order listed.
2. Pour into a pitcher and stir before serving. Can be stored in an airtight container for up to 12 hours (some live enzymes will be lost).

Lemon Lime Cooler

SERVES 2

1 bunch greens (kale, collards, romaine, spinach, chard, etc.)

1 bunch herbs (parsley, cilantro, and/or mint)

1 lemon, peeled

1 lime, peeled

2 cucumbers, ends removed

Optional: 1 green apple, cored (for added sweetness)

1. Juice the ingredients in the order listed.
2. Pour into a pitcher and stir before serving.

Homemade Organic Cashew Milk

SERVES 6 TO 10

1 cup raw cashews

6 cups water

Optional: 2 dates, pitted (for added sweetness)

Optional: 1 teaspoon vanilla extract, or seeds from one vanilla bean

1. Soak the cashews overnight (at least 6 hours) in 2 cups water.
2. Rinse and drain the soaked cashews.
3. Place the cashews, 4 cups water, and optional ingredients, if using, in a blender and blend on high for about 1 minute.
4. Pour the milk into an airtight container and store refrigerated for up to 4 days.

Maca Hot Chocolate

SERVES 2

2½ cups unsweetened nut milk (coconut, almond, or Homemade Organic
   Cashew Milk from the recipe on the previous page)

4 tablespoons raw cacao powder

1 tablespoon maca powder

2 dates, pitted

Pinch of sea salt

1. Combine all the ingredients in a blender and blend until smooth.

2. Pour into a small saucepan and slowly warm to desired temperature.

Breakfast

Quinoa Veggie Scramble

SERVES 4

2 tablespoons coconut or olive oil

2 cups chopped broccoli

2 cups chopped mushrooms

2 cups chopped tomatoes

4 cups spinach, stems removed and chopped

2 cups cooked quinoa

¾ teaspoon sea salt

Freshly ground black pepper

1. Heat the coconut or olive oil in a sauté pan on medium heat.
2. Add the broccoli, mushrooms, tomatoes, and spinach and cook for about 10 minutes, or until tender.
3. Add the quinoa, sea salt, and pepper to the pan and combine.
4. Allow to cook for another 2 to 3 minutes, or until the quinoa is warm. Serve immediately.

Perfect Porridge Parfait

SERVES 4

1 cup oat groats, rinsed and drained

1 cup Ezekiel cereal, muesli, or steel-cut or rolled oats

Sprinkle of cinnamon

4 teaspoons currants

16 ounces unsweetened almond milk

Optional: 4 teaspoons chia seeds

4 cups fresh or frozen fruit

1. In a "to go" glass container, place the oat groats, Ezekiel cereal or muesli or oats, cinnamon, currants, almond milk, and chia seeds, if using, and stir.

2. Top the mixture with fresh or frozen fruit and serve, or store in the refrigerator overnight or up to 3 days. Serve cold or, if desired, heat on the stove until warm.

Chia Seed Pudding

SERVES 4

4 cups diced fruit (e.g., pears and strawberries)

¼ cup currants, raisins, or goji berries

2 cups unsweetened nut milk

⅓ cup chia seeds

Juice and zest of 1 orange

1 tablespoon vanilla extract

¼ teaspoon cinnamon

½ cup shredded coconut

4 mint leaves, for garnish

1. Divide the diced fruit evenly among 4 bowls and top each with a sprinkle of currants, raisins, or goji berries.

2. Combine the nut milk, chia seeds, orange juice and zest, vanilla, and cinnamon in a small pitcher and stir. Pour ½ cup of the mixture over the fruit in each bowl.

3. Top the fruit bowls with shredded coconut.

4. Refrigerate for at least 30 minutes (or chill overnight).

5. Top each bowl with a mint leaf before serving. Can be made in advance and stored up to 3 days.

Mini Frittatas

SERVES 4

4 eggs, beaten

1 large red bell pepper, diced

½ small red onion, diced

3 sun-dried tomatoes, diced

3 tablespoons minced fresh basil

¼ teaspoon crushed red pepper flakes

¼ teaspoon paprika

¼ teaspoon sea salt

Freshly ground black pepper

½ teaspoon coconut oil

Optional: 1 to 2 ounces goat cheese

1. Preheat the oven to 375°F.
2. In a large bowl, mix all the ingredients, except the coconut oil, until combined.
3. Grease a muffin pan with the coconut oil. Pour the mixture into the pan.
4. Bake for 10 to 14 minutes, or until the frittatas are golden on top.
5. Let stand for at least 5 minutes and serve.

Walnut Breakfast Bars

MAKES 8 BARS

1 teaspoon coconut oil

1 cup rolled oats

¾ cup flour of choice, preferably almond or spelt

¼ cup ground flaxseeds

1 teaspoon cinnamon

¼ teaspoon sea salt

¼ cup honey

¼ cup coconut sugar

⅓ cup mashed very ripe banana

¼ cup coconut oil, melted

2 large eggs

½ cup chopped raw walnuts

¼ cup apricot preserves

1. Preheat the oven to 350°F.

2. Lightly grease an 8-by-8-inch baking pan with the 1 teaspoon coconut oil.

3. In a medium bowl, combine the oats, flour, flaxseeds, cinnamon, and sea salt.

4. In a large bowl, mix the honey, coconut sugar, banana, melted coconut oil, and eggs until combined. (For a vegan option, combine 2 tablespoons ground flaxseeds and 6 tablespoons water and let sit for 10 minutes. Use this mixture instead of eggs.)

5. Add the flour mixture to the liquids and stir just until combined.

6. Stir in the walnuts and pour the batter into the prepared pan.

7. Bake for 30 to 35 minutes, or until a toothpick inserted into the center comes out clean.

8. Near the end of the baking time, pour the apricot preserves into a small saucepan and bring to a boil.

9. When the bars come out of the oven, brush the preserves on top. Cool completely and cut into 8 bars. Store in a sealed container for up to 3 days. These can also be frozen for up to 1 month.

Carrot Cake Pancakes

SERVES 4

1⅓ cup flour of choice (almond, spelt, etc.)

2 tablespoons rolled oats

1 cup peeled and finely chopped carrots

1⅓ cup unsweetened nut milk

2 tablespoons coconut oil

1 teaspoon cinnamon

½ teaspoon nutmeg

1 teaspoon vanilla extract

1 teaspoon aluminum-free baking powder

½ teaspoon sea salt

Optional: 4 tablespoons maple syrup

Optional: 4 tablespoons butter

1. In a blender, place the flour, oats, carrots, nut milk, 1 tablespoon of the coconut oil, cinnamon, nutmeg, vanilla, baking powder, and sea salt and blend until combined.
2. In a small skillet, melt the remaining coconut oil over medium heat.
3. Pour the batter into the pan and cook for about 3 to 4 minutes on each side.
4. Top with maple syrup and butter, if desired.

Breakfast Burritos

SERVES 4

2 tablespoons coconut oil

2 sweet potatoes, peeled and chopped

1 cup chopped onion

1 cup chopped red bell pepper

2 cups chopped spinach

Dash of cayenne pepper

Sea salt and freshly ground black pepper

8 eggs, beaten (or ½ cup hempseeds, if vegan)

4 large sprouted grain tortillas

1. Melt 1 tablespoon of the coconut oil in a large skillet over medium heat. Add the sweet potatoes to the skillet and allow them to cook for about 10 minutes, or until tender.

2. When the sweet potatoes are tender, add the onion, red bell pepper, spinach, cayenne, sea salt, and pepper. Allow the vegetables to cook, stirring occasionally, for another 5 to 7 minutes, or until tender.

3. Melt the remaining coconut oil in a separate skillet over medium heat. Add the eggs and cook, stirring occasionally, for about 5 minutes. They should have the consistency of scrambled eggs. If you are making the vegan version, skip this step.

4. Add the vegetables to the scrambled eggs. If you are making the vegan version, instead add the hempseeds to the vegetables once they are fully cooked.

5. Place each tortilla on a plate, scoop the scrambled eggs with vegetables or hempseeds with vegetables onto each tortilla, wrap up tightly, and serve immediately.

Cinnamon Raisin French Toast Crunch

SERVES 4

4 eggs

1 cup unsweetened almond milk

2 teaspoons vanilla extract

¼ teaspoon sea salt

¼ teaspoon nutmeg

¾ teaspoon cinnamon

Coconut oil or butter to grease the pan

8 slices cinnamon raisin bread

½ cup raw walnuts, toasted and chopped

2 apples, cored and thinly sliced

1 tablespoon coconut oil or butter

¼ cup maple syrup

1. The night before, in a bowl beat together the eggs, milk, vanilla, sea salt, nutmeg, and cinnamon.

2. Grease a 9-by-13-inch baking dish with coconut oil or butter.

3. Arrange 4 slices of bread in the dish, breaking up pieces to fit in every nook and cranny.

4. Pour half of the batter on top.

5. Layer ¼ cup walnuts and one of the sliced apples on top.

6. Repeat the process, ending with apples and walnuts on top.

7. Cover and refrigerate the dish overnight, or for at least 8 hours.

8. In the morning, preheat the oven to 350°F.

9. Cover the dish with aluminum foil and bake for 30 to 40 minutes.

10. In a small pot, heat the maple syrup with 1 tablespoon of coconut oil or butter until the oil is melted. Drizzle over the French toast and serve immediately.

Blueberry Lemon Hempseed Muffins

SERVES 4

1 cup almond flour

1 egg, beaten

1 ripe banana, mashed

¼ teaspoon baking soda

Dash of sea salt

½ teaspoon vanilla extract

1 tablespoon coconut oil

2 tablespoons hempseeds

Juice and zest of ½ lemon

½ cup blueberries

1. Preheat the oven to 350°F.

2. Place all the ingredients except the blueberries in a bowl and mix well with a wooden spoon or stand mixer.

3. Once the batter is smooth, fold in the blueberries.

4. Grease a muffin or mini-muffin pan with coconut oil or line the pan with unbleached paper cups.

5. Divide the batter evenly among the muffin cups.

6. Bake for 25 minutes, or until a toothpick inserted into the center comes out clean.

7. Remove from the oven and place the pan on a cooling rack. Allow the muffins to cool for 10 minutes before serving. Leftover muffins can be stored in an airtight container for up to 3 days.

Lunch

On the Go Pasta Salad

SERVES 4

1 tablespoon coconut oil

1 cup mushrooms, thinly sliced

2 Roma tomatoes, chopped

1 bell pepper, chopped

½ cup pine nuts

Sea salt and freshly ground black pepper

2 cups sprouted macaroni or spiral noodles, cooked and chilled

2 fresh basil leaves, chopped

4 tablespoons olive oil

½ cup Kalamata olives, pitted and sliced

1. In a large skillet over medium heat, melt the coconut oil and sauté the mushrooms, tomatoes, bell pepper, and pine nuts for 5 to 6 minutes, or until tender.
2. Season with sea salt and pepper and allow to cool completely.
3. In a mixing bowl, combine the cooked macaroni or noodles, cooled vegetables, basil, olive oil, and olives.
4. Serve immediately or refrigerate for up to 2 days.

Avocado Sauté Mushroom Wrap

SERVES 4

4 cups mushrooms, finely chopped

1 cup finely chopped white onion

4 cups spinach, chopped

¼ cup aged balsamic vinegar

Sea salt and freshly ground black pepper

2 tablespoons coconut oil

4 sprouted grain tortillas

2 avocados, pitted and peeled

1. In a small mixing bowl, combine the mushrooms, onion, spinach, balsamic vinegar, sea salt, and pepper.

2. Heat the coconut oil in a sauté pan over medium heat and add the vegetables to the pan. Allow them to cook for 5 to 10 minutes, or until tender.

3. Place the tortillas on a serving plate and spread ½ avocado evenly over each wrap.

4. Spoon the sautéed vegetables over the avocado and wrap the tortillas tightly.

Spicy Tomato Kale Soup

SERVES 4

1 teaspoon olive oil

½ white onion, chopped

3 carrots, peeled and chopped

2 cloves garlic, minced

1 teaspoon sea salt

½ teaspoon freshly ground black pepper

½ teaspoon crushed red pepper flakes

1 tablespoon chopped fresh rosemary

1 tablespoon chopped fresh basil

1 tablespoon chopped fresh sage

1 bay leaf

1 quart vegetable broth

2 cups water

24-ounce can crushed tomatoes

15-ounce can cannelloni beans, strained and rinsed

1 bunch kale, stems removed and chopped

1. Heat the olive oil over medium heat in a large pot.

2. Add the onion and carrots and cook for 4 to 5 minutes.

3. Add the garlic and cook for another 2 minutes.

4. Add the salt, pepper, red pepper flakes, herbs, broth, water, and tomatoes to the pot and bring to a boil.

5. Once the soup is at a boil, reduce to a simmer and add the beans.

6. Simmer the soup for 25 minutes.

7. Discard the bay leaf and puree the soup, using a hand blender.

8. Add the chopped kale and stir to combine. Serve hot; store leftovers in the refrigerator for up to 3 days.

Chicken Salad Sandwich

SERVES 4

Champagne vinaigrette:

2 tablespoons chopped shallots

1 teaspoon Dijon mustard

2 teaspoons honey

2 cloves garlic

¼ cup champagne vinegar

Sea salt and freshly ground black pepper

½ cup olive oil

Optional: ½ cup Greek yogurt

Chicken salad:

12 ounces cooked chicken, diced

½ red onion, thinly sliced

½ green apple, cored and thinly sliced

¼ cup chopped parsley

¼ cup goji berries, chopped

Sea salt and freshly ground black pepper

4 slices sprouted wheat bread

8 leaves Bibb lettuce

½ cup almonds, chopped

To make the vinaigrette:

Combine the shallots, mustard, honey, garlic, vinegar, sea salt, and pepper in a blender and blend until smooth. Slowly blend in the oil to form a creamy vinaigrette. Transfer to a bowl and add the Greek yogurt, if using. Mix until combined.

To make the chicken salad:

1. In a large bowl, combine the vinaigrette, chicken, onion, apple, parsley, and goji berries. Season with sea salt and pepper as desired.

2. Serve each sandwich open-faced on a slice of sprouted wheat bread layered with a lettuce leaf, and top with the chopped almonds.

Open-Faced Crunchy Veggie Sandwich

SERVES 4

1 medium cucumber, chopped

2 celery stalks, chopped

4 carrots, chopped or grated

2 avocados, pitted, peeled, and chopped

¼ cup chopped raw walnuts

¼ cup olive oil

Sea salt and freshly ground black pepper

8 slices sprouted wheat bread

2½ tablespoons whole grain mustard

8 lettuce leaves

1. In a medium bowl, combine the cucumber, celery, carrot, avocados, walnuts, olive oil, sea salt, and pepper.

2. Toast the bread and spread each slice with mustard. Add lettuce to each slice and divide the salad evenly among the slices of bread.

Melt-in-Your-Mouth Kale Salad

SERVES 4

2 bunches kale, stems removed

Juice of 2 lemons

2 tablespoons olive oil

2 teaspoons honey

Sea salt and freshly ground black pepper

⅔ cup currants (or chopped raisins)

1 cup pine nuts, toasted

½ cup grated Parmesan

1. In a food processor, process the kale into small pieces.

2. In a large bowl, combine the lemon juice, olive oil, honey, sea salt, and pepper.

3. Add the chopped kale, currants, pine nuts, and Parmesan to the bowl.

4. Stir the ingredients together and serve.

Salad Dressings

Tahini Dressing

SERVES 10 TO 12

Juice of 1 large lemon

1 clove garlic, minced

½ cup water

½ cup raw tahini

1 teaspoon maple syrup or honey

1 tablespoon plus 1 teaspoon apple cider vinegar

1½ teaspoons low-sodium tamari

1 teaspoon ground coriander

1 teaspoon cumin

2 tablespoons hempseed or olive oil

¼ teaspoon sea salt

1 tablespoon raw sesame seeds

1. Combine the lemon juice, garlic, and water in a blender and puree for 15 to 30 seconds.

2. Add the remaining ingredients and puree until smooth.

3. Store for up to 1 week in an airtight container in the refrigerator. Shake before serving.

Maple Mustard Dressing

SERVES 10

¾ cup olive oil

¼ cup apple cider vinegar

¼ cup whole grain mustard

1 tablespoon maple syrup

½ teaspoon sea salt

½ teaspoon freshly ground black pepper

1. Whisk all the ingredients together in a bowl or process in a blender until smooth.

2. Store for up to 1 week in an airtight container in the refrigerator. Shake before serving.

Carrot Ginger Dressing

SERVES 6 TO 8

4 carrots, cut into chunks

½ white onion, quartered

4-inch piece of gingerroot, peeled and chopped

2 tablespoons white miso paste

¼ cup rice wine vinegar

2 tablespoons honey or coconut palm sugar

3 tablespoons dark toasted sesame oil

2 tablespoons olive oil

¼ cup water

½ teaspoon sea salt

½ teaspoon freshly ground black pepper

1. In a blender, process all the ingredients until smooth.

2. Store for up to 1 week in an airtight container in the refrigerator. Shake before serving.

Dinner

White Bean Chili

SERVES 4

2 tablespoons olive oil

1 medium onion, diced

1 red bell pepper, diced

1 medium carrot, diced

5 cloves garlic, minced

1 teaspoon smoked paprika

Dash of cayenne pepper

½ teaspoon cinnamon

1 teaspoon cumin

1 teaspoon turmeric

8 large tomatoes, diced, or a 14-to-18-ounce can diced tomatoes

Two 15-ounce cans chickpeas, rinsed and drained

4 cups vegetable broth

Sea salt and freshly ground black pepper

1 medium zucchini, diced

1. Heat the olive oil over medium heat in a large soup pot.

2. Add the onion, bell pepper, carrot, and garlic and sauté until the vegetables are tender.

3. Add the spices and cook for one minute.

4. Add the tomatoes, chickpeas, and vegetable broth and bring to a boil. Season with sea salt and pepper.

5. Turn down to a simmer and cook for about 20 minutes. Add a little water if more liquid is needed.

6. Add the zucchini and cook for about 20 minutes more. Serve hot; store leftovers in the refrigerator for up to 3 days.

Mac 'n' Cheese

SERVES 4

8 ounces 100% organic sprouted whole wheat or spelt pasta

½ head cauliflower, chopped

6 ounces mild goat's milk or cheddar cheese

1 tablespoon butter

Sea salt and freshly ground black pepper to taste

Optional: Dash of nutmeg

1. Bring 4 cups water to a boil in a large pot on high heat.
2. Add the pasta and cook until it is *al dente* or firm, following the package directions.
3. While the water is heating up for the pasta, steam the cauliflower in a steamer basket placed in a large pot filled with 1 or 2 cups boiling water for 5 to 7 minutes.
4. Shred the cheese with a grater or a food processor.
5. Grate the cauliflower by hand or pulse in a food processor.
6. Mix the grated cheese, cauliflower, butter, and seasonings with the drained pasta and stir to combine. Serve hot; store leftovers in the refrigerator for up to 3 days.

For Vegan Mac 'n' Cheese, replace the cheese with the following:

¾ cup nutritional yeast

Juice of ½ lemon

1 tablespoon tahini

2 tablespoons cashews

½ tablespoon Dijon mustard

½ tablespoon coconut oil

½ tablespoon garlic powder

½ tablespoon onion powder

⅛ teaspoon cayenne pepper

¼ to ½ cup unsweetened nut milk (if you have a nut allergy, substitute ½ to 1 cup water or coconut milk)

Sea salt and freshly ground black pepper

1. In a blender, process the nutritional yeast, lemon juice, tahini, cashews, Dijon mustard, coconut oil, garlic and onion powder, cayenne, nut milk, sea salt, and pepper until smooth. Pour the mixture into the bowl with the cauliflower, seasonings, and pasta and stir.

Masala Burgers

SERVES 4

½ cup quinoa, cooked

1 sweet potato, baked with skin removed, and mashed

1 egg, slightly beaten, or 1 tablespoon flaxseeds mixed with 2 tablespoons water

2 tablespoons chopped cilantro

1 small onion, diced

2-inch piece gingerroot, peeled and minced

1 clove garlic, minced

½ teaspoon sea salt

½ teaspoon garam masala (can be found in most local groceries)

½ teaspoon curry powder

¼ teaspoon mustard seeds

⅛ teaspoon cayenne pepper

Melted coconut oil for brushing the burgers

2 cups spinach

1. Preheat the oven to 400°F.

2. Combine all the ingredients except the coconut oil and spinach in a large bowl.

3. Form the mixture into 8 patties.

4. Place the patties on a large baking sheet covered with parchment paper.

5. Brush the tops of the burgers with coconut oil.

6. Bake for 15 minutes, then flip the burgers and brush with coconut oil again.

7. Bake for another 15 minutes, or until golden brown. Serve on top of the spinach.

Chicken with Sautéed Kale

SERVES 4

2 tablespoons coconut oil

4 cups kale, shredded

Juice of 2 lemons

Sea salt and freshly ground pepper

1 cup cashews

16 ounces chicken, baked (or ½ cup cooked white beans)

1. In a large skillet over medium heat, melt the coconut oil and sauté the kale with the lemon juice for 4 to 5 minutes. Season with salt and pepper.

2. Transfer the kale to a serving plate and sprinkle with cashews.

3. Top the kale with warm chicken or white beans.

Miso Soup with Black Rice Noodles

SERVES 4

8 cups water

1 sheet nori (dried seaweed), cut into large rectangles

½ cup chopped mushrooms and/or cubed firm organic tofu

5 ounces black rice noodles

½ cup red or white miso paste

¾ cup chopped green onions

Sea salt

1. In a large pot, bring the water to a low boil.

2. Add the nori, mushrooms and/or tofu, and noodles and lower the heat to a simmer for 5 to 7 minutes.

3. In the meantime, put the miso paste in a small bowl, add a little warm water, and whisk until smooth.

4. Add the green onions and miso to the soup and stir to ensure that the soup doesn't clump. It's important not to boil the miso; you don't want to kill the beneficial bacteria.

5. Heat at just below simmering point for 3 more minutes and serve immediately, or store and serve cold later. The soup can be stored in the refrigerator up to 2 days.

Moroccan Veggie and Chickpea Soup

SERVES 4

2 tablespoons olive oil

1 medium onion, diced

1 red bell pepper, diced

1 medium carrot, diced

5 cloves garlic, minced

1 teaspoon smoked paprika

Dash of cayenne pepper

½ teaspoon cinnamon

1 teaspoon cumin

1 teaspoon turmeric

8 large tomatoes, diced, or a 14-to-18-ounce can diced tomatoes

4 cups cooked chickpeas, or two 15-ounce cans chickpeas, rinsed and drained

4 cups vegetable broth

Sea salt and freshly ground black pepper

1 medium zucchini, diced

1. Heat the olive oil over medium heat in a large soup pot.

2. Add the onion, bell pepper, carrot, and garlic and sauté for 5 to 6 minutes, until the vegetables are tender.

3. Add the spices and cook for 1 minute.

4. Add the tomatoes, chickpeas, and vegetable broth and bring to a boil. Season with sea salt and pepper.

5. Turn down to a simmer and cook for about 20 minutes. Add extra water if more liquid is needed.

6. Add the zucchini and cook for about 20 minutes more. Serve hot. Leftovers can be stored in the refrigerator for up to 3 days.

Vegetable Lasagna

SERVES 4

1 tablespoon extra virgin olive oil

½ onion, chopped

2 garlic cloves, chopped

24-ounce can strained or crushed tomatoes

½ teaspoon crushed red pepper flakes

½ teaspoon sea salt

1 egg

15-ounce container ricotta

1 tablespoon dried Italian herbs, or ¼ cup fresh basil, chopped

1 large zucchini, sliced ½ inch thick

1 large yellow squash, sliced ½ inch thick

2 cups baby kale, spinach, or other dark leafy greens

½ cup Parmesan, shredded

½ cup goat mozzarella or cheese of choice, shredded

1. Preheat the oven to 375°F.

2. Heat the olive oil in a large sauté pan over medium heat and sauté the onion for 5 minutes.

3. Once the onion is tender, add the garlic and sauté for 2 more minutes.

4. Add the tomatoes, red pepper flakes, and salt and bring to a boil, then reduce to a simmer.

5. Allow the sauce to cook for at least 10 minutes. (Alternatively, you can use your favorite jarred tomato or marinara sauce.)

6. In a bowl, combine the egg, ricotta, and herbs and stir well.

7. Spread about ⅓ of the cooked tomato sauce on the bottom of a large baking dish.

8. Layer the zucchini on top of the sauce.

9. Spread ½ the ricotta mixture on top of the zucchini.

10. Layer with ⅓ more tomato sauce.

11. Layer the yellow squash on top of the tomato sauce.

12. Spread the remaining ricotta mixture on top of the squash.

13. Layer the greens on top of the ricotta.

14. Top with the remaining sauce and shredded cheese.

15. Cover with aluminum foil and bake the lasagna for 30 to 40 minutes, until the sauce is bubbly and the cheese slightly browned.

16. Allow the lasagna to rest for 10 minutes before serving.

Black Bean and Sweet Potato Soup

SERVES 4

1 tablespoon coconut oil or olive oil

1 onion, chopped

2 cloves garlic, minced

2 sweet potatoes, peeled and chopped

1 cup mushrooms, sliced

1 tomato, diced

2 cups spinach, stems removed and chopped

6 cups vegetable broth

2 cups cooked black beans

1 teaspoon cumin

1 teaspoon coriander

1 teaspoon curry powder

Sea salt and freshly ground black pepper

Toppings:

12 sprigs cilantro

1 avocado, pitted, peeled, and sliced

1. In a large soup pot, heat the coconut oil and sauté the onions and garlic for about 5 minutes.

2. Add the sweet potatoes, mushrooms, tomatoes, and spinach and sauté for 5 to 10 minutes.

3. Add the vegetable broth, black beans, cumin, coriander, curry, sea salt, and pepper and stir to combine.

4. Bring the ingredients to a boil, then lower the heat and simmer for about 20 minutes, or until the sweet potatoes and other vegetables are tender.

5. Pour the soup into serving bowls and top each with cilantro sprigs and sliced avocado.

   If you do not wish to serve 4, store the remaining soup in an airtight container in the refrigerator for up to 3 days, or freeze for up to 1 month.

Ginger Garlic Salmon

4¼ cups mirin (Japanese cooking wine, available in the Asian section of the grocery store)

2 to 3 tablespoons coconut palm sugar or maple syrup

½ cup low-sodium tamari or soy sauce

2 tablespoons minced peeled gingerroot

4 cloves minced garlic

1½ pounds wild salmon filets, with skin on

Optional: 4 scallions, chopped

1. Combine all the ingredients except the salmon and scallions in a small sauté pan over medium to high heat. Bring to a boil, then simmer for 5 to 7 minutes, stirring occasionally.

2. Let the marinade cool. Place the salmon in an ovenproof glass dish with the marinade. Be sure that bits of ginger and garlic are on the skinless side.

3. Marinate the salmon in the refrigerator for at least 1 hour and at most 6 hours.

4. Preheat the oven to 425°F.

5. Place the glass dish of salmon in the oven with the skinless side facing up. (The skin will stick to the dish and leave you with all the good fish.)

6. Bake for 15 to 20 minutes.

7. Let the fish rest for 2 to 5 minutes and top with chopped scallions if using. Serve immediately.

Turkey Meatballs with Spaghetti Squash

SERVES 4

1 spaghetti squash

½ cup water

1 pound ground turkey

¼ teaspoon dried oregano

¼ teaspoon garlic powder

¼ teaspoon dried rosemary

¼ teaspoon dried thyme

¼ teaspoon dried sage

½ teaspoon sea salt

Freshly ground black pepper

1 egg, beaten

24-ounce jar of tomato or marinara sauce

½ cup shredded Parmesan

1. Preheat the oven to 350°F.
2. Cut the spaghetti squash in half and scrape out all the seeds.
3. Place the squash facedown on a large baking sheet. Add the water, cover with foil, and bake for 45 minutes.
4. While the spaghetti squash is cooking, combine the remaining ingredients, except the tomato sauce and cheese, in a large bowl.
5. Form meatballs (about 2 tablespoons each) with your hands and place them on a greased cookie sheet.
6. Bake for 20 minutes alongside the spaghetti squash, turning halfway through.
7. Remove the meatballs from the oven and place in a sauté pan with the tomato sauce.
8. Warm the sauce thoroughly.
9. Remove the spaghetti squash from the oven and scrape out the flesh.
10. Divide the spaghetti squash among 4 bowls and top each with sauce and meatballs.
11. Sprinkle with Parmesan and enjoy.

Quick and Easy Home-Baked Pizza

SERVES 4

4 large sprouted wheat tortillas

½ cup tomato or pizza sauce

4 cloves garlic, minced

1 cup chopped onions

1 cup chopped green bell peppers

1 cup chopped broccoli

20 black olives, pitted and sliced

Crushed red pepper flakes

Optional: 4 ounces shredded mozzarella

Optional: 1 ounce shredded Parmesan

1. Preheat the oven to 450°F.
2. Put the tortillas on a large baking sheet and place in the oven for 3 to 4 minutes. Once the tortillas have started to crisp slightly at the edges, remove from the oven.
3. Spread the sauce over each tortilla and sprinkle on the garlic. Top with the remaining ingredients or experiment with toppings, being careful not to overload the crust. If using cheese, sprinkle it on top.
4. Bake for 10 minutes. Serve hot.

Mexican Casserole

SERVES 4

1 teaspoon olive oil

1 small onion, chopped

2 medium zucchini, chopped

1 green bell pepper, chopped

1 tomato, chopped

1 tablespoon chili powder

1 teaspoon cumin

15-ounce can black beans, rinsed and drained

15-ounce can kidney beans, rinsed and drained

2 cloves garlic, minced

2 jalapeños, seeded and minced

14-ounce can tomato sauce

8 small sprouted corn tortillas

2 ounces goat's milk cheddar cheese, shredded

Lime wedges

Sour cream or plain yogurt

1. Preheat the oven to 350°F.

2. Heat the olive oil over medium heat in a large skillet.

3. Add the onion and sauté for about 3 minutes.

4. Add the zucchini, green peppers, tomato, and spices to the skillet and cook for another 5 minutes.

5. Add the beans, garlic, and jalapeños and cook for another 2 minutes.

6. Turn off the heat and set aside.

7. Cover the bottom of a large baking dish with ½ the tomato sauce.

8. Place 4 of the corn tortillas over the sauce.

9. Add ½ the vegetable and bean mixture to the dish.

10. Add another layer of tortillas and then the rest of the vegetable and bean mixture.

11. Pour the remaining sauce over the top.

12. Top the casserole with shredded cheese and cover with foil.

13. Bake for at least 30 minutes, until the sauce starts to bubble.

14. Serve each portion with a lime wedge and a dollop of sour cream or plain yogurt.

Eggplant Parmesan

SERVES 4

1 large eggplant

3 tablespoons olive oil

1 large onion, chopped

3 cloves garlic, minced

8 ripe tomatoes, diced

½ teaspoon crushed red pepper flakes

½ cup chopped fresh basil

½ teaspoon sea salt

1 cup quinoa, cooked

3 ounces crumbled goat cheese

¼ cup shredded Parmesan

1. Preheat the oven to 400°F.

2. Slice the eggplant into ½-inch-thick pieces, coat lightly with 1 tablespoon of the olive oil, and place on a large baking sheet.

3. Bake the eggplant slices for 10 to 15 minutes, until slightly golden. Remove from the oven and lower the temperature to 350°F.

4. In a large skillet, heat the remaining 2 tablespoons oil over medium heat. Add the onion and sauté for about 5 minutes.

5. Once the onion is tender, add the garlic and sauté 2 more minutes.

6. Add the tomatoes, red pepper flakes, half the basil, and the sea salt. Allow the tomatoes to cook for at least 10 minutes and then mash them with a potato masher or fork.

7. Spread ½ the tomato sauce across the bottom of a large baking dish.

8. Layer the ingredients in this order: eggplant slices, quinoa, and remaining sauce. Top with the cheese and remaining basil.

9. Cover with foil and bake for 30 to 40 minutes. Serve hot. Store leftovers in the refrigerator for up to 3 days.

Grilled Chicken with Rhubarb-Cucumber Slaw

SERVES 4

1 red Anaheim chili pepper, seeded

2 cloves garlic

2 scallions, sliced

1 tablespoon low-sodium tamari

3 tablespoons olive oil

16 ounces skinless, boneless chicken breasts

1 cup diced rhubarb

½ cucumber, sliced and then halved

2 tablespoons chopped cilantro

2 teaspoons honey

1 tablespoon apple cider vinegar

Sea salt and freshly ground black pepper

1. In a food processor, pulse the red chili pepper, garlic, and scallions until chopped. While the processor is running, drizzle in the tamari and 2 tablespoons of the olive oil until a paste forms.

2. Spread the paste over the chicken and marinate for 20 minutes in the refrigerator.

3. Heat 1 teaspoon of the oil in a sauté pan over medium-high heat. Cook the chicken for 4 to 5 minutes on each side, or until cooked all the way through.

4. In a medium bowl, combine the rhubarb, cucumber, cilantro, honey, remaining olive oil, and vinegar.

5. Serve the chicken topped with the rhubarb-cucumber slaw.

Veggie Sloppy Joes

SERVES 4

1 tablespoon olive oil

½ cup diced green bell pepper

½ cup mushrooms, chopped

½ onion, chopped

½ jalapeño, seeded and diced

1 clove garlic, minced

2 tomatoes

4 cups cooked lentils

½ cup tomato paste

1 tablespoon soy sauce

2 tablespoons chili powder

1 tablespoon paprika

1 teaspoon dried oregano

1 teaspoon dried basil

Sea salt and freshly ground black pepper

4 sprouted burger buns

Shredded red cabbage, for garnish

Pickle slices, for garnish

1. Heat the olive oil in a large sauté pan over medium heat.

2. Add the bell pepper, mushrooms, onion, jalapeño, and garlic to the pan and sauté for 5 to 10 minutes, or until the vegetables are tender.

3. Meanwhile, in a blender, process the tomatoes until smooth.

4. To the skillet add the cooked lentils, tomato paste, blended tomatoes, soy sauce, chili powder, paprika, oregano, basil, sea salt, and pepper and combine.

5. Sauté the ingredients for 5 minutes, or until the mixture thickens.

6. Fill each bun with sloppy joe mixture and top with shredded red cabbage and pickles.

"Fast Foods" and Snacks

Organic Homemade Frappuccino

SERVES 2

3 cups brewed coffee, chilled

1 cup almond milk

4 tablespoons raw cacao powder

4 pitted dates

2 frozen bananas

20 ice cubes

1. Place all the ingredients in a blender, blend well, and serve chilled.

Superfood Popcorn

SERVES 4

½ cup popcorn kernels

3 teaspoons coconut oil

2 tablespoons hempseeds

½ teaspoon sea salt

4 teaspoons red palm oil, grass-fed butter, or ghee, melted

1. In a large pot, stir together the popcorn kernels and coconut oil, cover, and place over high heat.
2. Let the popcorn pop until you only hear a couple of pops per second.
3. Pour the popcorn into a large bowl.
4. Using a blender or food processor, blend the hempseeds and sea salt until fine.
5. Top the popcorn with the melted red palm oil, butter, or ghee and the hempseed and sea salt mixture.

Creamy Kale and Artichoke Dip

SERVES 4

½ bag frozen artichoke hearts, thawed and chopped

2 cups finely chopped kale, spinach, Swiss chard, or collards

1 clove garlic, minced

⅛ teaspoon freshly grated nutmeg

⅛ teaspoon cayenne pepper

½ teaspoon sea salt

½ teaspoon freshly ground black pepper

½ cup sour cream or Greek yogurt

1½ tablespoons mayonnaise

1½ tablespoons Parmesan or manchego, plus more for topping if desired

Coconut oil for greasing the pan

1. Preheat the oven to 375°F.
2. Combine all the ingredients except the coconut oil in a large bowl. Mix well.
3. Grease a medium baking dish with the coconut oil and put in the dip mixture.
4. Top with additional cheese, if desired.
5. Cover with aluminum foil and bake for 40 to 45 minutes.
6. Remove from the oven and let sit for at least 5 minutes before serving with homemade pita or tortilla chips (see next recipe).

Pita or Tortilla Chips

SERVES 4

5 whole wheat pitas or small sprouted corn tortillas

1 tablespoon coconut oil

¼ teaspoon paprika

¼ teaspoon sea salt

1. Preheat the oven to 400°F.

2. Cut the pitas or tortillas into triangles with a pizza cutter.

3. Combine the triangles with the coconut oil, paprika, and sea salt in a large bowl.

4. Place the triangles on a baking sheet and bake for 8 to 10 minutes, until crisp.

5. Let cool and enjoy.

Fast-Food Burritos

SERVES 4

8 small sprouted corn tortillas

Two 15-ounce cans black beans, rinsed and drained

Chili powder, to taste

½ onion, chopped

2 cups homemade or organic salsa

½ cup shredded goat cheese

Optional: avocado, romaine, organic sour cream, lime wedges

1. Preheat the oven to 375°F.

2. Place the tortillas on a sheet of parchment paper on a baking sheet.

3. Place ¼ cup black beans on each tortilla.

4. Sprinkle chili powder on top of the beans (1 to 2 shakes).

5. Put about 1 tablespoon onion on top of the beans.

6. Top each burrito with 1 tablespoon salsa.

7. Sprinkle each burrito with a handful of shredded cheese as well as optional toppings, if desired.

8. Roll and wrap each tortilla tightly.

9. Bake the burritos for approximately 10 minutes. (You can also prepare them up until the point of baking and then store them in a Ziploc bag in the freezer until ready to use.)

Note: Cooking time varies. Fresh burritos take 10 minutes to bake, while defrosted burritos take 20 minutes and frozen burritos take 30 minutes.

Warm and Heavenly Kale Tacos

SERVES 4

8 sprouted corn tortillas

2 shallots or ½ small onion, chopped

1 tablespoon coconut oil

2 cloves garlic, minced

¼ teaspoon sea salt

Freshly ground black pepper

½ head red cabbage, shredded

1 large bunch kale, chopped

2 tomatoes, diced

1 avocado, pitted, peeled, and sliced

Optional: ½ cup crumbled feta

2 cups sprouts

1 lime, sliced

1. Preheat the oven to 325°F and warm the tortillas.

2. In a large skillet, sauté the shallots or onion in the coconut oil over medium heat for 2 to 3 minutes.

3. Add the garlic and cook another 1 minute or so.

4. Add the sea salt, pepper, and cabbage and cook for 2 to 3 minutes.

5. Add the kale and cook until slightly wilted, 3 to 4 minutes. Remove from the heat.

6. Divide the kale and cabbage mixture among the corn tortillas and top with diced tomato, sliced avocado, feta (if using), sprouts, and a squeeze of lime.

Chickpea Curry Wraps

SERVES 4

1½ cups dried chickpeas, or two 15-ounce cans chickpeas, rinsed and drained

1 red bell pepper, seeded and chopped

½ cup chopped cilantro

½ cup raisins

4 cups baby spinach

4 large sprouted wheat tortillas

Dressing:

Juice of 1 lime

2 teaspoons curry powder

2 teaspoons honey

¼ cup olive oil

Sea salt and freshly ground black pepper

1. If using dried chickpeas, soak them in water overnight for at least 6 hours. Drain and rinse the soaked chickpeas and place them in a large pot. Cover with 2 to 3 inches of cold water. Bring the chickpeas to a boil over high heat; then lower the heat and simmer, covered, until softened, about 1½ hours.

2. In a large bowl, combine the cooked or canned chickpeas, red bell pepper, cilantro, and raisins.

3. In a separate small bowl, whisk together the dressing ingredients.

4. Add the dressing to the chickpeas and stir well. Let sit for 30 minutes in the refrigerator to develop flavors, or cover and refrigerate to eat later.

5. Add ½ the chickpeas to each tortilla and top each with 1 cup baby spinach. Roll tightly and enjoy.

Sweet Potato Fries

SERVES 4

4 large sweet potatoes, cut into strips

2 tablespoons coconut oil

½ teaspoon sea salt

Optional: crushed red pepper flakes and lime

1. Preheat the oven to 375°F.

2. Soak the potato strips in water for at least 10 minutes.

3. Rinse the potatoes and dry thoroughly.

4. Toss the potatoes with the coconut oil and sprinkle with sea salt.

5. Arrange the potatoes on a baking sheet and bake for about 25 minutes, turning halfway through.

6. The fries should be slightly brown when done. Toss with red pepper flakes and a squeeze of lime for a kick.

Sweets

Forever Cookies

MAKES 20 COOKIES

1 ripe banana

4 pitted dates

4 pitted prunes

¼ cup coconut oil, melted

1 teaspoon vanilla extract

2 cups rolled oats

⅔ cup nut meal

½ cup unsweetened coconut flakes

½ teaspoon cinnamon

½ teaspoon sea salt

1 teaspoon aluminum-free baking powder

7 ounces organic dark chocolate, chopped into pieces, or ½ cup dried unsweetened cherries

1. Preheat the oven to 350°F.
2. In a food processor, combine the banana, dates, prunes, coconut oil, and vanilla and blend until smooth.
3. In a large bowl, mix all the other ingredients well.
4. Scrape the contents of the food processor into the bowl and stir until the dough is moist and the ingredients well incorporated.
5. Place the dough in the refrigerator or freezer for at least 15 minutes.
6. Scoop out 2 tablespoons of the dough at a time and shape into balls. Place on a parchment-lined baking sheet.
7. Bake the cookies for 12 to 15 minutes.
8. Cool the cookies on a rack for at least 5 minutes before serving; otherwise, they will fall apart.

Note: This dough can be eaten raw. Press the dough into a log in a large Ziploc bag and freeze. You can enjoy slices of cookie dough anytime!

Almond Chocolate Freezer Fudge

MAKES 20 PIECES

1 cup almond butter

4 tablespoons coconut oil

1½ tablespoons maple syrup

½ teaspoon sea salt

4 ounces dark chocolate, chopped

1. Cream the almond butter, coconut oil, maple syrup, and sea salt together in a bowl.

2. Scoop the mixture into a parchment-lined small baking dish (8 by 8 inches).

3. Top with the chopped chocolate, cover, and freeze for at least 2 hours.

4. Remove from the freezer and carefully lift the ends of the parchment paper to remove the fudge.

5. Cut into 1-inch squares and store in the freezer in layers separated by parchment paper.

Homemade Coconut Milk Ice Cream (3 Flavors)

SERVES 10

Base:

13½-ounce can full-fat coconut milk

3 frozen bananas or ½ cup coconut palm sugar

Pinch of sea salt

For almond pistachio flavor:

1½ teaspoons almond extract

1 teaspoon vanilla extract, or seeds from one vanilla bean

½ cup toasted and chopped almonds and pistachios

For mint chocolate chip flavor:

2 teaspoons peppermint extract

⅓ cup raw cacao nibs or chocolate chips

For cookies and cream flavor:

1 tablespoon vanilla extract

10 cacao einkorn cookies (or other cookie of choice), broken into pieces

1. Combine the base ingredients in a blender and blend until smooth.
2. Add the liquid flavorings (the extracts or, if using, the vanilla bean seeds) to the blender and blend again.
3. Pour the mixture into an ice cream machine and turn it on.
4. Mix for at least 20 minutes, or until ice cream forms.
5. Stir in the dry ingredients (nuts, cacao nibs, or cookies).
6. Serve immediately. If the ice cream is stored in the freezer, put it back into the ice cream maker before serving to make it smooth and creamy again.

Homemade Liquid Stevia Extract

1 cup of stevia leaves (washed)

Organic vodka

1. Dry stevia leaves by putting them in the sun for 12 hours, or in a dehydrator.
2. Place dried leaves in a glass jar and pour in enough organic vodka to cover leaves.
3. Steep leaves in vodka for exactly 24 hours.
4. Filter out the leaves using a strainer.
5. To remove alcohol, cook the liquid on a stovetop burner on low for twenty minutes (but do not boil).
6. Transfer remaining liquid to a glass dropper bottle and store in your refrigerator for up to ninety days.

Congratulations!

I NOW PROCLAIM YOU to be a true Food Babe. You have completed my three-week habit change program. And hopefully, you've been following my 21-Day Eating Plan.

How do you feel? How do you look? Take some time to reflect on all the positives that you've experienced in these past three weeks. Maybe you're thinner. Maybe you're more energetic. Perhaps your sleep is better. Perhaps you feel healthier, with fewer aches and pains. How about your mood? What has changed for the better in your life?

I hope you understand this, too: The food industry is trying to lead us like sheep into eating processed, fake, chemical-filled foods. Big Food does not want us to pay any attention to ingredients, and I don't think they give a damn about what those ingredients are doing to our collective health.

But you do not have to be blindly guided by Big Food anymore... because you know the Food Babe Way.

My hope is that you want to walk this "way" for the rest of your life.

JOIN THE FOOD BABE ARMY: HOW TO START A PETITION

As a member of the Food Babe Army, you will be on the front lines of the movement that is sweeping the food industry by storm and creating a better food system for us all. Be a part of this change! You'll also be the first to know about major foodbabe.com campaigns and investigations, along with future petitions and news about the great strides we are taking. Sign up completely free here: foodbabe.com/subscribe.

Want to change the food system and the world? Here are five easy steps to start a petition:

1. *Decide what you want to change.* Pick something specific. Target one company or organization, rather than trying to make sweeping changes all at once. For instance, my petition to remove azodicarbonamide from bread at Subway was focused on that additive. I could have petitioned to overhaul the entire Subway menu, but that wouldn't have been as effective.

2. *Determine who's responsible for making the change.* Find out who has the power to make this change happen and target them. Compile a list of contact information for key individuals in the organization you will be petitioning. (Hint: Company websites and the networking platform LinkedIn are a great source of this type of information.)

3. *Gather all the facts.* Extensively research the reasons why this change needs to be made. Why is the current situation so bad? What research studies back up your claims? What are the benefits of making this change? Do you have any personal stories that you can include in the petition? After you feel satisfied with your research, summarize the facts in writing.

4. *Reach out for help.* Do you belong to any organizations that would help you with the petition? Do you have friends in the blogosphere with similar interests and goals? If you plan on using a petition platform like Change.org, contact them for help in advance. They may have someone who can help get the word out or devise a strategy for you.

5. *Post your petition.* You can post it on your own blog and/or platforms like Change.org, Care2.com, or SumOfUs.org. Once you have it posted, share it with everyone you know on e-mail and on social media. Send it to news organizations once you have some signatures, so they know it could be a story. And most important, don't give up. Companies assume you'll get tired and just stop campaigning. It took seven months of active pressure to get Kraft to start removing artificial food dyes, seven months for Chipotle to finally release their ingredients online, and nearly two years for Chick-fil-A to decide to go antibiotic-free. Changing the world does not happen overnight, but it can happen fast with resolve and commitment.

RECOMMENDED READING AND RESOURCES

Books

- *The American Way of Eating* by Tracie McMillan
- *The Beauty Detox Foods* by Kimberly Snyder
- *The Blood Sugar Solution* by Mark Hyman, MD
- *The China Study* by T. Colin Campbell
- *Conscious Eating* by Gabriel Cousens, MD
- *A Consumer's Dictionary of Food Additives* by Ruth Winter, MS
- *Cooked* by Michael Pollan
- *The Desire Map: A Guide to Creating Goals with Soul* by Danielle LaPorte
- *Eat Drink Vote: An Illustrated Guide to Food Politics* by Marion Nestle
- *Eating for Beauty* by David Wolfe
- *Eating on the Wild Side: The Missing Link to Optimum Health* by Jo Robinson
- *Eat to Live* by Joel Fuhrman, MD
- *The End of Dieting* by Joel Fuhrman, MD
- *Excitotoxins: The Taste That Kills* by Russell L. Blaylock, MD
- *Fast Food Nation* by Eric Schlosser
- *Fat Chance* by Robert H. Lustig, MD
- *The Fire Starter Sessions* by Danielle LaPorte

- *Food Journeys of a Lifetime* by National Geographic
- *Foodopoly* by Wenonah Hauter
- *Food Politics* by Marion Nestle
- *The Food Revolution* by John Robbins and Dean Ornish, MD
- *Food Rules: An Eater's Manual* by Michael Pollan
- *The 4-Hour Chef* by Timothy Ferriss
- *Grain Brain* by David Perlmutter, MD
- *The Green Beauty Guide* by Julie Gabriel
- *The Honest Life* by Jessica Alba
- *The Juice Lady's Guide to Juicing for Health* by Cherie Calbom, MS
- *The Juice Lady's Turbo Diet* by Cherie Calbom, MS
- *The Jungle* by Upton Sinclair
- *Man 2.0: Engineering the Alpha* by John Romaniello and Adam Bornstein
- *No More Dirty Looks* by Siobhan O'Connor and Alexandra Spunt
- *The Omnivore's Dilemma: A Natural History of Four Meals* by Michael Pollan
- *The Omnivore's Dilemma: Young Readers Edition* by Michael Pollan
- *Pandora's Lunchbox* by Melanie Warner
- *The Real Food Revolution* by Tim Ryan
- *Revive* by Frank Lipman, MD
- *Rich Food Poor Food* by Mira Calton and Jayson Calton
- *Salt Sugar Fat: How the Food Giants Hooked Us* by Michael Moss
- *Spiritual Nutrition* by Gabriel Cousens, MD
- *Spontaneous Happiness* by Andrew Weil, MD
- *Ultraprevention* by Mark Hyman, MD, and Mark Liponis, MD
- *The Unhealthy Truth* by Robyn O'Brien
- *VB6* by Mark Bittman
- *The Whole Heart Solution* by Joel Kahn, MD
- *Wildly Affordable Organic* by Linda Watson

Cookbooks

- *100 Days of Real Food* by Lisa Leake
- *Against All Grain* by Danielle Walker

- *The Art of Simple Food* by Alice Waters
- *The Art of Simple Food II* by Alice Waters
- *Crazy Sexy Kitchen* by Kris Carr
- *Eating the Alkaline Way* by Natasha Corrett and Vicki Edgson
- *Eat Taste Heal* by Thomas Yarema, Daniel Rhoda, and Johnny Brannigan
- *The Family Cooks* by Laurie David and Kirstin Uhrenholdt
- *It's All Good* by Gwyneth Paltrow
- *Living Raw Food* by Sarma Melngailis
- *The Oh She Glows Cookbook* by Angela Liddon
- *Rainbow Green Live-Food Cuisine* by Gabriel Cousens, MD
- *Raw Food/Real World* by Matthew Kenney and Sarma Melngailis
- *The Sprouted Kitchen* by Sara Forte
- *Superfood Kitchen* by Julie Morris
- *Superfood Smoothies* by Julie Morris
- *Super Natural Every Day* by Heidi Swanson
- *True Food: Seasonal, Sustainable, Simple, Pure* by Andrew Weil, MD, and Sam Fox
- *Vegetarian Traditions* by George Vutetakis

Magazines

- *Dr. Oz The Good Life* — doctorozmag.com
- *Experience Life* — experiencelife.com
- *Modern Farmer* — modernfarmer.com
- *Natural Health* — naturalhealthmag.com
- *Organic Eats* — organiceatsmag.com
- *Yoga Journal* — yogajournal.com

Restaurant Guides

- *Clean Plates* — cleanplates.com
- *Eat Well Guide* — eatwellguide.org
- *Happy Cow* — happycow.net
- *Organic Highways* — organichighways.com
- Pressed Organic Juice Directory — pressedjuicedirectory.com

Food Co-ops

- Coop Directory Service — coopdirectory.org
- Cooperative Grocer Network — cooperativegrocer.coop
- Local Harvest — localharvest.org/food-coops

Farmers' Market/Local Food Resources

- Farmers Market Coalition — farmersmarketcoalition.org
- Farm Plate — farmplate.com
- Local Harvest — localharvest.org/farmers-markets
- Real Time Farms — realtimefarms.com

Shopping Websites

- Abe's Market — abesmarket.com
- Azure Standard — azurestandard.com
- Door to Door Organics — doortodoororganics.com
- Full Circle — fullcircle.com
- Green PolkaDot Box — greenpolkadotbox.com
- Local Harvest — localharvest.org/csa/
- Nutiva — nutiva.com
- SPUD (Sustainable Produce Urban Delivery) — spud.com
- Thrive Market — thrivemarket.com
- Urban Organic — urbanorganic.com

Food Advocacy Groups

- Cancer Prevention Coalition — preventcancer.com
- Center for Food Safety — truefoodnow.org
- Center for Science in the Public Interest — cspinet.org
- Cornucopia Institute — cornucopia.org
- Environmental Working Group — ewg.org
- Food & Water Watch — foodandwaterwatch.org
- Food Democracy Now — fooddemocracynow.org
- Food Integrity Now — foodintegritynow.org
- Friends of the Earth — foe.org

- GMO Inside — gmoinside.org
- Institute for Responsible Technology — responsibletechnology.org
- Just Label It — justlabelit.org
- NOFA-NY — Northeast Organic Farming Association of New York — nofany.org
- NRDC — Natural Resources Defense Council — nrdc.org
- Only Organic — onlyorganic.org
- Organic Consumers Association — organicconsumers.org

Food Information Websites

- Center for Nutrition Studies — nutritionstudies.org
- Environmental Working Group — ewg.org
- Food Facts — foodfacts.com
- Fooducate — fooducate.com
- Labelwatch — labelwatch.com
- Living Maxwell — livingmaxwell.com
- Non-GMO Project — nongmoproject.org
- Organic Authority — organicauthority.com
- Seafood Watch — seafoodwatch.org
- Sustainable Table — sustainabletable.org
- Truth in Labeling — truthinlabeling.org

Natural Health and Healing Organizations

- Ann Wigmore Natural Health Institute — annwigmore.org
- Burzynski Clinic — burzynskiclinic.com
- Deepak Chopra — deepakchopra.com
- Dr. Cousens' Tree of Life Center US — treeoflifecenterus.com
- Gerson Institute — gerson.org
- Hippocrates Health Institute — hippocratesinst.org

Food News

- Helena Bottemiller Erich on Politico — politico.com/reporters/HelenaBottemillerErich.html
- Candice Choi on AP — bigstory.ap.org/content/candice-choi

- Food Navigator — foodnavigator.com
- Grist — Food — grist.org/food
- Huffington Post — Food — huffingtonpost.com/taste/
- Huffington Post — Healthy Living — huffingtonpost .com/healthy-living
- Natural News — naturalnews.com
- NY Times Health — nytimes.com/health
- Rodale — rodale.com
- Stephanie Strom on NY Times — topics.nytimes.com/top/ reference/timestopics/people/s/stephanie_strom/index.html
- Take Part — takepart.com

Health Blogs

- 100 Days of Real Food — 100daysofrealfood.com
- 101 Cookbooks — 101cookbooks.com
- Dr. Josh Axe — draxe.com
- Bruce Bradley — brucebradley.com
- Cherie Calbom — The Juice Lady — juiceladycherie.com
- Drew Canole — fitlife.tv
- Kris Carr — kriscarr.com
- Deliciously Organic — deliciouslyorganic.net
- Eating Rules — eatingrules.com
- Elana's Pantry — elanaspantry.com
- Food Renegade — foodrenegade.com
- Green Kitchen Stories — greenkitchenstories.com
- Green Lemonade — greenlemonade.com
- Dr. Mark Hyman — drhyman.com
- Inspired Bites, Robyn O'Brien on *Prevention* — blogs.prevention .com/inspired-bites
- Joyous Health — joyoushealth.com
- Dr. Frank Lipman — drfranklipman.com
- The Lunch Tray — thelunchtray.com
- Mama Natural — mamanatural.com
- Mamavation — mamavation.com

- Dr. Joseph Mercola — drmercola.com
- Mind Body Green — mindbodygreen.com
- *Mother Jones*, Tom Philpott — motherjones.com/tom-philpott
- My New Roots — mynewroots.com
- Naturally Savvy — naturallysavvy.com
- *New York Times*, Mark Bittman — bittman.blogs.nytimes.com
- Oh She Glows — ohsheglows.com
- Paleo Hacks — paleohacks.com
- Kimberly Snyder — kimberlysnyder.net
- Sprouted Kitchen — sproutedkitchen.com
- Underground Wellness — undergroundwellness.com
- Andrew Weil, MD — drweil.com
- Well + Good NYC — wellandgoodnyc.com
- Wellness Mama — wellnessmama.com
- The Whole Journey — thewholejourney.com
- Jason Wrobel — jasonwrobel.com/blog

CORPORATE BUCKS TRY TO DEFEAT MANDATORY GMO LABELING

HERE'S A RUNDOWN OF exactly how much certain corporations have spent during the past twelve months to make sure that our foods do not carry GMO labels. These numbers reflect data up to November 19, 2014.

Company	Washington Prop I-522	California Prop 37	Colorado Prop 105	Oregon Prop I-92	Total Contributions
ABBOTT NUTRITION	$185,025	$334,500	$190,000	$160,000	$869,525
B&G FOODS, INC.		$40,000			$40,000
BASF PLANT SCIENCE	$500,000	$2,040,000			$2,540,000
BAYER CROPSCIENCE	$591,654	$2,000,000			$2,591,654
BIMBO BAKERIES USA	$137,460	$422,900	$270,000	$230,000	$1,060,360
BIOTECHNOLOGY INDUSTRY ORGANIZATION		$502,000	$26,323	$10,750	$539,073
BRUCE FOODS CORPORATION	$4,364	$38,500			$42,864
BUMBLE BEE FOODS	$52,365	$420,600	$50,000	$45,000	$567,965
BUNGE NORTH AMERICA	$137,896	$248,600			$386,496
BUSH BROTHERS & COMPANY	$23,565				$23,565
C. H. GUENTHER & SON, INC.		$24,700			$24,700
CAMPBELL SOUP COMPANY	$384,888	$598,000			$982,888
CARGILL	$143,133	$249,963	$135,000	$111,000	$639,096
CLEMENT PAPPAS & COMPANY	$30,547	$100,100			$130,647
CLOROX	$17,455	$39,700			$57,155
COCA-COLA	$1,520,351	$1,690,500	$1,385,000	$1,170,000	$5,765,851
COLORADO BIOSCIENCE ASSOCIATION			$688		$688
COLORADO CORN GROWERS ASSOCIATION			$5,060		$5,060

COLORADO FARM BUREAU			$13,456		$13,456
COLORADO LEGISLATIVE SERVICES			$3,375		$3,375
COLORADO SUGARBEET GROWERS ASSOCIATION			$500		$500
CONAGRA FOODS	$828,251	$1,176,700	$250,000	$350,000	$2,604,951
COUNCIL FOR BIOTECHNOLOGY INFORMATION		$375,000		$12,827	$387,827
CROPLIFE AMERICA		$9,500			$9,500
DEAN FOODS CO.	$174,553	$253,950			$428,503
DEL MONTE FOODS COMPANY	$125,677	$674,100			$799,777
DESCHUTES COUNTY FARM BUREAU				$500	$500
DOLE PACKAGED FOODS COMPANY		$175,000			$175,000
DOW AGROSCIENCES	$591,654	$2,000,000	$306,500	$1,157,150	$4,055,304
DUPONT PIONEER	$3,880,159		$3,000,000	$4,518,150	$11,398,309
E. I. DUPONT DE NEMOURS & CO.		$5,400,000			$5,400,000
FARIBAULT FOODS, INC.		$76,000			$76,000
FARMERS ALLIANCE FOR INTEGRATED RESOURCES			$1,537		$1,537
FLOWERS FOODS, INC.	$205,099	$182,100	$250,000		$637,199
GENERAL MILLS, INC.	$869,271	$1,230,300	$820,000	$695,000	$3,614,571
GODIVA CHOCOLATIER, INC.		$42,700			$42,700
GOYA		$56,700			$56,700
GROCERY MANUFACTURERS ASSOCIATION		$2,002,000	$101,400	$155,000	$2,258,400
H. J. HEINZ COMPANY		$500,000			$500,000
HERO NORTH AMERICA		$80,800			$80,800
HERSHEY COMPANY	$360,450	$518,900		$320,000	$1,199,350
HIGHWAY SPECIALITIES, LLC				$750	$750
HILLSHIRE BRANDS COMPANY	$282,775	$85,900			$368,675
HIRZEL CANNING COMPANY		$100,900			$100,900
HORMEL FOODS CORPORATION	$76,803	$467,900	$85,000	$85,000	$714,703
HOUSE-AUTRY MILLS, INC.		$1,500			$1,500
IDAHOAN FOODS, LLC		$10,000			$10,000
INVENTURE FOODS, INC.		$15,600			$15,600
KELLOGG COMPANY	$322,050	$790,700	$250,000	$500,000	$1,862,750
KNOUSE FOODS COOPERATIVE, INC.	$20,946	$167,600	$25,000	$20,000	$233,546
KRAFT		$2,000,500	$1,030,000	$870,000	$3,900,500
LAND O'LAKES, INC.	$144,878	$153,300	$900,000	$760,000	$1,958,178
MARS INCORPORATED		$498,350			$498,350
MCCAIN FOODS USA, INC.		$53,400			$53,400
MCCORMICK & COMPANY	$148,369	$248,200		$130,000	$526,569
MEAD JOHNSON NUTRICIAN COMPANY		$80,000	$50,000	$50,000	$180,000

MICHAEL FOODS				$30,000	$30,000
MONDELÉZ INTERNATIONAL	$210,336	$181,000		$720,000	$1,111,336
MONSANTO	$5,374,411	$8,112,867	$4,755,578	$5,958,750	$24,201,606
MOODY DUNBAR, INC	$2,619	$5,000			$7,619
MORTON SALT		$21,400			$21,400
NESTLÉ USA, INC. AND AFFILIATED ENTITIES	$1,528,206	$1,461,600			$2,989,806
NIAGARA BOTTLING			$10,000		$10,000
NORTHWEST FOOD PROCESSORS ASSOCIATION				$709	$709
NUTRITION EDGE COMMUNICATIONS			$8,800		$8,800
OCEAN SPRAY CRANBERRIES	$80,295	$409,100	$80,000	$35,000	$604,395
OREGON FARM BUREAU				$300	$300
PEPSICO	$2,352,966	$2,485,400	$1,650,000	$2,350,000	$8,838,366
PINNACLE FOODS GROUP, LLC	$175,425	$266,100			$441,525
PIONEER HI-BRED RESEARCH CENTER			$38,500		$38,500
POST FOODS, LLC		$5,150			$5,150
REILY FOODS COMPANY		$18,400			$18,400
RICH PRODUCTS CORPORATION	$34,911	$248,300		$30,000	$313,211
RICHELIEU FOODS, INC.		$5,200			$5,200
ROCKY MOUNTAIN FOOD INDUSTRY ASSOCIATION			$1,830		$1,830
SARA LEE CORPORATION		$343,600			$343,600
SARGENTO FOODS, INC.		$10,000			$10,000
SHEARERS FOODS, INC.	$36,656		$35,000	$30,000	$101,656
SMITHFIELD FOODS, INC.		$683,900	$200,000		$883,900
SNACK FOOD ASSOCIATION		$10,000			$10,000
SNYDER'S-LANCE, INC.				$5,000	$5,000
SOLAE, LLC		$62,500			$62,500
STARLITE MEDIA, LLC		$41,785			$41,785
SUNNY DELIGHT BEVERAGES COMPANY	$30,547	$139,700	$25,000	$25,000	$220,247
SYNGENTA CORPORATION		$2,000,000			$2,000,000
THE HERSHEY COMPANY			$380,000		$380,000
THE J. M. SMUCKER CO.	$349,978	$555,000	$345,000	$295,000	$1,544,978
TREE TOP, INC.		$110,600			$110,600
UNILEVER		$467,100			$467,100
WELCH FOODS, INC.	$41,893	$167,000	$35,000	$30,000	$273,893
WM. WRIGLEY JR. COMPANY		$123,350			$123,350
GRAND TOTAL CONTRIBUTIONS	**$21,977,881**	**$46,111,715**	**$16,713,547**	**$20,860,886**	**$105,664,029**

BIBLIOGRAPHY

Part One: Those Tricky Sons of...

Introduction

Center for Science in the Public Interest. Food Dyes, A Rainbow of Risks. Online: cpinenet.org/new/pdf/food-dyes/rainbow-of-risks.pdf. 2010.

Winter, Ruth. *A Consumer's Dictionary of Food Additives.* New York: Three Rivers Press, 2009.

Chapter 1: We've Been Duped

American Heart Association. 2011–2012 Annual Report: 17–18.

Kindy, Kimberly. Food Additives on the Rise as FDA Scrutiny Wanes. *Washington Post,* www.washingtonpost.com/national/food-additives-on-the-rise-as-fda-scrutiny-wanes/2014/08/17/828e9bf8-1cb2-11e4-ab7b-696c295ddfd1_story.html?wpisrc=nl_hdtop, August 17, 2014.

Neltner, T., et al. Conflicts of interest in approvals of additives to food determined to be generally recognized as safe: out of balance. *Journal of the American Medical Association—Internal Medicine* 173 (2013): 2032–2036.

Nueman, W. FDA and Dairy Industry Spar Over Testing of Milk. *New York Times,* www.nytimes.com/2011/01/26/business/26milk.html?_r=0, January 25, 2011.

Tobacman, J. K. Review of harmful gastrointestinal effects of carrageenan in animal experiments. *Environmental Health Perspectives* 109 (2001): 983–994.

Ye, J., et al. Assessment of the determination of azodicarbonamide and its decomposition product semicarbazide: investigation of variation in flour and flour products. *Journal of Agricultural Food Chemistry* 59 (2011): 9313–9318.

Chapter 2: We Are the Chemicals We Eat—The Sickening 15

American Cancer Society. Known and Probable Human Carcinogens. Online: www.cancer.org/cancer/cancercauses/othercarcinogens/generalinformationaboutcarcinogens/known-and-probable-human-carcinogens, updated October 17, 2013.

American Chemical Society. Soda warning? high-fructose corn syrup linked to diabetes, new study suggests. *ScienceDaily*, August 23, 2007.

American Nutrition Association. Free glutamic acid (MSG): sources and dangers. *Nutrition Digest* 37.1 (2001).

Bellinger, D. A strategy for comparing the contributions of environmental chemicals and other risk factors to neurodevelopment of children. *Environmental Health Perspectives* 120 (2012): 501–507.

Benbrook, C. M., et al. Organic production enhances milk nutritional quality by shifting fatty acid composition: a United States-wide, 18-month study. *PLOS ONE* 8 (2013): e82429.

Blaser, M. *Missing Microbes: How the Overuse of Antibiotics Is Fueling Our Modern Plagues.* New York: Henry Holt, 2001.

Bray, G. A. Fructose: should we worry? *International Journal of Obesity* 32, Supplement 7 (2008): S127–S131.

Carwile, J. L., et al. Canned soup consumption and urinary bisphenol A: a randomized crossover trial. *JAMA*, online November 22, 2011.

Centers for Disease Control and Prevention. Antibiotic Resistance Threats in the United States. Online: www.cdc.gov/drugresistance/threat-report-2013/pdf/ar-threats-2013-508.pdf#page=14, 2013.

Centers for Disease Control and Prevention. Trans Fat: The Facts. www.cdc.gov/nutrition/everyone/basics/fat/transfat.html, 2014.

Environmental Working Group. EWG's Dirty Dozen Guide to Food Additives: Generally Recognized as Safe — But Is It? www.ewg.org/research/ewg-s-dirty-dozen-guide-food-additives/generally-recognized-as-safe-but-is-it, November 12, 2014.

Glover, M., and Reed M. Propylene glycol: the safe diluent that continues to cause harm. *Pharmacotherapy* 16 (1996): 690–693.

Grandjean, P., and Landrigan, P. J. Neurobehavioural effects of developmental toxicity. *Lancet Neurology* 13 (2014): 330–338.

Gutierrez, D. Farm-raised tilapia fish may increase inflammation. *Natural News*, December 11, 2008.

Hamblin, J. The toxins that threaten our brains. *Atlantic*, March 18, 2014.

Handa, Y., et al. Estrogen concentrations in beef and human hormone-dependent cancers. *Annals of Oncology* 20 (2009): 1610–1611.

He, K., et al. Association of monosodium glutamate intake with overweight in Chinese adults: the INTERMAP Study. *Obesity* 16 (2008): 1875–1880.

Ley, R. E., et al. Microbial ecology: human gut microbes associated with obesity. *Nature* 444 (2006): 1022–1023.

Onishchenko, G. G., et al. [About the human health safety estimation of ractopamine intake together with the food] *Vestnik Rossiĭskoĭ Akademii Meditsinskikh Nauk* 6 (2013): 4–8.

Park, A. NYC's Trans Fat Ban Worked: Fast-Food Diners Are Eating Healthier. Online: www.healthland.time.com/2012/07/17/nycs-trans-fat-ban-worked-fast-food-diners-are-eating-healthier, July 17, 2012.

Stanfield, M. *Trans Fat: The Time Bomb in Your Food, the Killer in Your Kitchen.* London: Souvenir Press, 2008.

Tate, P. L., et al. Milk stimulates growth of prostate cancer cells in culture. *Nutrition and Cancer* 63 (2011): 1361–1366.

Trasande, L., et al. Infant antibiotic exposures and early-life body mass. *International Journal of Obesity* 37 (2013): 16–23.

Chapter 3: Cut Out the Chemical Calories

Baillie-Hamilton, P. F. Chemical toxins: a hypothesis to explain the global obesity epidemic. *Journal of Alternative and Complementary Medicine* 8 (2002): 185–192.

Estruch, R., et al. Primary prevention of cardiovascular disease with a Mediterranean diet. *New England Journal of Medicine* 368 (2013): 1279–1290.

Holtcamp, W. Gut check: do interactions between environmental chemicals and intestinal microbiota affect obesity and diabetes? *Environmental Health Perspectives* (March 2012): 120–123.

Katz, D. L., and Meller, S. Can we say what diet is best for health? *Annual Review of Public Health* 35 (2014): 83–103.

Lustig, R. H. Fructose: metabolic, hedonic, and societal parallels with ethanol. *Journal of the American Dietetic Association* 110 (2010): 1307–1321.

Penza, M., et al. Genistein affects adipose tissue deposition in a dose-dependent and gender-specific manner. *Endocrinology* 147 (2006): 5740–5751.

Stahlhut, R. W., et al. Concentrations of urinary phthalate metabolites are associated with increased waist circumference. *Environmental Health Perspectives* 115 (2007): 876–882.

Tang-Péronard, J. L., et al. Endocrine-disrupting chemicals and obesity development in humans: a review. *Obesity Reviews* 12 (2011): 622–636.

Part Two: 21 Days of Good Food and Good Habits

Day 1 — Cleanse Daily with My Morning Lemon Water Ritual

Alleger, I. Getting in tune with nature. *Townsend Letter for Doctors and Patients,* April 1, 2004.

Bacaj, A. Amazing uses for apple cider vinegar. *Gerson Healing Newsletter,* September 1, 2013.

Nick, G. L. Medicinal properties in whole foods: the Capsicum fruit. *Townsend Letter for Doctors and Patients,* June 1, 2002.

Ostman, E., et al. Vinegar supplementation lowers glucose and insulin responses and increases satiety after a bread meal in healthy subjects. *European Journal of Clinical Nutrition* 59 (2005): 983–988.

Schnepers, A. Pucker up for lemons and limes: tart, refreshing and healthful. *Environmental Nutrition,* August 1, 2005.

Whang, S. *Reverse Aging.* Miami: JSP Publishing, 1998.

Day 2—Be a Lean, Green Drinking Machine

Hamilton, A. *Squeezed: What You Don't Know about Orange Juice*. New Haven: Yale University Press, 2010.

Klotter, J. Nutrients and organic produce. *Townsend Letter for Doctors and Patients*, January 1, 2012.

Meyerowitz, S. Don't mow it—eat it! *Better Nutrition*, December 1, 1998.

Robinson, J. Breeding the Nutrition Out of Our Food, *New York Times*, www.nytimes.com/2013/05/26/opinion/sunday/breeding-the-nutrition-out-of-our-food.html?pagewanted=all&_r=0, May 25, 2013.

Shaughnessy, D. T., et al. Inhibition of fried meat–induced colorectal DNA damage and altered systemic genotoxicity in humans by crucifera, chlorophyllin, and yogurt. *PLOS ONE* 6 (2011): e18707.

Stenblom, E. L., et al. Supplementation by thylakoids to a high carbohydrate meal decreases feelings of hunger, elevates CCK levels and prevents postprandial hypoglycaemia in overweight women. *Appetite* 68 (2013): 118–123.

Day 3—Stop Drinking with Your Meals

Dennis, E. A., et al. Water consumption increases weight loss during a hypocaloric diet intervention in middle-aged and older adults. *Obesity* 18 (2010): 300–307.

Orci, T. Are tea bags turning us into plastic? *Atlantic*, www.theatlantic.com, April 8, 2013.

Day 4—Be Aware of What's in Your Water

Balan, H. Fluoride—the danger that we must avoid. *Romanian Journal of Internal Medicine* 50 (2012): 61–69.

Environmental Working Group. Fighting for Safer Tap Water. www.ewr.org, December 2010.

Fenichel, P., et al. Bisphenol A: an endocrine and metabolic disruptor. *Annales d'Endocrinologie* 74 (2013): 211–220.

Jha, S. K., et al. Fluoride in groundwater: toxicological exposure and remedies. *Journal of Toxicology and Environmental Health* 16 (2013): 52–66.

Day 5—Ease Back on Dairy Foods

Cancer Weekly. Study findings from University of Osnabrueck provide new insights into prostate cancer, December 18, 2012.

Cornucopia Institute. A Shopping Guide to Avoiding Organic Foods with Carrageenan. www.cornucopia.org, May 2012.

Food & Beverage Close-Up. Study finds organic milk from pasture-fed cows to be higher in beneficial nutrients. June 9, 2008.

Key, T. J. Diet, insulin-like growth factor-1 and cancer risk. *Proceedings of the Nutrition Society* 3 (2011): 1–4.

Macdonald, L. E., et al. A systematic review and meta-analysis of the effects of pasteurization on milk vitamins, and evidence for raw milk consumption and other health-related outcomes. *Journal of Food Protection* 74 (2011): 1814–1832.

Melnik, B. C. et al. The impact of cow's milk–mediated mTORC1-signaling in the initiation and progression of prostate cancer. *Nutrition & Metabolism* 9 (2012): 74.

Outwater, J. L., et al. Dairy products and breast cancer: the IGF-1, estrogen, and bGH hypothesis. *Medical Hypotheses* 48 (1997): 453–61.

Qin, L. Q., et al. Estrogen: one of the risk factors in milk for prostate cancer. *Medical Hypotheses* 62 (2004): 133–142.

Day 6—No More Big Gulps!

American Academy of Environmental Medicine. Genetically Modified Foods Position Paper. Online: www.aaemonline.org/gmopost.html, 2008.

Bernstein, A. M., et al. Soda consumption and the risk of stroke in men and women. *American Journal of Clinical Nutrition* 95 (2012): 1190–1199.

Center for Science in the Public Interest. It's Sweet . . . But Is It Safe? www.cspinet .org, December 31, 2013.

Consumer Reports. Is there a health risk in your soft drink? Stronger regulations for caramel coloring in food and beverages are needed, www.consumerre ports.org, January 2014.

Food and Drug Administration. Serious Concerns over Alcoholic Beverages with Added Caffeine. FDA Consumer Updates. Online: www.fda.gov/ForConsum ers/ConsumerUpdates/ucm233987.html, November 17, 2010.

Fowler, S. P., et al. Fueling the obesity epidemic? Artificially sweetened beverage use and long-term weight gain. *Obesity* 16 (2008): 1894–1900.

Gardner, H., et al. 2012. Diet soft drink consumption is associated with an increased risk of vascular events in the Northern Manhattan Study. *Journal of General Internal Medicine* 27 (2012): 1120–1126.

Halade, G. V., and Fernandes, G. Study on the relationship between oral exposure to aspartame and fasting glucose and insulin levels in 40 diabetes-prone mice. Presented at the American Diabetes Association's Scientific Sessions, June 25, 2011.

Horowitz, B. Bromism from excessive cola consumption. *Journal of Toxicology—Clinical Toxicology* 35 (1997): 315–320.

Israel, B. Brominated battle: soda chemical has cloudy health history. *Scientific American*, December 11, 2011.

Jih, D., et al. Bromoderma after excessive ingestion of Ruby Red Squirt. *New England Journal of Medicine* 348 (2003): 1932–1934.

National Toxicology Program. Toxicology and carcinogenesis studies of 4-methylimidazole (Cas No. 822-36-6) in F344/N rats and B6C3F1 mice (feed studies). *National Toxicology Program Technical Report Series* 535 (January 2007): 1–274.

Nettletone, J. A., et al. Diet soda intake and risk of incident metabolic syndrome and type 2 diabetes in the Multi-Ethnic Study of Atherosclerosis (MESA). *Diabetes Care* 32 (2009): 688–694.

Swithers, S. E. Artificial sweeteners produce the counterintuitive effect of inducing metabolic derangements. *Trends in Endocrinology and Metabolism* 24 (2013): 431–441.

White, A. S., et al. Beverages obtained from soda fountain machines in the U.S. contain microorganisms, including coliform bacteria. *International Journal of Food Microbiology* 137 (2010): 61–66.

Day 7—Love Your Liver

Alcohol and Tobacco Tax and Trade Bureau, U.S. Treasury. Limited Ingredients, www.ttb.gov/ssd/limited_ingredients.shtml.

Anheuser-Busch website: www.tapintoyourbeer.com.

Donaldson, S. What's in Your Beer? Fish Bladder and Antifreeze Ingredient? Online: www. abcnews.go.com/Health/food-babe-petitions-beer-makers-disclose -additives/story?id=24085296, July 11, 2014.

Mak, Tim. Europeans Recall Fireball Whiskey Over a Sweetener Also Used in Antifreeze. *The Daily Beast,* www.thedailybeast.com/articles/2014/10/28/frat house-favorite-fireball-whiskey-recalled-in-europe.html, October 28, 2014.

Sunday Mirror. Reasons Why Drink Is Ruining Your Diet; Whether You're Trying to Lose Weight or Just Eat Healthily, Over-Indulging in Alcohol Can Undo All Your Good Work, August 3, 2003.

Day 8—Pass on Fast Food

Demeyer, D. The World Cancer Research Fund report 2007: a challenge for the meat processing industry. *Meat Science* 80 (2008): 953–959.

Feskens, E. J., et al. Meat consumption, diabetes, and its complications. *Current Diabetes Reports* 13 (2013): 298–306.

Frazier, D. A. The link between fast food and the obesity epidemic. *Health Matrix* 17 (2007): 291–317.

Kat-Chem, Ltd., Budapest. Azodicarbonamide. Online: www.kat-chem.hu/en/ prod-bulletins/azodikarbonamide, 2014.

Klotter, J. MSG & obesity. *Townsend Letter for Doctors and Patients,* November 1, 2004.

Yang, C., et al. Most plastic products release estrogenic chemicals: a potential health problem that can be solved. *Environmental Health Perspectives* 119 (2011): 989–996.

Day 9—Detox from Added Sugar

Ahmed, S. H., et al. Food addiction. *Neuroscience in the 21st Century,* 2013, 2833–2857.

Hansen, N. Eating lots of carbs, sugar may raise risk of cognitive impairment, Mayo Clinic study finds. *Mayo Clinic News Network,* www.newsnetwork .mayoclinic.org, October 16, 2012.

Hyman, M. *The Blood Sugar Solution 10-Day Detox Diet: Activate Your Body's Nat-ural Ability to Burn Fat and Lose Weight Fast.* New York: Little, Brown, 2014.

Public Health and Medical Fraud Research Cooperative. Truvia—New Low Cal-orie Sweetener (Toxin), www.qualityassurance.synthasite.com, 2008.

Vegetarian Journal. Decoding sugar packaging: which sugars aren't processed with bone char?, April 1, 2013.

Day 10 — Eat Meat Responsibly

The Animal Welfare Institute, www.awionline.org.

Brownstone, S. Can Silicon Valley Make Fake Meat and Eggs That Don't Suck? *Mother Jones*, www.motherjones.com, December 2, 2013.

Campbell, T. C., et al. Diet, lifestyle, and the etiology of coronary artery disease: the Cornell China study. *American Journal of Cardiology* 82 (1998): 18T–21T.

Consumer Reports News. How about some heavy metals with that protein drink? www.consumerreports.org, June 2, 2012.

Day 11 — Eat Raw More Than Half the Time

Fontana, L. Low bone mass in subjects on a long-term raw vegetarian diet. *Archives of Internal Medicine* 165 (2005): 684–689.

Franceschi, S., et al. Role of different types of vegetables and fruit in the prevention of cancer of the colon, rectum, and breast. *Epidemiology* 9 (1998): 338–341.

Jung, S. K., et al. The effect of raw vegetable and fruit intake on thyroid cancer risk among women: a case-control study in South Korea. *British Journal of Nutrition* 109 (2013): 118–128.

Koebnick, C., et al. Long-term consumption of a raw food diet is associated with favorable serum LDL cholesterol and triglycerides but also with elevated plasma homocysteine and low serum HDL cholesterol in humans. *Journal of Nutrition* 135 (2005): 2372–2378.

Mommers, M., et al. Consumption of vegetables and fruits and risk of ovarian carcinoma. *Cancer* 104 (2005): 1512–1519.

Spiller, G. A., et al. Effect of a diet high in monounsaturated fat from almonds on plasma cholesterol and lipoproteins. *Journal of the American College of Nutrition* 11 (1992): 126–130.

Tang, L., et al. Consumption of raw cruciferous vegetables is inversely associated with bladder cancer risk. *Cancer Epidemiology Biomarkers & Prevention* 17 (2008): 938–944.

Day 12 — Break Some Bread — and Other Carbs

Dixit, A. A., et al. Incorporation of whole, ancient grains into a modern Asian Indian diet to reduce the burden of chronic disease. *Nutrition Reviews* 69 (2011): 479–488.

Organics.org. Bleached vs Unbleached Flour. Online: www.organics.org/bleached-vs-unbleached-flour/, December 26, 2013.

Van de Vijver, L. P., et al. Whole grain consumption, dietary fibre intake and body mass index in the Netherlands cohort study. *European Journal of Clinical Nutrition* 63 (2009): 31–38.

Day 13 — Balance Your Healthy Fats

Apte, S. A., et al. A low dietary ratio of omega-6 to omega-3 fatty acids may delay progression of prostate cancer. *Nutrition and Cancer* 65 (2013): 556–562.

Dona, A., and Arvanitoyannis, I. S. Health risks of genetically modified foods. *Critical Reviews in Food Science and Nutrition* 49 (2009): 164–175.

Kang, J. X., and Liu, A. The role of the tissue omega-6/omega-3 fatty acid ratio in regulating tumor angiogenesis. *Cancer Metastasis Review* 32 (2013): 201–210.

Mozaffarian, D., et al. Trans fatty acids and cardiovascular disease. *The New England Journal of Medicine* 354 (2006): 1601–1613.

Skerrett, P. J. FDA gets with the evidence, proposes that trans fats are not "safe." *Harvard Health Publications*, www.health.harvard.edu/blog/fda-gets-with-the -evidence-proposes-that-trans-fats-are-not-safe-201311086854, November 8, 2013.

Day 14—Supplement with These 10 Superhero Foods

Gonzales, G. F., et al. Lepidium meyenii (Maca): a plant from the highlands of Peru—from tradition to science. *Forschende Komplementärmedizin* 16 (2009): 373–380.

Puga, G. M., et al. Increased plasma availability of L-arginine in the postprandial period decreases the postprandial lipemia in older adults. *Nutrition* 29 (2013): 81–88.

Ranilla, L. G., et al. Evaluation of indigenous grains from the Peruvian Andean region for antidiabetes and antihypertension potential using in vitro methods. *Journal of Medicinal Food* 12 (2009): 704–713.

Day 15—Know Thy GMOs!

American Academy of Environmental Medicine. Genetically Modified Foods. www.aaemonline.org/gmopost.html, 2009.

Aris, A., and Leblanc, S. Maternal and fetal exposure to pesticides associated to genetically modified foods in Eastern Townships of Quebec, Canada. *Reproductive Toxicology* 31 (2011): 528–533.

Bøhn, T., et al. Compositional differences in soybeans on the market: glyphosate accumulates in Roundup Ready GM soybeans. *Food Chemistry* 153 (2014): 207–215.

Campbell, A. W. Glyphosate: its effects on humans. *Alternative Therapies in Health and Medicine* 20 (2014): 9–11.

Consumer Reports Food Safety and Sustainability Center, GMO report, www .greenerchoices.org/pdf/CR_FSASC_GMO_Final_Report_10062014.pdf, October 2014.

de Vendômois, J., et al. A comparison of the effects of three GM corn varieties on mammalian health. *International Journal of Biological Sciences* 5 (2009): 706–726.

Joensen, L., and Ho, M. Argentina's GM woes. (Thinking ecologically.) *Synthesis/ Regeneration*, December 22, 2003.

Mesnage, R., et al. Cytotoxicity on human cells of Cry1Ab and Cry1Ac Bt insecticidal toxins alone or with a glyphosate-based herbicide. *Journal of Applied Toxicology* 33 (2013): 695–699.

Thongprakaisang, S., et al. Glyphosate induces human breast cancer cells growth via estrogen receptors. *Food and Chemical Toxicology* 59 (2013): 129–136.

Day 16—Dine Out the Food Babe Way

Fujioka, K., et al. The effects of grapefruit on weight and insulin resistance: relationship to the metabolic syndrome. *Journal of Medicinal Food* 9 (2006): 49–54.

McMillan, T. *The American Way of Eating: Undercover at Walmart, Applebee's, Farm Fields and the Dinner Table*. New York: Scribner, 2012.

Day 18 — Change Your Little Grocery Shop of Horrors

Blatt, B. "Unacceptable Ingredients." How Many of the Groceries Sold at Walmart Would Be Banned by Whole Foods? www.slate.com, February 18, 2014.

Environmental Working Group. "Clean 15" and "Dirty Dozen," www.ewg.org.

Day 19 — Cook Outside the Box

Group, E. F. *Health Begins in the Colon*. Houston: Global Healing Center, 2007.

Moritz, A. *Cancer Is Not a Disease — It's a Survival Mechanism*. Brevard, NC: Ener-Chi Wellness Press, 2008.

Schardt, D. Microwave myths. *Nutrition Action Healthletter*, www.cspinet.com, April 2005.

Vallejo, F., et al. Phenolic compound contents in edible parts of broccoli inflorescences after domestic cooking. *Journal of the Science of Food and Agriculture* 83 (2003): 1511–1516.

Day 20 — Fast Every Day

Cahill, L. E., et al. Prospective study of breakfast eating and incident coronary heart disease in a cohort of male U.S. health professionals. *Circulation* 128 (2013): 337–343.

Cousens, G. *Conscious Eating*. Berkeley, CA: North Atlantic Books, 2000.

Heilbronn, L. K., et al. Alternate-day fasting in nonobese subjects: effects on body weight, body composition, and energy metabolism. *American Journal of Clinical Nutrition* 81 (2005): 69–73.

Horne, B. D., et al. Randomized cross-over trial of short-term water-only fasting: metabolic and cardiovascular consequences. *Nutrition, Metabolism, and Cardiovascular Diseases* 23 (2013): 1050–1057.

Junger, A. *Clean: The Revolutionary Program to Restore the Body's Natural Ability to Heal Itself*. New York: HarperCollins, 2012.

Klotter, J. Intermittent Fasting for Weight Loss. *Townsend Letter*, February 1, 2014.

Mattson, M. P., and Wan, R. Beneficial effects of intermittent fasting and caloric restriction on the cardiovascular and cerebrovascular systems. *Journal of Nutritional Biochemistry* 16 (2005): 129–137.

Pan, J. W., et al. Human brain beta-hydroxybutyrate and lactate increase in fasting-induced ketosis. *Journal of Cerebral Blood Flow and Metabolism* 20 (2000): 1502–1507.

Day 21 — Travel Organically

Szentmihályi, K., et al. [Mineral content of some herbs and plant extracts with anti-inflammatory effect used in gastrointestinal diseases]. *Orvosi Hetilap* 154 (2013): 538–543.

ACKNOWLEDGMENTS

WITHOUT MY HUSBAND, FINLEY, there would be no Food Babe. No amount of words can express how much I love you for always believing in me. Thank you for changing the world with me.

This book is written in memory of my mother-in-law, Diane, who taught me grace, compassion, and how to look at the bright side of any situation. Thinking about you gives me courage every single day.

I am forever grateful for my mom and dad, who have protected me tirelessly, from the moment I was born. I'll never forget the lessons I've learned from you both, especially understanding how to stand up for myself and how to be unconventional without worrying about what other people think.

Thank you to my brother, Yog, and sister-in-law, Judy, and my two nephews, Ian and Dylan, for cheering me on, putting up with my food police mentality, and always keeping me in check. I owe so much gratitude to my grandparents, who continue to encourage me to hold on to my roots.

Thank you to my father-in-law, Finley, for his humorous one-liners and career advice, and to Laura, Summers, Taylor, Henry, and all of my wonderful aunties, uncles, and cousins. Reeva, thank you for being the little sister I never had and for making yourself available for the intense web chats and phone calls out of the blue.

Thank you to Sushila Melvani and the Sri Aurobindo Society in Pondicherry, India, for looking after me, praying for me, and sending blessings throughout my life. If it hadn't been for my closest girlfriends begging me to start a blog and get on social media, this train wouldn't ever have left the station.

I love you, Nicole, Anamore, Vicky, Marianne, Ruba, Liz, Gimar, Amy, Lee, and Heather. Thank you to my friends in the corporate world — Ed, Rachel, Wes, Larry, Diane, and Rob — who inspired me to investigate, follow my heart, and preach.

To my two brilliant agents, Steve Troha and Scott Hoffman: Thank you for showing me the way for my first (and second!) book. Thank you to Tracy Behar, my editor, for believing in this book and me from the very first sight. I feel so at home with the whole Little, Brown team because of your unwavering support and guidance. Thank you to Michelle Aielli and Cathy Gruhn, for helping me through the media mayhem. To the talented and amazing Maggie Greenwood-Robinson, thank you for your encouragement and thoughtful insights, which made this book come together so beautifully. Thank you to Ryan Holiday, for your support, strategy, and intellect. Thank you to Sean Busher, my dear friend and photographer, his team, and Scooter, who worked tirelessly to get the perfect shot for the cover. Thank you to Derek Halpern, my mentor and friend, who always turns my frown upside down and inspires me to work even harder. Thank you to Dr. Mark Hyman for standing up to Big Food, for fighting with me, and for writing a beautiful and inspiring foreword for this book.

Without my Food Babe team, this train would come to a screeching halt — thank you, Pam, Kim, Janet, Lexi, Krista, and Lindsey for your incredible, passionate work.

Thank you to Max Goldberg for your incredible advocacy and friendship and for encouraging me early in this journey to attend product shows and meet the company leaders behind them.

To my dear friend and mentor, Lisa Leake, thank you for showing me you can do what you love and change the world.

To all the amazing activists who inspire me daily — John Roulac, Pulin Modi, Mark Kastel, Robyn O'Brien, Ken Cook, Heather White, Alicia Gravitz, Kris Carr, Gary Hirshberg, Dr. Josh Axe, Dr. Michael

Jacobson, Dr. Joseph Mercola, Mike Adams, Pamm Larry, Jeffrey Smith, Zuri Allen, Will Allen, Congressman Tim Ryan, John and Ocean Robbins, Leah Segedie, Bettina Siegal, Kari Hamerschlag, Melanie Warner, Ronnie Cummings, Birke Baehr, Rachel Parent, Dave Murphy, Lisa Stokke, Cheri Johnson, and many more.

When I think back on what shaped me the most to take on this role as investigator and outspoken activist, I can't help thinking of my debate coach, Barbara Miller, and debate partners Matt Lietzke and Wendi Wright. I'm forever grateful for your tough love and teachings.

Last but not least, thank you to all my inspiring readers. You are why I'm here with this message; without you I would be nothing. Your collective commitment to a better food system is powerful—more powerful than you can imagine.

INDEX

acesulfame potassium (Ace-K), 48, 64, 124
acetaldehyde, 134
acetoacetamide, 124
acid-alkaline balance, 68, 80–81, 121
acid reflux, 268
activism, 3–6, 13–14, 19–21, 27–28, 33, 225
additives, food, x, xi, 5, 11, 38–57; alcoholic
    beverages with, 129–38; bread and carbs
    with, 181–84; fast food with, 49, 147–50;
    in meat, 36, 48, 149–50; safety review of,
    34–37
aflatoxin, 199
agave nectar, 162–63
Agent Orange, 220
Ahmed, Serge H., 155
air travel, 270–77
alcoholic beverages, 56, 128–42, 239
Allen, Zuri, 30
allergies, 9–10, 53, 69, 232
almond butter, 191, 199, 274
almond milk, 40, 114
almonds, raw, 177–78
aluminosilicates, 134
aluminum, 55, 108
American Academy of Environmental
    Medicine, 120–21
American Heart Association, 32
Anheuser-Busch, 130–31, 139
animal by-products, 50, 52, 130, 135, 156
antibiotics, 12, 24–25, 36, 41–42
"antinutrients," 68
appetite suppression, 87, 99–100, 232
Applebee's, 228–29
arsenic, 56, 70, 104, 108

artificial sweeteners, 48, 64, 123–25, 134, 157
ascorbic acid, 81, 121, 134
aspartame, 48, 123, 157
Ayurveda, 96–97
azodicarbonamide, xi, 52; bread with,
    25–26, 33, 182; fast food with, 149

Bacillus thuringiensis (Bt), 182, 194, 216–17
bacteria, 24–25, 109, 122, 201–2
Baillie-Hamilton, Paula F., 59
baking powder, 289
bean pastas, 187–88
beans, 47, 68, 243
bean sprouts, 211–12
beer, 129–34, 138–39
beet sugar, 157, 159
Bellinger, David, 55
benzene, 121
benzoic acid, 121, 136
beta-agonists, 40
beverages, 242; alcoholic, 56, 128–42, 239;
    recipes for, 291–96; *see also* juices; water
BHA/BHT (butylated hydroxyanisole/
    butylated hydroxytoluene), x, 36,
    48–49, 136
bioflavonoids, 210
bisphenol A (BPA), 45–47, 60, 106, 130
Bittman, Mark, 256
Blaser, Martin J., 41
Blatt, Ben, 247
blenders, 89, 274
blogging, 13–14, 20–21, 23, 28
Blumberg, Bruce, 59
bone char, 156

BPA (bisphenol A), 45–47, 60, 106, 130
brain health, 55, 267
bread, 181–90, 289; azodicarbonamide in, 25–26, 33, 149, 182; dough conditioners in, 52, 182; in local grocery stores, 275; recommendations for, 185–90, 243; refined flour in, 44–45, 181–83; whole grain, 183–84, 189–90, 243, 248
breakfast, 61, 267; eating plan for, 282–86; foods for, 242–43; recipes for, 297–304
breast cancer, 39–40, 43, 112, 178, 219
Breast Cancer Fund, 39–40
brewing chemicals, 129–34
bromated vegetable oil (BVO), 107, 125, 136–37
Bt (Bacillus thuringiensis), 182, 194, 216–17
Buck, Peter, 32–33
bulk foods, 257
Burger King, 8, 259
butter, 196–98, 232, 289
buying local, 167–68, 225, 253
BVO (bromated vegetable oil), 107, 125, 136–37

cacao, raw, 204
caffeine, 84, 120, 137
calcium, 111
calcium propionate, 182
calcium sodium EDTA, 129
calories, 23, 37, 41, 58–65; see also obesity; weight loss
cancer, 35–36, 43, 48–49, 174, 263; dairy and, 35, 111–12; fats and, 193; food dyes and, 4, 118–19; meat and, 39–40, 165, 167; raw foods and, 178; wheatgrass and, 88
canned foods, 45–47, 289
canola oil, 193
caramel coloring, 52, 119, 129, 131, 138
carbohydrates, 67, 181–90
carcinogens, 4, 35–36, 43, 48–49, 174, 263
carrageenan, 35, 52–53, 115, 130, 133
Carson, Rachel, ix
car travel, 270–77
cashew milk, 114, 295
cayenne pepper, 80–82
celery juice, 108
celiac disease, 70
cellulose, 149

Center for Science in the Public Interest (CSPI), 30, 124, 135, 149, 263
cereal, 242–43, 248, 289
"certified organic," 44; see also organic foods
chain restaurants, 227–38
Change.org, 30, 107, 338
cheese, 28–31, 113–14, 289
Cheesecake Factory, 227, 229
chemicals, x, xi, 19; carcinogenic, 4, 35–36, 43, 48–49, 174, 263; fattening, 59–63; freedom from, 12–14; Sickening 15, 38–56; in specific diets, 63–74; see also additives, food; ingredients
chewing gum, 50, 97–98
chia seeds, 205–6
chicken, 24–25
Chick-fil-A, 5, 10, 22–26, 49, 145, 338
Chili's, 229–30
Chinese food, 234–35
Chipotle, 5, 21–22, 338
chlorine, 106–8, 183
chlorophyll, 86–87
chlorpyrifos, 56, 84
chocolate, 158, 289
cholesterol, 177–78
chromium, 108
cilantro, 55
citric acid, 94
CLA (conjugated linoleic acid), 115, 197
Clinton, Bill, 27
Coca-Cola, 107, 119, 161
coconut palm sugar, 157, 159
coconut water, 108
coffee, 83–84, 90, 256–57
colorectal cancer, 87, 150, 178
community-supported agriculture (CSA), 168, 253
condiments, 166, 244–45
conjugated linoleic acid (CLA), 115, 196
Consumer Reports, 119, 173
coolers, 274–75
corn, 22, 132, 216–17, 220
corn syrup, 130, 132, 157; see also high-fructose corn syrup
Cornucopia Institute, 30, 53, 114, 203–4
corporations, x; activism against, 3–6, 13, 19–21, 27–28, 33, 225; FDA and, 34–37; GMO labeling and, 221, 346–48; nutrition information from, 153

Costco, 241
cottonseed oil, 194
crab, imitation, 236
cruciferous vegetables, 55, 208
CSA (community-supported agriculture),
    168, 253–54

dairy foods, 110–17; adulterated, 111–12;
    antibiotics in, 12, 36, 42; cutting back on,
    110, 167, 256; labels on, 168–71; options
    for, 112–15, 251, 289; see also milk
dandelion, 55, 179, 276
DATEM, 52, 182
DDT/DDE
    (dichlorodiphenyltrichloroethane/
    dichlorodiphenyldichloroethylene), 56
DeLuca, Fred, 32–33
deserts, food, 153
desserts, 244, 333–35
detoxification, 73, 79, 266; drinks for,
    80–84, 86–87; heavy metal, 55; post-
    travel, 273, 275–76; sugar, 155–64
dextrose, 130, 132, 161
diabetes, 121, 123, 150, 167, 189
diets, 58, 63–74; analysis of, 61–63; detox,
    73; Food Babe Way, 74–76; gluten-free,
    69–71, 186; low-calorie, 64–65; low-
    carb, 67, 181; low-fat, 65–67;
    Mediterranean, 73–74; paleo, 68–69;
    pescetarian, 72; raw foods, 69; vegan,
    71–72, 165
diet soda, 48, 123–25
digestion, 81, 97–99, 268
diglycerides, 52, 182
dimethylpolysiloxane, 32, 49, 122, 149
dining out, 227–40; in chain restaurants,
    228–31; drinking fluids while, 97, 99; at
    parties and gatherings, 238–40; tips for,
    231–38, 256, 261; travel and, 270–77
dinner, 62, 267; eating plan for, 282–86;
    recipes for, 312–26
dinner parties, 238–40
distilled liquor, 136–38, 141, 239
Doctor's Associates Inc., 32–33
dough conditioners, 52, 182
Dr. Oz Show, The, 29
dyes, 11, 51–52; alcoholic beverages with,
    130–31, 136–38; artificial, 3–5; baked
    goods with, 183; Chick-fil-A and, 24–25;

macaroni and cheese with, 28–31;
    seaweed with, 237; soda with, 118–19

Earth Fare, 246
eczema, 9–10, 12
eggs, 168–69, 171, 251
Emanuel, Rahm, 27
endocrine disruptors, 218–19
energy drinks, 120
Environmental Protection Agency, 103, 216
Environmental Working Group, 43, 103–4,
    250, 255–56
erythritol, 48, 123–24, 161
estrogen, 39, 42–43, 60, 130, 219
ethanol, 56
Ethiopian food, 237
ethnic foods, 234–38
ethyl acetate, 84
excitotoxin, 51

Facebook, 23, 28, 30, 225
farmers' markets and co-ops, 168, 225, 253
fast foods, 145–54; additives in, 49, 147–50;
    making your own, 152–54; recipes for,
    327–32
fasting, 73, 266–69, 276
fat burning, 128–29, 266
fats and oils, 191–200, 289; adulteration of,
    192–93; diet low in, 65–67; healthier,
    197–200, 251; preservatives in, 48–49; in
    restaurant food, 232; trans, 49–50, 192,
    195; unhealthy, 193–96, 252; in veggie
    burgers, 174
FDA (Food and Drug Administration), 4,
    34–37, 45, 130, 161, 189, 195–96
fermented foods, 201–4
fiber, 88
fish, 55, 72, 171–72, 233
flavors, artificial and natural, x, 11, 50–51;
    baked goods with, 183; beer with,
    129–30, 133; tea with, 101
flour, 44–45, 181–84, 289
fluids: benefits of, 79; timing meals with,
    91, 96–102; see also beverages; juices;
    water
fluoride, 56, 103–4, 108
Food Additives Amendment, 34
Food Babe Army, x, 13–14
foodbabe.com, 13, 20

Food Babe Eating Plan, 21-Day, xii, 14–16, 56–57, 74–76, 281–87; snacks in, 286–87; week 1 of, 79, 282–83; week 2 of, 143–44, 283–85; week 3 of, 215, 285–86
Food Babe Feats, 215
fountain drinks, 121–22
freezer items, 244, 256
French food, 237
Frito-Lay, 241
frozen yogurt, 20–21, 116
fructose, 47, 60, 162–63; see also high-fructose corn syrup
fruits and vegetables: blending and juicing, 85–93; dried, 243; freezing, 256; growing, 254; label numbers on, 224; nutritional value of, 86; pesticides in, 42–43; raw, 177–80, 276; shopping for, 251, 253, 256–57
fungicides, 42–43

Gandhi, Mahatma, 240
gardening, 254
generally recognized as safe (GRAS), 34–37, 125, 195
General Mills, 225
genetically modified organisms. See GMOs
genistein, 60
ghee, 198–99
ginger tea, 100, 273–74
glucose, 47
glutamic acid, 54, 147–48; see also MSG
gluten, 69–71, 73, 181, 186
glycemic index, 159, 181, 189, 236
glyphosate, 43, 218–19
GMOs (genetically modified organisms), 12, 216–26; alcoholic beverages with, 130, 132, 134, 136, 140; animal feed with, 24–25; baked goods with, 182; butter and, 196–97; Chipotle and, 22; high-risk, 251; juice with, 94; labeling, 26–28, 197, 220–21, 224, 346–48; microwave popcorn and, 46; other names for, 218–20; pesticides in, 43; soda with, 120–25; Trader Joe's and, 249; veggie burgers with, 175
goat cheese, 113
goji berries, 205
Goldberg, Max, 30
golden berries, 209–10

Gonzales, Gustavo F., 209
government "action," 26–27, 34–37
grains, 181, 242–43; ancient, 186, 188; gluten-free, 70; intact, 189–90; sprouted, 52, 185, 188, 212–13; whole, 183–84, 189–90, 243, 248
grapefruit, 231
GRAS (generally recognized as safe), 34–37, 125, 195
green drinks, 85–95, 108, 282
green powder, 273
greens, blending and juicing, 85, 88–93
Grocery Manufacturers Association (GMA), 220–21
grocery stores, 168–71, 246–58, 275
growth hormones, 35–36, 39–40, 223

habits: forming new, 74–75, 215; soda-drinking, 120, 126
Hamilton, Alissa, 94
hangover hunger, 128–29
health problems, food-related, 6, 8–9, 12, 19, 153, 167, 217–18
Heart-Check certification, 32
heart disease: artificial sweeteners and, 123; dairy and, 111; fats and, 49, 192–93, 195; intact grain and, 190; meat and, 150, 167; nighttime eating and, 268
heavy metals, 54–56, 135, 173
hempseeds, 207–8
herbicides, 43, 218–20
herbs, dried, 251
hexane, 173–74, 193
high-fructose corn syrup (HFCS), 157; alcoholic beverages with, 130, 132, 137; Chick-fil-A and, 25; soda with, 118; weight gain and, 60
Hirshberg, Gary, 218
Ho, Chi-Tang, 47
holiday gatherings, 238–40
Holtcamp, Wendee, 59
homeostasis, 209
honey, 157, 160, 289
hop extract, 133
hormones, synthetic, 12, 35–36, 39–40, 111–12, 223
hydrogenation, 49–50, 192, 195–96
Hyman, Mark, xii, 155
hyperactivity, 28–29

IGF-1 (insulin-like growth factor 1), 68, 112
Indian food, 8, 235
ingredients, 289–90; disclosure of, 5,
    20–23; high-risk, 222–23; reading list of,
    37, 41; staple, 242–45; synthetic, 94;
    see also additives, food; labeling
insulin, 47, 92, 121, 181
International Agency for Research on
    Cancer, 49, 119
Internet shopping, 252–53, 255
inulin, 94, 162
Italian food, 237–38

Jack in the Box, 149
Jackson, Jesse, 26–27
Japanese food, 235–37
Johnson, Cheri, 30
juicers, 92–93
juices, 291–96; concentrated, 94; fasting
    with, 276; green, 85–93, 291–92; store-
    bought, 93–95
junk food, 6–10

kale, 55, 86–87
Kavanagh, Sarah, 107
Kessler, David, 51
kimchi, 202
King, Martin Luther, Jr., ix
kitchen cleanout, 241–45
kombucha, 203
Kraft Foods, 3–5, 28–31, 338

labeling, 5, 37, 41; of beer, 130–31; of bread,
    45; and GMOs, 26–28, 197, 220–21, 224,
    346–48; of juices, 93–95; of meat, dairy,
    and eggs, 168–71; of trans fats, 50
labels. *See* labeling
Land O'Lakes, 197
L-cysteine, 52, 149
lead, 55–56, 109
Leake, Lisa, 28, 30
lectin, 68
lemon juice, 80–81
lemon water ritual, 80–84, 282
leptin, 47
Let's Move initiative, 33
LinkedIn, 337
liqueurs, 141
liquor, distilled, 136–38, 141, 239

Little Caesars, 147
liver, 81, 128
Local Harvest, 225
lunch, 61–62; eating plan for, 282–86;
    recipes for, 305–9
Lustig, Robert H., 60

maca, 208–9
macaroni and cheese, 28–31
malic acid, 134
Malta Goya, 119
manganese, 56, 135
maple syrup, 157, 160
margarine, 192
marketing, deceptive, 20–21, 31–33
Matthews, Chris, 27
McDonald's, 7, 49, 149–50, 259
McMillan, Tracie, 228
Mead, Margaret, ix
meals: cooking from scratch, 224; drinking
    fluids with, 91, 96–102; ingredients for,
    242–45; *see also* Food Babe Eating Plan,
    21-Day
meat, 165–76, 289; additives in, 36, 48,
    149–50; antibiotics in, 12, 42; buying
    local, 167–68; eating less, 166–67, 256;
    factory-farmed, 166–67, 275; fake, 173–75;
    grass- *vs.* grain-fed, 168; growth
    hormones in, 39–40; labeling, 168–71;
    organic, 251; restaurant, 233; shopping
    list for, 175–76
medical associations, partnering with, 32
Mediterranean diet, 73–74
Mellow Mushroom, 147
mercury, 55–56, 72
methamidophos, 150
methylene chloride, 84
4-methylimidazole (4-MEI), 119, 129
Mexican food, 235
microwaves, 46, 263, 275
milk: goat, 113–14; hormones in, 12, 40;
    nondairy, 40, 114–15, 295; organic, 40,
    115; pasteurized, 111; raw, 110, 112–13;
    see also dairy foods
MillerCoors, 130–31
millet, 186, 188–89
miso, 202–3
Modi, Pulin, 30
money, saving, 254–57

monoglycerides, 52, 182
Monsanto, 35–36, 43, 194, 216, 218–19, 223, 225
MSG (monosodium glutamate), 51, 53–54, 147–48; ethnic foods with, 234; nicknames for, 54; veggie burgers and, 175; weight gain and, 60

National Toxicology Program, 36, 49, 59
Neltner, Tom, 36
neurotoxins, 54–56, 174
night eating syndrome (NES), 268
nitrates, 36, 48, 109, 150
Non-GMO Project verification label, 223–24
noodles, 187–88
nut butters, 191, 199, 274
nuts, 114–15, 239, 243

oats, 188–89, 272–73, 289
Obama, Barack, 26
Obama, Michelle, 27, 33
obesity, x, 58–59; antibiotics and, 41–42; food deserts and, 153; GMOs and, 121; gut bacteria and, 202; intact grain and, 190; microwaves and, 263; MSG and, 53; sweeteners and, 47–48, 118, 123–25, 155, 157
obesogens, 59–63
oils. See fats and oils
Olive Garden, 230–31
omega-3 and -6 fatty acids, 174, 192–95, 205, 207
organic foods, 44; alcoholic, 139–41; breads, 187; GMOs in, 223; marketing, 20–21; meat, dairy, and egg, 40, 115, 168–69, 198; pesticides in, 43; protein-rich, 233; shopping for, 250–57

packaging, 45–46, 146–47
paleo diet, 68–69
"partially hydrogenated" oils, 196
pasta, 181, 187–88, 243, 289
pasteurization, 94–95, 111
Pauling, Linus, ix
PCBs (polychlorinated biphenyls), 56
peanut butter, 199
Pepsi, 107, 118–19, 161
perchlorate, 103, 109
pescetarian diet, 72; see also seafood

pesticides, 42–43, 219; in beverages, 83–84, 100–101, 135; in fast food, 150; in water, 109
petitions, 13; how to start, 337–38; noteworthy, 28–29, 33, 107, 130–31
petroleum, 50–51, 109
PFAAs (perfluoroalkyl acids), 146
PFOA (perfluorooctanoic acid), 46, 146
phosphoric acid, 121
phytonutrients, 86, 206
pink slime, 150
pizza, 147–48, 238
plastics, 45, 101, 106, 146–47, 263
PLU (price lookup) numbers, 224
politics, GMOs and, 26–28
Pollan, Michael, 150, 262–63
popcorn, microwave, 46
potato, Russet Burbank, 150
preservatives, x, 48–49; baked goods with, 182; GRAS, 36; restaurant food with, 227; soda with, 121
probiotics, 41–42
Procter & Gamble, 50
produce. See fruits and vegetables; grains; nuts; seeds
propylene glycol, 49, 130, 133, 137
propyl gallate, 49
prostate cancer, 40, 111, 151
protein powder, 172–73, 274
proteins, 175–76, 233
PVPP (polyvinylpolypyrrolidone), 135

quinoa, 186, 188–89, 210–11

ractopamine, 40
Rahim, Ahmed, 101
raw foods, 69, 177–80, 276
rBGH (recombinant bovine growth hormone), 35–36, 39, 223
rebaudioside, 161–62
recipes, 288–335; beverage, 291–96; breakfast, 297–304; dinner, 312–26; fast food and snack, 327–32; ingredients in, 289–90; lunch, 305–9; salad dressing, 310–11; sweet, 333–35
restaurants: chain, 228–31; ethnic, 234–38; see also dining out
rice, 70, 188–89, 236, 290
Roberts, Susan, 239

Roulac, John, 30, 220
Roundup, 43, 218–19
Ryan, Tim, xi

saccharin, 48, 157
salad and salad dressings, 232, 310–11
saliva, 97–99
salmon, farmed, 72, 171–72, 233, 236
sauerkraut, 202
SCOBY (symbiotic culture of bacteria and
    yeast), 203
seafood, 55, 72, 171–72, 233
seeds, 114–15, 211–12, 243
Segedie, Leah, 30
sensitivities, food, 69, 232
Sheridan, Jameth, 121
shopping, 246–58
shower water, filtering, 105–6
shrimp, 172
silicon dioxide, 149
Silly Putty, x, 12, 32, 49, 122, 149
smoothies, 85, 88–89, 291–96
snacks, 62–63, 244, 286–87, 327–32; juice for,
    92; postworkout, 108; raw, 180; travel, 274
social media, 12–13, 23, 28, 30, 225
sodium benzoate, 121, 136
soft drinks, 118–27; alternatives to, 125–27;
    cancer and, 118–19; fountain, 121–22;
    GMOs and chemicals in, 120–25;
    sweeteners in, 47–48, 118, 123–25
sorbitol, 137
soup, 45–46, 232–33
soy, 22, 173, 216, 219–20
soy sauce, 236, 290
spices, 251, 263–64
spinach, 86–87
spirulina, 206
sports drinks, 107–8
sprouts, 52, 179–80, 185, 188, 212–13
staple foods, 242–45
Starbucks, 5, 83–84
stevia, 48, 160–62
storage, 256, 260–61
stress relievers, 208–9
Subway, 5, 31–33
sucralose, 48, 64, 134, 157
sucrose, 134, 137
sugar and sweeteners, 155–64, 290;
    alcoholic beverages with, 130, 132,

134–35, 137; animal bones and, 156;
    artificial, 48, 64, 123–25, 134, 157; baked
    goods with, 45, 182; good and bad, 156–57,
    159–64; green juice with, 91–92;
    hidden, 47, 157; natural, 158–59, 204;
    soda with, 118, 120; sports drinks with,
    107; see also high-fructose corn syrup
sulfites, 129, 133, 135, 140
sulfur dioxide, 135
sulfur-rich foods, 55
superfoods, 201–14
sweets, 244, 333–35; see also sugar and
    sweeteners

TBHQ (tertiary butylhydroquinone),
    23, 25, 46
TBT (tributyltin), 60
tea, 100–102, 256, 290
tempeh, 203
tequila, 141, 239
Thai food, 235
Thayer, Kristina, 59
THC (tetrahydrocannabinol), 207
tilapia, 172
tomato products, 46–47
Trader Joe's, 249–50
trans fats, 49–50, 192, 195
traveling, 270–77
tribromophenol, 135–36
tributyltin (TBT), 60
TVP (textured vegetable protein), 174–75

United Buying Clubs, 257
USDA organic standards, 44, 139–40,
    168–69, 223

vegan diet, 71–72, 165
vegetables. See fruits and vegetables
veggie burgers, 174–75
Vietnamese food, 237
Vilsack, Tom, 27
vinegars, 82–83, 290
vitamins, 71, 81, 111, 121, 134

Walmart, 241, 247–48
wasabi, 236
water, 103–9, 290; bottled, 106–7;
    contaminants in, 42, 103–4, 108–9;
    curbing appetite with, 99–100, 232;

filtered, 104–6, 125–26, 255; fluoridated, 56, 103–4; temperature of, 82–83, 99–100; for travel, 273; when to drink, 99–100
water bottles, 105
Watson, Linda, 256
weight loss, 57, 74–75; foods promoting, 82, 87, 231; water and, 99–100; *see also* obesity
wheat, 181–82
wheatgrass juice, 87–88, 276

white carbs, 181–83
Whole Foods, 247–48
Wigmore, Ann, 88
wine, 134–36, 139–40, 239

yeast, GMO, 136, 140
Yoforia, 20–21
yoga, hot, 276
yoga mat ingredient. *See* azodicarbonamide
yogurt, 20–21, 116, 203–4

ABOUT THE AUTHOR

FOR MOST OF HER life, Vani Hari ate whatever she wanted—candy, soda, fast food, processed food—until her typical American diet landed her where that diet typically does, in a hospital. Despite her successful career in corporate consulting, Hari decided that health had to become a priority. Her newfound goal drove her to investigate what is really in our food, how it is grown, and what chemicals are used in its production. The more she learned, the more she changed and the better she felt.

Encouraged by her friends and family, Hari started a blog called foodbabe.com in 2011. It quickly became a massive vehicle for change. In just the last three years, foodbabe.com has led campaigns against companies like Kraft, Starbucks, Chick-fil-A, and Subway that attracted more than 500,000 signatures and led to the removal of several controversial ingredients used by these major food companies. Through corporate activism, petitions, and social media campaigns, Hari and her Food Babe Army have become one of the most powerful populist forces in the health and food industries. Hari has been profiled in the *New York Times* and *USA Today* and has appeared on *Good Morning America*, CNN, *The Dr. Oz Show*, *The Doctors*, and NPR.

Join the Food Babe in her fight for better food and healthier living at foodbabe.com. Follow her on Twitter @thefoodbabe and on Facebook at facebook.com/thefoodbabe.